Mariel Hemingway's Healthy Living
from the Inside Out

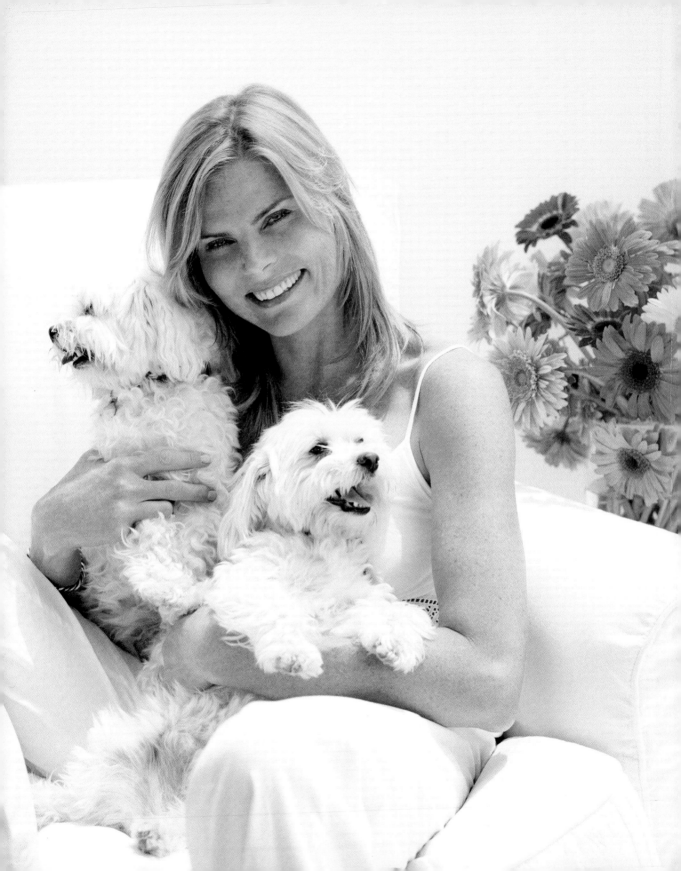

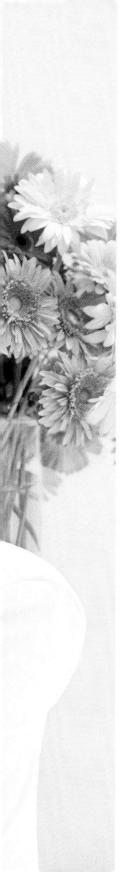

Mariel Hemingway's
Healthy Living
from the Inside Out

EVERY WOMAN'S GUIDE TO
REAL BEAUTY, RENEWED ENERGY,
AND A RADIANT LIFE

Mariel Hemingway

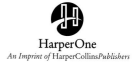

HarperOne
An Imprint of HarperCollins*Publishers*

This book is written as a source of information only. The information contained in this book should by no means be considered a substitute for the advice of a qualified medical professional, who should always be consulted before beginning any new diet, exercise, or other health program.

All efforts have been made to ensure the accuracy of the information contained in this book as of the date published. The author and the publisher expressly disclaim responsibility for any adverse effects arising from the use or application of the information contained herein.

MARIEL HEMINGWAY'S HEALTHY LIVING FROM THE INSIDE OUT:
Every Woman's Guide to Real Beauty, Renewed Energy, and a Radiant Life.
Copyright © 2007 by Mariel Hemingway. All rights reserved. Printed in the United States of America.
No part of this book may be used or reproduced in any manner whatsoever without written permission
except in the case of brief quotations embodied in critical articles and reviews. For information address
HarperCollins Publishers, 10 East 53rd Street, New York, NY 10022.

HarperCollins books may be purchased for educational, business, or sales promotional use. For information please write: Special
Markets Department, HarperCollins Publishers, 10 East 53rd Street, New York, NY 10022.

HarperCollins Web site: http://www.harpercollins.com

HarperCollins®, ⬛®, and HarperOne™ are trademarks of HarperCollins Publishers.
first HarperCollins paperback edition published in 2008

ART DIRECTION BY BETH TONDREAU; DESIGN AND TYPESETTING BY BTDNYC
PHOTOGRAPHY BY BRIAN NICE
Photographs on pages v, 19, 12, 18, 20, 25, 91, 176, 198, 203, 210, 267 by Beth Tondreau

LIBRARY OF CONGRESS CATALOGING-IN-PUBLICATION DATA IS AVAILABLE.

ISBN: 978-0-06-089040-7

08 09 10 11 12 RRD (W) 10 9 8 7 6 5 4 3 2 1

For my husband Z,
my greatest and most cherished teacher.
In divine love forever.

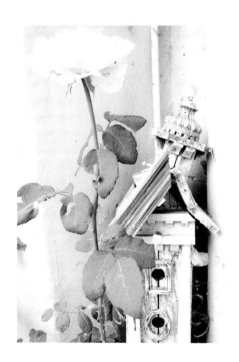

In deep appreciation, I thank the following people:
My amazing daughters Dree and Langley who guide me to the heart of living presently everyday;
my Guru Paramahansa Yogananda; His Holiness the Dalai Lama for his inspiration
in all aspects of my life; Sri Daya Mata, an exemplary model of a God-guided life;
Amely, thank you for giving me my voice; Patrick #2; Mike M.; Gareth; Gideon; Mark; Claudia;
KC, because if she gets this everyone will; Dr. Ron R; Tenzin; Hale; and Lee.
And finally I thank my five dogs for slowing my heart and making me smile!!!

Contents

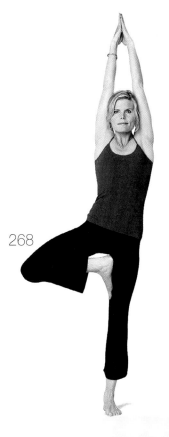

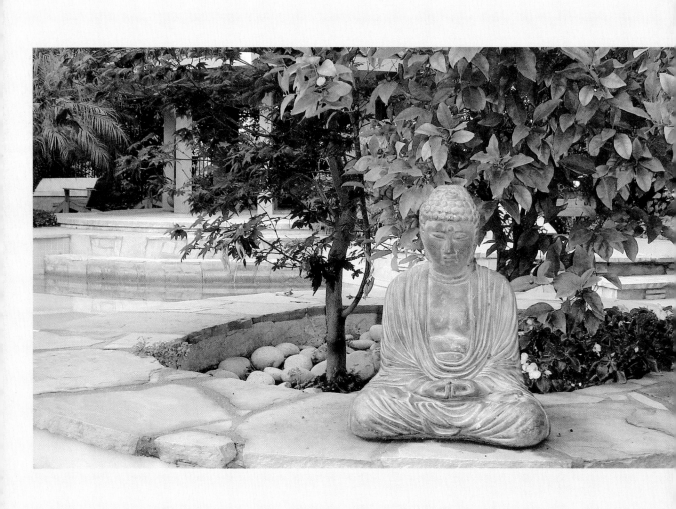

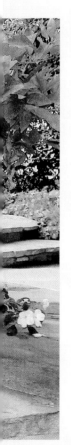

Mariel Hemingway's Healthy Living from the Inside Out

Introduction

QUESTION: WHICH OF THESE THINGS HAVE YOU DONE THIS WEEK?

    A. Switched on the TV news within five minutes of waking up.

    B. Eaten lunch while driving.

    C. Taken your cell phone into the bathroom.

    D. Used a strong cup of coffee as a pick-me-up.

    E. Looked in the mirror and had a mean thought about your body.

QUESTION: WHICH OF THESE THINGS HAVEN'T YOU DONE THIS WEEK?

    A. Laid the table for breakfast.

    B. Noticed what time the sun set.

    C. Driven with the radio and your cell phone switched off.

    D. Exercised.

    E. Looked in the mirror and had a loving thought about your body.

SOMETIMES LIFE'S MAJOR REVELATIONS come in such quiet moments, you almost miss them. Two years ago I was traveling down a quiet country road in the middle of New Zealand's South Island after a long, cold day on the set of an action movie. The gray springtime light was finally fading to darkness, and I was quietly thrilled to be in the car's passenger seat with the heat blasting at my feet, after a morning of shooting water scenes in the frigid ocean and an afternoon of throwing kung fu kicks on dry land. I was thinking about the healthy dinner I planned to cook and how I'd use my quiet night alone to rest and recharge when a hesitant voice from the driver's side broke the silence.

"Um, Mariel? Can I ask you a question?" It was Anna, the foxy nineteen-year-old local whose job as production assistant kept her racing around on my tail from dawn to dusk.

"Absolutely," I said.

"Well," she hesitated, as if slightly embar-rassed, "the rest of the crew and I are wondering something. How is it that at the end of the day you're the only person on set who isn't exhausted and cranky, who isn't clutching a coffee cup and eating cookies to keep going, and isn't getting sick?" She sneezed, then added in the most diplomatic way she could, "You're so much older—I mean, we're twenty years younger than you, at least. And you have three times our energy."

The question surprised me. For most of the two decades that I'd worked in the entertainment industry, I'd always been something of the kook on set—the health nut with the funny habits. I'd get teased for doing Sun Salutations during the long waits for my scenes or for bringing big vats of whey protein powder to the catering table at lunch. (Lovingly teased, I should add, but teased nonetheless.) Or the fact that I meditated daily and would wake up before our early call times to do it—that was doubly weird to most. Although I almost never talk about my practices, little clues to my lifestyle would pop up here and there, always setting me slightly apart. Anything smacking of what I call the yogic attitude—creating calm

from the inside out through food and exercise and quiet contemplation—was more or less not cool.

Yet here I was, after a good twenty years of following these lifestyle practices, suddenly finding that the very people who used to giggle at me were now coming to me with questions. Once Anna broke the ice, more curious inquiries followed. "How can I eat in a way that makes me feel better?" "Why am I so tired even when I get enough sleep?" "What will help get rid of this awful stomachache I get every time I'm anxious?" Movie sets have traditionally been far from health conscious. Working long hours under significant amounts of stress and often eating on the fly, people do what they can to stay alert all day and calm under pressure. Caffeine, sugar, cigarettes, and occasional tantrums to let off steam are the standard methods of self-maintenance,

AUTHOR'S NOTE: CAN MEN DO THIS PROGRAM? Of course! Most of the information in this book applies to everyone. I refer to my own experiences as a woman, wife, and mother throughout because that is what I know, but almost all the concerns and issues I speak of are universal. Men will get as much from this program as women will, so please keep reading!

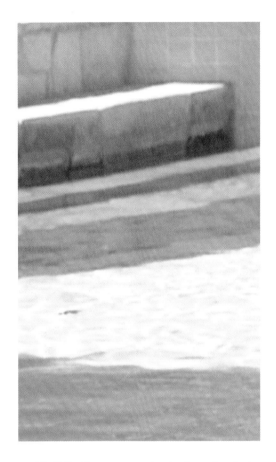

and half the time you survive by knowing that if you hang on a bit longer, you can fall apart when the job's done. In other words, it's a microcosm of society at large. So when my down-under colleagues started asking about my simple, preventive methods for keeping my body boosted, my mind calm, and my spirits high, it set me thinking.

If the veteran lighting guys with the Teflon stomachs are inquiring about my cod liver oil and the college-age interns want to know how long I meditate, I'll bet a pretty wide cross section of people are seeking the same thing: to learn how to slow down, take stock of how they feel, and take back some control of their health and of their lives.

■ ■ ■

I BELIEVE we all have the same problems, they just come in different wrapping paper. And the more I talk to people, not just on movie sets but also to my friends, colleagues, and even my children's acquaintances, the more it's clear that below the surface of our very different appearances, lifestyles, and interests lie some universal concerns. At the start of the twenty-first century, the desire to stay well and find some kind of inner peace is becoming more urgent. The rapid and often relentless pace of life has delivered unprecedented opportunity, but it's also brought on exhaustion, and what many of us want most is to redress the imbalance. We want to feel more rested and restored and to reconnect with lives that seem to be getting away from us. Above all, we want to learn how to live in balance: to be less susceptible to stress and sickness and to have health and peace of mind as the norm, not the exception, in our lives.

Almost every part of life now exists in a more accelerated form than ever before: food is faster, travel is quicker, and communication is more or less instant. Our environments are crowded with noise, media, and technology; "stuff" fills every corner of our homes (much of which, not surprisingly, becomes rapidly obsolete). We confront so many situations in the course of a day that we never get a chance to process everything before the next morning comes. Meanwhile, many of us feel a lingering undertow of frustration that makes it hard to find satisfaction in our present lives. It's as if a perpetual refrain is echoing in the backs of our minds: What else should I be doing? What's out there that might be better than this?

Partly, we bring the situation upon ourselves. The pressures to do more and achieve more with our time seem to grow every year, and we keep signing up for more. Work has become more intense, with jobs demanding more hours, more responsibilities, and more results. Yet we expect more of ourselves on the home front as well. Women in particular expect our relationships to be blissful and passionate, our homes to be immaculate and chic, and our children to be star athletes and scholarship students. Usually our standards for our physical appearances are excruciatingly high too. There's almost no way to do it all without going slightly nuts: we multitask our way through the demands as best we can, dividing our energy and our attention into fragments that inevitably add up to be less than the whole.

Our growing concerns about how to live better and be healthier are related to threats we can't quite name or see. Environmental and social hazards in the world are undeniably affecting our health, but sometimes we get just enough information to scare us but not enough to help us make good choices. We hear so much about toxic foods, disease-causing foods, and fattening foods that it's hard to know what we can and can't eat.

Almost everyone knows somebody who's living with cancer. How much of this epidemic, we wonder, is caused by pollutants that we knowingly consume through food and stimulants or unknowingly consume from our atmosphere? Meanwhile, natural things such as the sun have suddenly become controversial. Some say sun exposure will kill you while others say we need regular stints of it to create vitamin E. (As you'll read later, I think *moderate* exposure to sunlight is critical to good health.)

Modern life delivers a steady stream of small stresses that affect the way we feel every day. Some come from our individual lifestyle choices and some from the world at large—and it's a lot of work to process them all. A stress is any kind of strain on our system. It includes those toxins we consume through eating, breathing the air, and drinking the water because our organs have to work hard to eliminate them. It includes the screwy sleep patterns we fall into by working or hanging out until 1:00 A.M. because falling asleep too late can throw our hormones, and subsequently our appetite and moods, way out of kilter. Stress can even come from too much sedentary activity, including spending too much time in the car, because our bodies need to move in order to function at their best.

Factor in the array of mental and emotional challenges that most everyone has to deal with—from finances and family issues to the fears and insecurities we have about our talents, looks, and futures—and doesn't it make sense that these days our total stress loads are reaching maximum capacity?

The sheer amount of stress we face, combined with the speedy pace of our lifestyles, makes it hard to start and end each day with optimism and calm. Stress drives us to use certain foods and stimulants as crutches instead of figuring out a diet that creates a condition of optimal health. (Many of us use caffeine to get energized, but—hands up—who also relies on a strong cup of coffee to help them go to the bathroom? That's using food the wrong way.) Stress contributes to mild anxiety issues and attention problems and even to negative thought patterns and behavior. The fact is, we've strayed too far from simple principles of looking after ourselves well. We're consuming things that cloud our minds, we're holding stress in our bodies, and more often than not we're too rushed to reflect on our lives. The result is that we often feel like our lifestyles are controlling us and not vice versa.

If I've learned anything over my years of practicing healthy habits, it's that we can transform any of these situations, and ultimately transform our lives, through some simple choices. We already have everything we need to counter modernity's stresses and create a life in which, day to day, we feel great. We can remedy that maxed-out state and get more energy by day and better rest by night. We can build a core of joy and peace at our center that keeps us balanced no matter what craziness is going on outside us. We can take control of our moods, boost our sex drive, and even shed a lot of the ghosts that keep us stuck in old habits. Now more than ever, the onus is on each one of us to empower ourselves. And it's not hard to do if we just start bringing a little more awareness to the things we do each day.

You might be saying, "What? I can't control the quality of the air outside my home. I can't choose to commute to work by foot or bike. I can't cut my stressful boss/parent/kids out of my life." But that's not the point. When it comes to your health and wellness, there are indeed many things you can't control. The trick is to ask, *What can I control?* The answers are fairly simple: The food I eat. The way I exercise. My response to emotional stresses. My home environment. Making even small modifications in these four areas can be extraordinarily powerful—and, should you need it, deeply healing. That is what this book is about.

If you make just a few changes in these four areas, you will notice physical and mental payoffs right away. Eating one or two different foods can make a huge difference in your digestion and detoxification, boosting your energy, immune system, and spirits. Taking a short time-out to sit in total quiet helps you shed the stress that accumulates in your mind and body, and even in your face. (Try it; you'll be surprised how quickly furrowed brows start to smooth.) Bringing a few touches of warmth and sacredness into your home soothes your soul and makes you feel more grounded. We're not talking extreme makeovers or overnight transformations; those quick-fix approaches can rarely be sustained. Instead, try making one small change here, another small change there, and slowly you will discover what works for you. With time, you can change the look and feel of your whole life for the better. Remember, giant leaps are made of inches.

Another, subtler effect will quietly take place at the same time. By focusing on the day-to-day choices that you can control, you anchor yourself squarely into your life as it unfolds *right now*. You bring your attention again and again to the present moment, and you stop worrying about what happened in the past or what might happen in the future. In doing so, you slow down the rush and enjoy your time. And I've found that when you approach your life from this starting point, in place of frustration you more often touch fulfillment.

■   ■   ■

WE ALL HAVE our different reasons for seeking out a balanced life. When I started on my journey, I wasn't reacting to the environmental hazards of today or to the sheer pressure of work and life. I was just trying to survive.

My childhood was far from peaceful. In our house, outside the town of Ketchum, Idaho, life was lived at pendulum extremes—either chilly silence or flaming arguments, often back-to-back. As the son of Ernest Hemingway, my father had inherited a complicated burden: the genetic tendencies toward addiction and over-consumption; the pain of abandonment caused by the way his father lived and, most tragically, the way he died; and the guilt and self-doubt that come with being the child of a legend, fearing that nothing you can do will ever match what your parent achieved. My mother, by contrast, was very beautiful yet painfully bitter. Her first husband had died in World War II, and after she married my father, she resented him sorely for not being the man to whom she'd truly lost her heart. The two of them fought pretty much every day of my childhood. (I didn't find out that my mom had been married before until I was sixteen and stumbled across the fact by accident; that's what happens in the happy home of noncommunicators.)

I was the youngest of three daughters, and by the time I was old enough to be conscious of adult relationships, my parents had more or less given up trying to be great role models. My dad would depart to spend hours fishing in the nearby wilderness areas, and my mom eventually retreated more and more to her room. She got sick with cancer at the age of fifty-one years old, and as my two older sisters were entering their own phases of teenage trouble and rebellion, I became her young caretaker, quietly shuttling between her and my father, trying to stay out of the line of fire when they clashed. None of it was made easier by the fact that my family was always somewhat in the limelight. The enormity of my grandfather's myth meant everyone in town always knew our business. And when my middle sister, Margaux, became one of the first true "supermodels" in the late seventies, the drama increased exponentially. She jumped into the limelight at an early age, and she had to do battle with her demons in public, negotiating the ups and downs of celebrity and the temptations of drugs, food, and alcohol.

According to all I saw all around me as a child, being an adult meant a roller-coaster ride of major highs and devastating lows that inevitably led to sickness, craziness, or self-destructive behavior. I didn't want any of that in my own future, so, beginning in my early teens, I sought ways to achieve calm and control in my own body and mind through diets and workouts and what might be called inner work. I was using superclean food and tough daily exercise regimes as preventive measures even before the word *preventive* was in vogue. I wanted to insure myself against ever becoming sick, fat, or insane, and I set about undoing the extremism I'd inherited from my family—the running-with-the-bulls approach to life encoded deeply in the Hemingway DNA.

Ironically but not surprisingly, I took a pretty extreme approach to finding peace. I'd grown up pleasing people because it was the only

way to get attention in my house, so I turned that talent to health and well-being. For a good portion of my youth I was the perfect student of any challenging diet and the perfect patient to any nutritionist, doctor, or healer who said they knew what was best for my body and, to some extent, my mind and spirit too. Of course, I was also motivated by ego and fear about my appearance. I had entered the movie business at a young age, and throughout my late teens and twenties, I worked my butt off to stay skinny, svelte, and as sensational as a girl subsisting on celery and burned popcorn could be.

Even after I married my husband, Stephen, at the age of twenty-three and we had our two beautiful daughters, I struggled to allow myself to relax and enjoy life. If anything, having children intensified my commitment to keeping "clean and balanced" in body and mind. My biggest fear was that I would pass on the Hemingway clan's compulsive over-indulgence to my children. I ate less and exercised more, tightening the reins on all my health and beauty regimens. To put it bluntly, all my so-called healthy choices were motivated by panic. I kidded myself that I had the purest body on the block, but in reality I had built a lifestyle of deprivation, and my energy levels and immune function began to dip below par. Yet it was the only way I knew how to stay physically and emotionally consistent: withhold food from the emotional demons, or slay them with a tough workout. Of course, the messy emotions didn't go away—I was just too tired to deal with them.

What turned the tide for me were the practices of yoga and meditation, which I began to explore in my midtwenties and then got serious about in my late twenties. In yoga I found a challenge that couldn't be conquered with sheer discipline and sweat. Yoga practice didn't allow me to mindlessly burn through inner pain; instead, it gently turned me around to look at my pain and taught me to treat myself kindly enough to unravel some of my problems. I began to accept my body rather than constantly trying to dominate it. I became aware that it had its own systems of checks and balances: sophisticated biological systems that were able to keep my weight and moods in check if I let them. Yoga did its work on me—slowly. It forced me to peel back some of the armor in which I'd sheathed myself and examine the person inside. Eventually I began to surrender to its way. I began to observe myself not only during yoga class, but also when I was cooking dinner or getting irritated when there were crumbs left on the counter. It slowed my reaction time down and allowed me to become more conscious of who I was and how I was.

There was no sudden transformation or instant new start. But that yogic attitude I'd acquired led me to seek more peace in my life, and I learned some simple meditation. When I began carving out time to sit in silence on a daily basis, I got much better at observing and reflecting on all the events in my world. It was almost as if I was a concerned friend watching from the sidelines, asking, "Why the heck are you doing all that harsh stuff to your body?" In fact, I was becoming a kinder friend to myself in everything I did. This style of conscious living had major benefits. It allowed me to achieve things more calmly and easily and to be motivated by what was actually good for me rather than being driven by my emotions, which more often than not led to screwed-up and destructive behavior. It led me to start making healthy choices throughout my life—in my diet, in my relationships, and at home with the family.

Over time, living my life with more awareness and kindness powerfully transformed me as a woman, wife, mom, actor, and friend.

But it took until my late thirties before I truly mellowed out and learned to trust my own instincts rather than rely on a squadron of experts. I realized with something of a shock that I could be the expert on me. I'd certainly spent enough time in study and had accumulated tons of experience—so why *wouldn't* I know what was best for me?

I began to listen to what my body needed in terms of food, movement, rest, and emotional release, and I learned that if I made sure to structure my life so that every day included a few reasonably easy routines, I could create a consistency that allowed me to feel good every day, without highs and lows, without the scary pendulum swings I'd come to believe were a deeply embedded part of my personality.

Most important, I learned something huge: how to do things in moderation. A *sustainable,* lifelong healthy path didn't have to be bereft of treats and fun, nor did it have to come with a dose of shame. I no longer feared that I'd lose all my good work if I ate too much one day, or did a gentle workout instead of going for the burn, because I knew that now my choices were in tune with what I needed. I'd gradually developed the sensitivity to understand how my nutritional, physiological, and emotional needs changed from day to day, week to week, and year to year.

To be fair, some of my practices today might still seem a bit extreme. I don't eat sugar in any form whatsoever, including alcohol, because when I was younger I had addictive tendencies and it's proven better for me just to clear it out of my system. Occasionally I do an eight-hour meditation as part of my spiritual practice. But these are things I've discovered work well for me and make me feel good. That's what matters. Each person must find a way that suits who she is and how she likes to live. I still enjoy consulting professionals about my health and my home from time to time, but these days if my intuition overrides what they tell me, I let my gut be my guide.

The result of finding my own way? My physical health has gotten better and better, to the point that I rarely get a cold or flu today and feel fantastic for my age because I've found ways to let my body function at a high level of efficiency. I've also lightened up enormously in my expectations of myself and those around me because I discovered that I could enjoy life, not just police it. (I also stopped trying to police my kids and husband so much, which has infinitely improved our relationships.)

Today, the simple but reliable protocols I follow in four important areas—diet, yoga and exercise, meditation, and caring for my home environment—are the cornerstones of my life. I know that when I do my work in all of them—for example, by eating in a way that makes me feel great and shedding any stress with some silent contemplation—I know that I've done the best I can to ensure I start and end the day feeling grounded and peaceful. Whatever happens in between, I can't necessarily control: bills pile up, work gets hectic, teenage daughters have teary meltdowns, PMS strikes, my husband gets cranky (occasionally). But by cultivating calm and balance at my core, I can observe, listen, and take a breath before I respond.

■　■　■

IT'S FUNNY, for the first two decades that I practiced yoga and ate whole foods and put some attention into the energy of my home, skeptics would complain it was all too crunchy or new agey for them. They'd joke, "I don't own Birkenstocks, so take that tofu away! Stop talking about the feng shui of your kitchen, you hippie!" Today people are equally skeptical but for the opposite reason. These simple practices have acquired such a chichi image that they often seem way out of reach. Anytime you see yoga represented in the media, it's so pristine and perfect, you think you're allowed to do it only if you wear tight white Lycra and own an infinity pool. Likewise, the organic food movement has become so trendy, you'd be forgiven for thinking you're doing it right only if your idea of a quick snack is a mélange of baby beets in at least four different shades of pink.

I don't do my downward dogs next to an infinity pool. Sometimes I do them in my bedroom with the window open. If I'm working on a film I unroll my mat and do them in a cramped RV (and bang my toes up against the ceiling when I go into handstand). My house doesn't look or sound like a Zen temple either. For better or worse, it's filled with color, people, and the odds and ends of life—including teenagers' skateboards and five furry dogs. And while I eat vast quantities of vegetables, there is a limit. Mélanges of anything are pretty much out.

My basic lifestyle practices are my tools. They're pragmatic and functional, and they get dirty from daily use.

It's important to take the preciousness out of these practices. For one thing, these tools are neither fancy nor out of reach. Walking, yoga, sitting in silence, cooking your own wholesome food, bringing warmth and comfort into your home—they're simple things that are free or reasonable in cost, and you shouldn't have to go far to do them.

But there's another reason to make these tools part of daily life. Whenever we get too precious about our journey to health and balance and start thinking we need to be 100 hundred percent pure in every activity we do, we fall into a dangerous trap. We start thinking we have to aim for perfection. And the first thing you need to know about any of this stuff is, *Throw out perfection!* Neither you nor I nor the most advanced yoga practitioner nor spiritual swami is ever going to get there. And why would any of us want to? I guarantee that what feels perfect today probably won't feel perfect tomorrow because for anyone, but

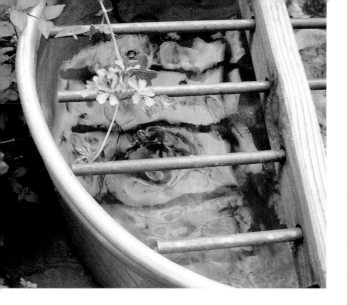

particularly for women, our circumstances, our bodies, our energies, and our interests are always changing. (If you don't agree, try doing a sweaty, muscle-testing workout on that day of the month when you feel fragile and teary from PMS and get back to me.)

Furthermore, most women's lives come with built-in limitations. Who has time for a ninety-minute power hike five times a week plus hours of spiritual reflection plus a full-time job plus, if you're a mom, making your own meals along with meals for everyone else in the family, not to mention doing the laundry and school runs too? If we tried to follow to the letter all the guidelines that we see in those yoga-by-the-infinity-pool magazines, we'd end up as frazzled and exhausted as we were before. The not-perfect approach is moderate yet still powerful. When you approach exercise with deep, focused intention, *a twenty-minute workout will be as effective as forty minutes done with less attention.* An *incredibly nutritious* breakfast smoothie can be whipped up in the time it takes for the kettle to boil. And

you definitely don't need to do thirty minutes of sitting in silence to feel a change; *try sitting for three.*

Limitations can be used to our advantage. You learn a good life skill: to work with what you have and not to sweat it if you don't achieve exactly what you set out to do. If you practice having a peaceful mind while you're folding the sheets, that's a type of meditation. If you exercise by chasing kids around a playground, it's okay: your body and mind can still get some release. Women don't always have the luxury of stopping the world so they can get off (though we can learn how to put the world on pause). In general, we have to keep things moving. We are good at making our world work, and that's why choosing to make it work with peace is so rewarding.

This nonperfect approach helps us stay open-minded, flexible, and curious. To experiment and keep trying new things. The mantra to keep in mind? Forget about reaching perfection. Discover what is perfect for you *today.*

■ ■ ■

NOT LONG AGO I appeared on *Larry King Live* to talk about the legacy of suicide on a family, a subject with which I am quite familiar. Several times during the show Larry said, "You are the rock of your family." I thought about that afterward; people have called me many things, but never a rock. It was a huge compliment because I've worked hard for that sense of inner strength. In fact, I've had to work harder than ever for it the older I've become.

I remember thinking I'd nailed it when I reached my late thirties. I'd been through a lot, but I'd done my work, so as I approached my fourth decade, surely it was time to kick back and glide. Wrong! That's when some of the rockiest stuff hit. My husband battled, and beat, life-threatening cancer twice, undergoing eight surgeries in the process. My dad passed away at the same time that my husband was diagnosed. My daughters hit their own rocky period—the middle teen years. And I've had to face all the thorny questions that any woman of my age faces after bringing up two kids and seeing them approach adulthood, such as wondering how to reconnect to my own femininity. Not to mention dealing with the issue of being a woman over forty in Hollywood, redefining myself and my career. Yet time after time, when I've needed to dig deep into my reserves of energy and calm, I've found what I needed.

That's why I know for certain that my tools really work. They've been put to the test in a big way in the last few years. They've worked for me in the middle of unrest at home, and they've worked for me on faraway film sets, where it's a challenge to implement any routine at all.

Being pleased with how these practices work on the road and surprised at the interest they pique in other people, I began to wonder, How can I guide others to start on their own journey to a more balanced, healthful way of being? How can I translate what I've learned over the years into a program that anyone can follow—not a strict, make-it-or-break-it regime but the opposite, a fun, personal investigation?

I also wondered how to bring different areas of practice—food, exercise, silence, and home—together into one whole life. Because even though there are scores of books on each of the subjects separately, none of them ever shows the reader how to bring it all together.

That's why I wrote *Healthy Living from the Inside Out.* It's a creative, inventive way to begin building the better life you want and revealing the better you. Together we can explore some new options that will help you sail through a stressful world without having to overhaul every aspect of your life. Instead, you'll make changes much more organically, by discovering how some simple, healthful lifestyle practices can be incorporated into the busy life you already have.

Most significantly, this book is a guide to building *your own individualized lifestyle.* I am not an authority on everybody's life; I'm the authority only on my own. The goal of this program is to help you become intimate with your needs, your tastes, and your interests. As a result, you will find your own tools. Nobody's downward dog will look quite the same as yours. Nobody's meal will taste the same as yours. Nobody's bedroom will feel the same as yours. And therein lies the beauty of this program. When you truly observe what works for you and what pleases you, rather than just following a bunch of laws that a book dictates, you prove to yourself that the capacity for greatness lies within you. You become empowered.

Making changes is an experiment, not an exact science. It's an art, not a how-to. You become the creator of your own journey to wellness when you listen to what you need. You become the artist of your own life when you discover routines and rituals that reflect who you are and what you believe. You become the sculptor of your own body too. When you are eating and moving and behaving with more awareness of your body's needs, you naturally shed the extras that you no longer need—weight comes off, the body takes its shape, stress leaves tight muscles, the skin glows, and you smile a lot more. People will ask you, "What are you doing differently?"

Of course, when you embark on this journey, it helps to have a map. That's why you will start with this four-week program, with exercises and routines to complete each day and week. Commit to doing them on this schedule for the first four weeks; you can get free-form later. Having guidelines to follow at first is helpful because we are *training the body and the mind to try new patterns and break old ones that no longer serve us.* That's how we absorb new habits into our lives. It's how the new behaviors become second nature.

Within the program, you always have options. You can pick between certain tasks each day or week, thereby beginning the practice of asking yourself, "What is perfect for me today?" You can also repeat the program for a second thirty-day stint, selecting the options you missed the first time around. Or pick the book up again a few months from now, and do it as a refresher. No matter where you are in your life, the Quickstart 30-Day Program can always help you renew and recharge yourself when life has gotten too busy or too complicated. My hope is that you'll keep the book on your shelf to dip into anytime you need some inspiration or information. Consider it a whole-person handbook, a resource guide for your healthy, balanced life.

Take a moment to check in with your attitude as you start. Remember, this program isn't about changing your life entirely; it's about helping you get more out of the life you have: more health, more peace, more pleasure. So decide to make your life your test lab for four weeks. Try a few new things, test them out, and see for yourself how they make you feel. It's that easy. So be curious, be playful! Use this program as an opportunity to be new. Don't stick to the same routine every day, don't eat the same foods every day, alter your habits, twist things just a little, turn yourself upside down, do a yoga pose you haven't done before, think about something you haven't thought about for years. If you can bring this playfulness and curiosity to the work, you are already well on your way.

■ ■ ■

The Quickstart 30-Day Program

Becoming a better you is achieved through the discipline of caring for these four avenues: food, exercise, silence, and home. We will explore each area separately, and along the way you will see how they connect into a single whole. The choices you make in one area support the choices you make in another without your having to think about it.

Food (Nourish):

Food affects you physically, mentally, and emotionally, and everyone has slightly different food needs. When you learn what works for your unique body, and know how to make tasty natural foods part of your diet, you will use food in a positive way to boost your body and mind and correct imbalances of weight, mood, and energy.

Exercise (Move):

Exercise is pivotal to feeling and looking your best. Not only will you use it to strengthen and condition your body, you also will use it to heighten your awareness of how you feel in body, mind, and spirit. In this program we'll use yoga and simple hiking to transform not just your physique, but your mental and emotional state as well.

Silence (Observe):

The ultimate benefits of life come from being quiet and taking the time to recognize how you feel inside. When you bring silent reflection into your life, you slow down the rush, observing your actions, and then you can make powerful changes with calmness and clarity.

Home (Restore):

It's important to create the conditions for success. No matter where you live or how much you've got, you can make your home a haven that supports your quest for a balanced life— a place where you can rest and recharge, a sacred space to reflect and heal. Doing this not only brings harmony to your own existence, it also promotes harmonious interactions with your family and friends.

Each of the four sections is made up of four steps that will simplify these complex subjects. Each section gives you the seeds of new practices: doable and maintainable actions that anyone can work into their day. You are going to learn how to do things differently than you've done them before—eating, exercising, even breathing! Even if you already know something about diet, about yoga, or about shifting the feel of your home, simply commit to learning a new way for a few weeks, and be open to seeing the results.

REMEMBER, this program is *not* about becoming an expert in these four areas. A balanced life doesn't come from being a know-it-all about every nuance of Ashtanga yoga. It comes instead from knowing what you need so that you can keep learning and evolving for months and years to come. That's why I am big on asking yourself questions. The project of building a balanced, better lifestyle rests on self-awareness. It means paying attention to the little things from moment to moment and constantly making inquiries: "Why have I got this headache again—do I need to eat something nutritious and cut out the black tea?" "Why am I so anxious—do I need to blast up a steep hill and let it go?" "Why am I unsettled in my house—do I need to spend an afternoon clearing out some clutter?" This is the opposite approach to the typical health book, which offers a one-size-fits-all solution to every tricky situation. But I guarantee that this habit of observing and asking questions will produce powerful results. Sometimes you will need to try a few different things until something works, for example, to help you get on a good sleep pattern or to get your diet working right. Answering these questions is how you build your own set of tools.

Much of this inquiry will take you into emotional terrain. That's important. True change requires that we look critically at our current habits and honestly evaluate whether our old ways of doing things serve us anymore. Often the only thing that gets in the way of implementing better habits is our attitude. We resist ditching patterns that might be keeping us stuck because they're safe and reliable. They allow us to act on autopilot. This program will encourage you to confront those safety nets and to jettison the autopilot. Just try *not* doing the habit that you do mindlessly (that last cup of coffee to get you going or that third glass of wine to wind down after a hectic day), and then simply see how you feel.

Sometimes that simple change is where bigger change starts: the realization that "I could pick something else." Other times we see with clarity that there are emotional triggers causing us to make bad choices. The beauty of observation and self-inquiry is that when we understand the trigger, we can disarm it and eventually forget it ever existed.

To me, this inward investigation is the most important aspect of the journey. Sometimes a new food or exercise regime that you follow for a few weeks is no more than a Band-Aid: a temporary fix-it applied to the surface. But when new lifestyle habits are combined with self-knowledge and self-acceptance, they will change you at the core.

I know what it's like to feel imprisoned by bad habits. Or to feel mired in old patterns from the past. But let me share something. At the end of this sentence, slam the book shut, let it fall into your lap, pause for ten seconds, then begin reading again.

That's how easy as it is to change your life. Emotions, bad habits, and old patterns don't have glue; they're not stuck or nailed to you. They're just ideas. If they feel stuck to us, it's because we're holding onto them. We can decide to simply let them go.

There's just one thing I ask of you before you read further. When you decide to commit to doing the 30-Day Program, please also commit to being kind to yourself. Remember, our goal is to always find our way back to a manageable middle ground. That's what we are training to do because that's how we stay healthy. I'm against making big resolutions because they always come loaded with guilt. Being kind and moderate rather than all-or-nothing about this program means that if you decide morning time is your meditation time, and it doesn't work out one morning, don't give up on your whole day. You can still find five minutes to sit quietly before you go to sleep. Moderation means creating a structure for your day and at the same time forgiving yourself and being aware and accepting of all that happens in your day. To this end, my only requirement of you before you embark on the program is that you make a contract to be a friend to yourself.

First Exercise: A Contract with Yourself

Throughout the 30-Day Program, you will be asked to write a weekly e-mail to yourself in which you can set your intentions for the week ahead, reflect on how you are feeling, observe what works for you and what doesn't, and record what changes are occurring. Writing down thoughts makes a journey become real. It helps to clarify your purpose and your progress, and it can serve as motivation later when you look back and see proof of the changes you've made so far. No one else will read it, there are no grades, and there is no right or wrong way to do it. Simply release the thoughts that come to you, and keep them tucked away. Below is the first e-mail you need to write. Type it up, fill in the blanks, and send it to a dedicated folder in your in-box. It may make you smile or even smirk, but I ask you to write it anyway. Add to it any extra thoughts that come up, and then send it to yourself. This e-mail lays out the intentions of graceful acceptance and loving-kindness that I believe are integral to the entire program.

I, _____, agree to be kind to myself through the four weeks of following these suggestions. I agree to put myself first. To treat myself with the compassion and patience I would treat a close friend. To drop the harsh criticism I put on myself when I look in the mirror or eat something bad or am not perfect at everything I do. For four weeks, I_____, agree to act like I am my own best friend. If I catch myself thinking mean thoughts about myself, I pledge to ask myself: "Would I say that to my best friend?"

■ ■ ■

EMBARKING ON THIS PROGRAM may make other people raise their eyebrows. Not everyone in your family or among your friends may support you when you eat new foods, take more time for yourself, or change old habits. Your changes might bring up for them things they wish they were doing. Believe me, it can be frustrating when you want to change your life and other people want you to stay the same. Just be brave enough to say, "You know what? I'm going to be different. For thirty days I choose to do things differently. My family might look at me strangely. My workmates may look at me strangely. But who cares?"

Maybe they're not supportive. All you need to do is figure out how much time and space you need each day to do your practices, then set your boundaries and stick to them.

This work is far from selfish. When you take care of yourself, you can better take care of others. What you do to transform your own lifestyle, your own habits, and maybe even your own consciousness will radiate out and affect those around you. You can't take anyone else on the trip, and I definitely don't advise making your partner, spouse, or kids do what you're doing. But in my experience, one person making changes profoundly alters the rest of the family's choices and the way they feel about themselves—even if it takes a while.

Now inhale deeply, and take stock of where you are and what you want to achieve. Know that in our do-more, be-more culture, the fact that you've picked up this book and are interested in making some small changes to feel better is enough. Know that with one small modification to your day, you can change the way you feel. Know that one small change will make you feel so good, it will inspire the next small change. Know that six months from now, you will feel like a different person entirely. Take a moment and envision that different person. How does she look? What has changed in her body, her energy, and her attitude? Feel how she feels, take a look at her world, and embrace everything about her. The journey toward that person starts right now.

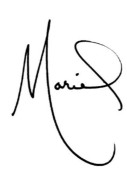

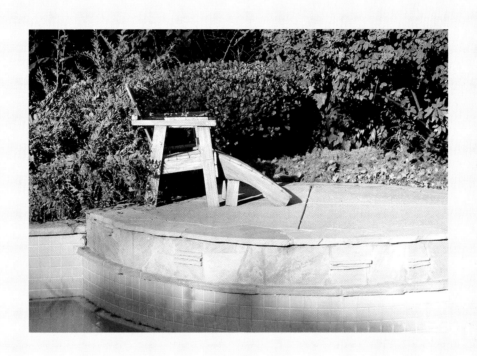

PART ONE

Food

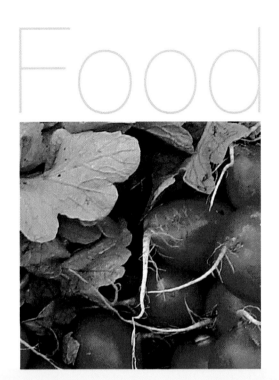

Silence

Exercise

Home

Food

QUESTION: HOW FAST DO YOU LIKE YOUR FOOD?

Consider if you ever do any of the following three things. Then simply ask yourself, next time you're about to repeat the habit, "Could I make a different choice—one that is more careful and more calming?"

Scenario A. Do you reheat the coffee or tea that you brewed earlier in the day?

Scenario B. Do you grab a sandwich from the same deli or fast-food joint every day for lunch?

Scenario C. Do you use the microwave to heat a meal at night?

COULD YOU:

A. Throw out the excess hot drink after you've had the morning cup and leave it at that? Warmed-up cups of old coffee or tea are just sad. Try making just the amount you need in the morning. Later in the day when you want a hot drink, try hot water and lemon.

B. Find about seven minutes in the morning to make lunch and take it with you? Throw the extra piece of fish or free-range chicken you cooked the night before into a container as part of a colorful salad recipe. Not only are you in control of what you eat, you'll save that seven minutes later when you're not standing in line, and you'll have more time to eat lunch calmly.

C. Veto the microwave, at least for the thirty days you're on this program? Going slower has its benefits. When you get home from work, put your meal in the oven at a low temperature, and go take a bath or shower. When you're finished your food will be warm, not zapped, and you will feel a lot calmer while you eat. It's part of making the act of eating just a bit more sacred.

CREATING BALANCE THROUGH FOOD doesn't have to mean a radical overhaul, crash diet, or detox. Simply bring your attention to the small things, and you are well on your way to building a better way of eating.

■   ■   ■

ACHIEVING A WHOLE-BODY, balanced way of eating has been one of the biggest challenges of my life. I love food and, in equal measure, have hated the way I love food. I've done everything. I've been vegetarian, then a vegan, then a vegan who practiced the restrictive art of food combining. I've gorged on fat-free carbs, then fat- and carb-free foods (basically, I ate anything with a high air content), and at one point I pledged loyalty to liquid food, and liquid only, during daylight hours. (That was a weird period.) It took a lot of trial and even more error throughout my teens, twenties, and thirties to learn how to eat well without obsessing and without panicking. Or to put it another way, how to be health-happy, not health-crazed.

The simple, moderate, and powerful way of eating I follow today makes me feel amazing. Where once I considered food my adversary, something that existed to trip me up and make me fat or addicted, now it's my ally. Food is the linchpin to my well-being—physical, mental, and emotional. That's why I consider eating well to be not just the foundation of a balanced life, but also a pragmatic way to practice being grounded, conscious, and self-aware.

That may surprise you, because the positive power of food is often overlooked. In fact, these days it almost sounds bizarre to say that food can actively help you slow down and find your calm. When you look around at what's offered, doesn't it sometimes seem like it's the thrill that counts? Everything is about big flavors: exciting taste sensations that blow your mind! Fast delivery: power up with on-the-go, instant, high-octane foods and drinks, and just feel the rush! Big promises: eat this and lose ten pounds in twenty days! Even if you're not a fan of convenience foods and ready-made meals, chances are you almost always

consider, "What's quicker?" when it comes to ordering out or preparing food at home.

Yet when you resist the temptation to speed and give yourself just a little more time to consider what you eat, you can make changes that will lead you to the healthy, balanced way of eating you seek. You can reprogram yourself to get deeper satisfaction from food instead of constantly wanting more. You can use food to nourish, nurture, and heal; you can boost your metabolism to shed excess weight and let your best shape be revealed. Get curious about how food affects your body and mind, and you open the door to a whole new way of using it. Today, each time I prepare a meal or select something off a menu, I am making a deliberate choice. I'm asking, "How shall I use food to make myself feel great today?" It's a powerful place to be. I choose the food rather than it choosing me.

That's why eating is an excellent place to start this program. Not only does improving what you eat make you feel and look better, it also gives you an entrée into the subtler practices I want to share, such as observation and self-inquiry. When you start inquiring about food, you develop the ability to know yourself in a much deeper way. "Why do I feel the way I do?" "What from my past may be driving my behavior in the present?" By asking and answering your own questions, you are reconnecting to that teacher inside, the part of you that is smarter than you realize.

■   ■   ■

THERE ARE SO MANY GREAT REASONS to care deeply about what we eat.

Becoming well-nourished will empower us to resist illness, it will lessen our chances of acquiring degenerative diseases, and it will slow down the aging process. (Yes, that does mean we can eat our way to fewer wrinkles.) It will keep us on an even keel emotionally and help our minds stay sharp and clear. It will give us sustained and steady energy by day and help us sleep better at night. And most important, it will bring new levels of pleasure and presence to our lives.

There are even more good reasons to tailor your nutrition with a few custom details to suit your specific needs. When your eating is in balance with your individual physical needs, you may be surprised at how small annoyances begin to clear up, like skin problems, allergies, or that irksome tendency to get cranky by midafternoon. When the balance is wrong, you may be off in all sorts of ways: tired and droopy even after you eat, irritable and bloated, or stricken with headaches or constipation, which can affect your whole outlook on life. Bad food can also, as we'll see, pull you into a cycle of negative thoughts about yourself.

Because we have to eat several times a day anyway, modifying the way you eat is one of the most accessible and rewarding things you can do to control the way you look and feel.

So why is it such a challenge to find a way to eat that is simple, moderate, and powerful? It's not because we don't care about food. As a society, we're obsessed with it. But we're mainly obsessed with how to stop eating so much of it, not how to eat smart.

Maybe it comes from a fear of what we don't understand. Almost every week we hear of a new scientific study: eat this, avoid that,

don't even look at the other. One side says, eat plenty of red meat like your cave-dwelling ancestors, cut out all grains, and watch the weight fall off. The other says, eat plants as much as possible, and run, don't walk, from any animal product. One side says, eat like a Frenchwoman, with full cream and red wine! The other says, choose Japanese—all fresh fish and miso. If you start researching online, you'll soon reach information overload: saturated-fat lobbyists and low-fat lobbyists; the prochocolate camp and the antichocolate camp; the soy celebrators and soy defamers, all loudly beating on their drums and claiming absolute authority.

The only thing they can agree on: if you follow my rules, you'll be transformed!

Trying to navigate the miles of crowded supermarket shelves can be equally overwhelming. Processed products vie for your dollars and tempt your worst impulses (not to mention kids' worst impulses). Or sometimes the shiny boxes and colorful packets speak to your better instincts—that part of you that deep down wants to make good choices—by claiming to be "enriched" or "fortified," a marketing ploy that, let's be honest, hardly helps to clarify things.

Meanwhile, wandering around the mega-sized health food marts that are popping up nationwide can make you feel like Dorothy on the yellow brick road—dazzled but disoriented. New fruit juices you've never heard of advertise their ultrahigh antioxidant levels, but what, again, do antioxidants do? Farmed fish sits next to wild fish that's twice the price, but do I need to spend the extra? Organic coffee and nonorganic both smell delicious; if it's organic, does that mean it's good for me? (Sure, you could ask the checkout girl, but honestly, who wants to be the dork with all the questions?)

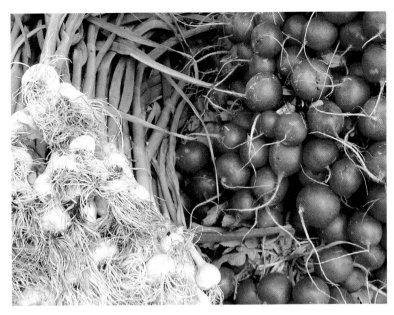

The torrent of information can make anybody feel too confused to take action. Unless your true passion is cooking or reading nutrition Web sites, you probably end up with much the same items in your cart that you had this time last week—and last year. And any dissatisfaction about the way you feel or the way you look? That's probably stayed the same as well. It's no wonder that the myth persists that healthy eating is hard.

The truth is that it *is* possible to clear a path through the latest intelligence and arrive at a manageable middle ground: a simple, affordable, and pleasurable way of eating that suits your body, temperament, and lifestyle and lets you maintain an optimal weight. It is possible to buy and prepare nutritious foods without having a PhD in the subject—and without breaking the bank. And I definitely know that it's possible to take any fear and loathing out of food—if that's what sometimes comes up for you—and replace it with pleasure and delight. The trick is to digest a reasonable amount of the factual information that all those studies and new products provide, and then try to reach a balance between your head and, not your heart exactly but something more primal, your gut instinct.

Of course, the diet experts with their provocative ideas do have some crucial information to share. Clearly, the way modern America eats today is deeply flawed, and the epidemics of obesity, diabetes, and other diseases with clear links to diet are only getting worse. Everyone could benefit from better understanding the role food plays in determining their lifelong health, and many of the books and articles that come out every month are revelatory. But I caution against expecting the latest best-selling diet book or trendy regime to suddenly turn you around. While the books' theories may be great, in practice they can often be those Band-Aids I mentioned: temporary fixes that don't stick for long.

Why not? Because trying to follow someone else's regime is incredibly hard: it puts you in a defensive, deprivation-focused mode, struggling not to want the things you've always wanted. It is hard to implement in a busy, imperfect life, where sometimes you just have to pick from the food available at your local lunch spot and give yourself a break. And it leads to this never-ending, emotional yo-yo game that women constantly play—critiquing themselves, hating their bodies, punishing themselves, and when they fall off the regime for a moment, throwing up their hands and going, "See, I can't do it!" (The evidence is in the numbers: according to the National Association of Eating Disorders, 45 percent of women are on a diet on any one day, and 95 percent of dieters regain any weight they lost within one to five years.)

There's another, subtler reason that I think it's wise to stop expecting the diet of the month to turn you into a paragon of health. It encourages you to constantly look outward, to experts, for the information that you should be gathering by looking inward. You can make your own diet dos and don'ts fairly easily when you start asking simple, basic things like, "How does this food make me feel?" "Am I more energetic, more upbeat, when I eat this several times a week?" "Do I feel sluggish and heavier when this food is in my daily diet?" As I learned when I finally let go of my own dependency on experts and advisers, so much of the knowledge we need to create a viable and sustainable eating plan is within us, if we just begin to trust ourselves.

Building sensitivity to what works for you is the key to creating what I think of as a "personal balance plan" when it comes to food. It's how new, healthy habits will stick with you for the long term: discovering the specific things that make you feel great rather than signing up for the latest fad. Because apart from some obvious no-no's that are bad for everyone—drive-through double cheeseburgers with supersize fries—the truth is that eating well doesn't come down to following strict,

one-size-fits-all nutritional rules or everyone buying the exact same ingredients for dinner. It comes down to tuning in to the question, "What is right for me today?"

QUESTION: FOR ME, FOOD IS:
   A. A sensory pleasure that brings me pleasure and delight.
   B. A fuel source that's utilitarian: it keeps me going.
   C. An emotional stabilizer that rewards and comforts me.

YOU MAY HAVE PICKED A, B, and C. But let's go straight to the core for a second and begin with a very basic idea.

   D. Food is a drug.

The way I see it, food—by which I mean everything we ingest, including beverages—is in many ways a drug. It can cause a powerful chemical effect in our body and can shift our emotional state or behavior profoundly for the better or the worse. And as many people know, it can be scarily addictive as well. Yet few of us think of food as a drug. Even though we take it for granted that an Advil or Midol will do something to the way we feel within fifteen minutes of popping it into our mouths, we can be oddly shortsighted about the impact of ordinary fodder like food and drink.

Why do we underestimate the effects of what we're ingesting? Sometimes it's because the feedback is not so fast. Food tends to operate at a slower speed than ibuprofen even though ultimately it effects change on a deeper level. Of course, some reactions may be just as speedy—think of the hit you get from an espresso or dark chocolate. Start visualizing all the food you eat as having a chemical and emotional pull on your whole body rather than just curing hunger pangs, and it helps you tune in to the bigger picture of food, mood, and health. Just like little colored pills, food comes with an obligation to use it responsibly. Every time you eat, you have the power to select something that might make you feel great or totally drag you down.

That's why food is the first thing I turn to when I'm in a funk. I ask myself, "What have I eaten today?" and do a brief inventory. If it checks out and I feel I'm well-nourished, only then do I question other factors, like family stress or the need to work out or take some quiet time, and I slowly untangle the source of the bad feelings. If I realize my food intake has sucked, I can remedy it with something that nourishes me.

Understanding the fundamental power of food is the key to using food in a balanced way. Knowing that *everything you eat can shift the way you feel* will motivate you as you experiment with some of the ideas in the food component of the 30-Day Program. First, you will cut out all the crap—those bad foods and drinks that may be throwing you off balance, clouding your thinking, and harming your body or are simply nutritionally void and stealing space from better foods. Second, you will tune in to what proportions of macronutrients— carbs, proteins, and fats—should be on your plate to best fuel your individual body chemistry. Third, you will introduce some "foods that boost" into your diet, things that I've found to deliver great nutritional value and that are relatively simple to buy and prepare on a routine basis. This is not about dipping into a recipe book every night, it's about having some easy standards at the ready so you can actually have a life. (Believe me, I eat the same things most days, so much so that my challenge is probably to mix things up a little more.)

And fourth, just as important as looking at what you eat, you will consider how and why you eat. Are you stuck in certain habits that hinder healthy eating? Do you need to give meals more significance and time? For some people—me included—eating comes wrapped in lots of complex emotional history. We do ourselves a favor when we peel back some of these layers and ask, "Am I holding on to old beliefs about food that no longer serve me, and are they getting in the way of my making some pretty simple changes?"

By spending some time on these four areas, you are creating an internal and external environment that makes it easier to find that elusive quality—moderation. Moderation means having a "personal balance" eating routine and knowing what works for you, but also deviating from the routine if circumstances require without hating yourself afterward. Eating in moderation also means enjoying some small indulgences—getting more satisfaction from high-quality treats, eaten less often, than a steady stream of addicting junk.

This "personal balance" approach does demand that each person take more responsibility for her diet. It's not a radical quick-fix. There's no promise of losing so many pounds in so many months or guaranteeing a bikini body by June. It's about building a balanced body chemistry and balanced expectations of food so that you can develop a long-term way of eating that will not let you down in times of stress and that is easy to modify as you get older or your life circumstances change. It's about blending information with intuition.

The change happens in an organic way. When you clear away some of the fuzz that comes from bad chemicals and emotional uncertainty, you develop a calmer, more commonsense approach to food. You can start to hear your natural desire for food that is fresh, nutritious, and in season, and you lose your taste for the dull, processed products that do little to boost your body. Cravings do lose their power, and your body's regulatory instincts—to eat only when hungry, to stop eating when full—are able to do their work. Remember that the body wants to stay in balance and that it has the capacity to regulate itself. You will find that when the "what" you eat is right for you, the "how much" starts to take care of itself. Working toward your personal balance with food can mean the end of weight-loss regimes—for good. Because when you supply your body with the right amount of nutrients it needs to achieve a state of optimum health, you allow your body to achieve and maintain the healthy weight that suits your frame.

I love experimenting with food because its effects reveal themselves right away. From one meal to the next, you can feel different—sometimes better, sometimes worse. Whatever the outcome, there's something empowering in understanding how *your small, everyday choices can start to change your life.*

In fact, I'm such a believer in the power of small, focused changes that the only thing we're going to work on at first is breakfast.

That's it. We're not going to worry about lunch or dinner or anything in between. We'll spend the first week of the Quickstart 30-Day Program seeing how small changes in the first meal of the day might make us feel better.

True good health is not a condition that is merely free of adverse symptoms. It's a state of dynamic well-being, one that is reminiscent of childhood exuberance and joy. When your body is functioning the way it's designed to function, you should be experiencing boundless energy all the time, a keen awareness of your surroundings, a very strong and positive emotional state, and a natural love and zest for life.

—WILLIAM WOLCOTT, *The Metabolic Typing Diet*

Building Basic Instinct

Nutrition can seem overly complex. So many factors are in play—the many different kinds of fats and sugars and minerals to keep in mind—that it can seem like you've lost out if you don't know every detail. But that's not the case. You already know more than you think you do. Want the proof? Glance at the following pairs of foods, and let your gut tell you which choice will create fresh and clean energy for your body and your mind.

1. White-bread bagel with Smucker's-style peanut butter and jelly or a soft-boiled organic egg, half an avocado, and a tomato
2. Arugula salad with four vegetables and grilled tofu or fried chicken and french fries
3. A mocha frappé and chocolate chip scone or raw cashew nuts, an organic Fuji apple, and green tea

It may seem like a kindergarten exercise, but notice how without having to think much about it, you had an immediate reaction to the foods you knew would feel clean and uplifting while filtering out the ones that would feel kind of cloggy (even if your habitual desires were trying to tell you something different.) This very elemental instinct is there to serve you. As you learn to listen to it more and make instant decisions based on what it tells you, eating right will become so simple it will eventually become second nature. (If you didn't have this immediate reaction, you will by Week 2 of the program.)

Despite the barrage of new trends and innovations that circulate through the nutrition world, remember that you will find your way to eating right by using common sense because underneath all the flashy science, the fundamental concepts never change. You eat food because you need the energy and vital nutrients to live. Natural foods that are close to their living state have the most life energy to give, whereas food products that are a long way off from their original state have less. It's a simple question to keep in mind as you make selections: "Does this look the way nature intended it to look?" If the components of the meal or snack in front of you have gone through various processes to get from the earth to your plate—being refined, processed, hydrogenated, homogenized, colored, enhanced, and so on—they have less vital energy to offer.

As irritating as it is, the old cliché "You are what you eat" is still true. If you want to run clean inside and feel clear in your mind and vibrant in your spirit, you need to pick foods that come from clean soils, clean water, and calm animals (when possible). You need to select whatever seems to be bursting with natural color, flavor, and aroma.

Start looking at all the foods you buy or order with that phrase in your head—"I am what I eat"—and you'll be surprised how your natural instinct starts speaking up more loudly.

At the core of the 30-Day Program, and hopefully the rest of your life, is a commitment to eating wholefully. That's my code word for healthy, whole foods that offer the best energy possible to our whole self: our bodies and our minds. "Whole foods" simply means foods that are closest to their natural state, not refined, processed, or chemically altered. They contain all the nutrients within themselves for optimal assimilation by our bodies, and eating them ensures us the highest amount of nutrients food has to offer.

(To the question of whether you can eat whatever you want and then pop a few vitamin pills on the side to pick up the slack, the answer is definitely no. You get more vitamins and minerals out of whole foods in their natural state because many of those nutrients exist in their whole-food form as a complete package with important cofactors that allow the body to absorb them. We'll talk about supplements more later; for now, know there's no good reason to cheat on your foods.)

Exercise: Check Your Food for Vital Stats

Only 46 percent of American meals contain a fresh product. More shocking: as recently as five years ago, 90 percent of the money spent on food was spent on processed food. That means a lot of food from cans, boxes, and vacuum-packed containers going into our bodies. Think for a moment about what's in your cupboard, fridge, and freezer. A good test is to check how many of the items will spoil in the next ten days or so. How many could be there in one month, or three . . . or six? (Quick clue: if many things have expiration dates over two weeks into the future, or in the case of frozen food, if it went through several processing stages before being frozen, your vital-energy stock will drop.) In this program we will weed out the feeble foods and begin to replace them with bumper fodder.

The Imbalances

What's the biggest health threat facing us today? Malnourishment. That sounds ironic given the fact that we consume more calories per capita than ever before. But we've been operating on some erroneous ideas about weight and health at the same time that our access to cheap food has grown. The result is that today we consume far more grains and complex carbohydrates than our bodies can process and have forsaken natural saturated fats, which are critical in *moderate* amounts, for the industrialized, hydrogenated fats that our bodies were not designed to consume. The result is that in tiny increments, we've been digging our way into subpar levels of health.

Malnourishment comes from misinformation about what hurts and what heals. You can be malnourished by overeating: consuming too much of the wrong food and too little of the food that boosts. You can be malnourished by undereating, of course. And most surprisingly, perhaps, you can be malnourished just by being somewhere in the middle of the spectrum. For the majority who are in between the two extremes, unbelievably, even the simple act of following the government-produced food pyramid or the Standard American Diet (called, ironically enough, sad for short) will leave you less than well-nourished and more susceptible to sickness, weight gain, and depleted energy.

Here are the common imbalances that will be redressed as you start following the advice in this program. You'll learn more about each one as you read on and discover what alternatives are available that can send your vitality and wellness to new levels. But keep them in mind as you start to think about what you eat each day. Simply redressing a few of these imbalances will make a huge change in the way you look and feel.

Top 7 Mistakes of the Modern Diet

1. Too much sugar from sugary foods, grains, and starches
2. Not enough nutrient-dense, "naturally occurring" food
3. Not enough water
4. Too much bad fat, not enough good fats
5. Too few healthy bacteria to support intestinal and immune health
6. Too many chemicals from preservatives, pesticides, and food enhancers
7. Forgetting that eating is an act of self-nurturing and behaving like it's just a tiresome necessity

The Hallmarks of the 30-Day Food Philosophy

- **SLOW**—avoid convenience foods, cut out on-the-go eating, opt for simple foods, not instant anything.
- **KIND**—operate with an attitude of acceptance, not panic; give yourself permission to enjoy treats.
- **MODERATE**—aim for a sustainable middle ground where good-quality food serves your body and pleases you.

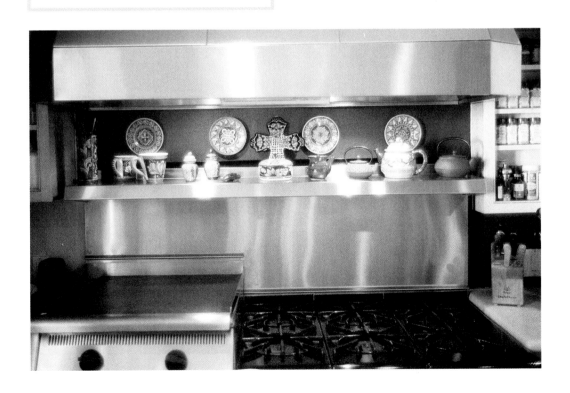

Cut the Crap

QUESTION: WHICH OF THE FOLLOWING STATES HAVE YOU EXPERIENCED?

■ You've eaten a bunch of sugary treats, perhaps over the holiday period, and you've got that wired, buzzy feeling in your head and your body feels sluggish and gross.

■ You're not sure if you want to eat real food now; perhaps you'll skip dinner.

■ You ate dinner from your local Chinese food take-out joint, or maybe you picked up some fast food and a soda, and now you have a slight headache and a thirsty, itchy feeling in your body. You take an aspirin.

■ You drank a strong cup of coffee or black tea to set yourself up for an afternoon of work that you don't feel like doing. For a while you are jolted wide awake, then later you feel inexplicably tired or bummed out.

THE FIRST STEP in building greater sensitivity toward our food is to filter out some of the bad stuff in our system. In fact, this is where a lot of the work in building a good diet goes: clearing the clutter, getting rid of the unnecessary junk that only serves to trip us up. It's like priming a blank canvas so that we can get creative. Your internal environment needs to be calm and tranquil in order for you to observe with any effectiveness how your food choices affect the way you feel. If there are lots of polluting foods and stimulants in your system, you experience a kind of chemical noise, and it's hard to find that peace.

These noisy foods have a negative impact on you physically and psychologically. Moreover, eating them makes it hard to feed yourself the healthful foods you need. Because these loud substances are often the ones with the big kick and big flavor, they drown out the subtle messages your body is sending you about what, when, and how much to eat, and they create a kind of false satisfaction. When you're full of sugar or your appetite is suppressed by caffeine, you're diverted from nutritious food and thereby contributing to malnourishment.

Noisy foods can be the first thing to throw us out of balance because, to put it frankly, they can make us feel bummed out. It's easy to recognize when you see an extreme example, like that friend who's depressed but is always clutching a Styrofoam cup of coffee and smoking cigarettes. But in small ways, at different points in our day or week, we all suffer from poor choices. I used to see it in my teenage daughters. Though they eat well most of the time, once in a while one of them was bottomed out, despondent, and unable to get any traction on her life. I'd ask what she'd eaten so far that day, and inevitably the answer would be "Starbucks and a muffin." Or a giant bag of trail mix loaded with salt, sugar, and preservatives. Not only was she feeding the funk with her choices, she was depriving herself of the beneficial nutrients that might help build a bridge out of the blues. My maternal advice? "Go eat a hard-boiled egg and some turkey slices for protein right now." If you can get the nonsense noise out of your system, you will stop a lot of negativity. (And if you are contemplating taking anxiety medication for moderate depression or anxiety, or even sleeping pills to help you wind down, it behooves you to first take a serious look at your diet and cut the crap out.)

You don't have to be a zealot when it comes to cutting back on noisy foods. Trying to be militant and cutting out all at once everything that may possibly have some negative effects is more likely to cause frustration and feelings of failure, not success. All you need to do is agree to experiment for this four-week period. How does it feel to cut back on caffeine or replace all salty snacks with tart fruit? Could you agree to cut out sugary treats? Simply observe how you feel without these overstimulating or agitating foods and drinks in

your body. You not only will get back in touch with the body's own natural regulations and limits so that you find eating balanced meals more easy, you will also set yourself up for success not just with food but with all aspects of your lifestyle.

Does all this mean you should never eat white chocolate and macadamia cookies again? Some, like my friend the nutritional expert Ron Rosedale, do see diet in such tough terms. I think it's not so black-and-white. I believe that everything is on the planet for a reason. What point is there in eating if you don't get pleasure, delight, and fun from food? If you have a favorite treat, keep it in your life. But we are working to get to that place of moderation. By the fourth week of this program, you will have cleaned out your diet considerably and have a cleaner slate. Then you can add back some of the treats you love once in a while and appreciate them in small, potent doses.

WHAT IS NOISY FOOD?

You can lower the strain placed on your body by reducing your intake of the big three polluters: sugars, chemicals, and caffeine. If you do only one thing, cutting down on the foods that keep you riled up will effect surprisingly big changes in the way you look and feel. Why do I consider them "noisy"? Because they disrupt the internal calm that you can find when you follow a clean, quiet diet. It goes back to the food-as-drug idea. Think of food as a powerful chemical that, once eaten, enters the bloodstream and causes activity to occur throughout our bodies, including our brains. Some foods, particularly whole foods, which have gone through minimal processes in getting from the earth to your plate, filter into the bloodstream slowly and quietly and get on with doing the work of nourishment that nature intended. Other substances, usually ones that have been refined and are several steps removed from an original state, storm their way in, disturbing the peace and forcing the body to react urgently to keep blood sugar levels and hormones under control.

Often they are not substances that our body has evolved, over millions of years, to use as fuel. Early humans did not snack on hydrogenated oils or MSG or, for that matter, on slabs of fluffy Wonder bread. As for sugar and caffeine, they may be naturally occurring substances, but the forms we consume them in and the amounts we ingest are not natural. Eating these foods prompts your body to go into an emergency mode in order to keep the subtle ebb and flow of bodily functions in balance. Hormones are released to slow down the rush of sugar into the blood. The liver goes into overdrive to process chemicals such as colorants or preservatives. No wonder it can feel like you're on a roller coaster of high energy and low mood after eating noisy foods—everything's tipping around inside as your body tries to clean up the spill.

If this toxic load builds up because you ingest a steady supply of sugar, caffeine, or highly processed foods, then your natural system of checks and balances gets disturbed, your detox centers get overworked, and your metabolism—the system that converts food into energy efficiently and keeps your weight regulated—gets totally confused.

Not surprisingly, the foods that create the most noise are often the ones that are most addicting. They deliver exciting, big reactions—big tastes, big rushes, big highs. If not addictive, then at the very least they still work as crutches—things that can be relied upon to instantly shake up your mood or to supply sweet, sedating comfort. Noisy foods have a strong chemical and emotional pull because, just like a drug, they act quickly to change the way you feel. But their help is deceptive. Just as popping a painkiller to cure a symptom means you don't stop to consider the root cause of the pain, so using these fast-acting foods can muffle any hidden imbalances. Rather than asking, "What's out of balance in my diet that I'm flagging at 4:00 P.M.?" you have a double latte. Instead of inquiring, "What's out of balance in my diet that makes me crave sugar even after a full meal?" or even, "Why do my taste buds lust for salty, cheesy, fast food?" you munch on a snack that gives quick relief. In this way you prevent yourself from getting to the source of an *imbalance that you can rectify with smart eating.*

That's why it can be so challenging to kick the habit of certain foods and drinks. They become a crutch that you rely on too much. And until you actively turn down the volume by reducing your intake of these foods (and thereafter replace them with nutritionally rich ones), you will remain at a distance from the natural regulations that keep you well.

Yet the rewards are great because getting calm on the inside is the first step to self-acceptance. As I've found from personal

Taste Inflation

Another good reason to cut the crap and move toward a simpler, more natural diet: you get much more pleasure out of food. Why? Because habitually consuming foods with artificially high sugar and salt levels, with additives like MSG to give everything a kick, or with any kind of "Frankenfood" flavor combo (think of the bizarre unions of flavors found in chips, dips, and processed treats) will dull the sensitivity of your taste buds and change your expectations of how food should taste. Sweet, salty, fatty tastes are the booming bass notes in a flavor; they can drown out subtler sensations. When your diet is full of these extremes, you lose the ability to register subtler flavors, like the sweetness of a blueberry or the delicacy of a real peach instead of peach-flavored iced tea. That's the reason people sometimes complain, "Healthy food is boring!" It's not the food that's boring, it's that their ability to perceive subtle flavors has fled.

Strip away some of the crap—the sugar, salt, fake food additives, and yucky fats in fried foods—and your ability to taste adjusts again to the way it should be. At first, foods may seem lacking in sweetness or saltiness. Yet in short order, as you eat a more diverse diet, new flavors, aromas, and textures reveal themselves to your tongue. It effects a powerful transformation: you start to want less and less of the bad stuff until you almost forget you ever loved it. My husband is a great example. He was a junk food addict for most of his life. He loved Twinkies, pizza, and fries, and he scoffed at my vegetables. When cancer forced him to reevaluate his diet and habits, which also included high levels of stress and some cigarettes, he switched to my way of eating. The magic happened quickly: his taste buds sparked back into life, and he began to love the tastes and flavors of better food. Today he lives for my breakfast smoothies. He finds fresh berries to be fabulously sweet. He loves these nonfake, subtly sweet treats. Believe me, if his taste buds can transform, anybody's can.

experience, if you can create a state of inner chemical calm, you can start to relax and treat yourself more kindly. You'll be better able to look at your life from a calm and reasonable place and implement changes that support you instead of sinking into those funks where self-defeating thoughts keep you stuck—where you're hating your body or hating your life or critiquing every small effort you make to change. When you have peace inside your body at the most basic level, you are laying the groundwork for a much more positive state of mind.

The 7 Most Common Noisy Foods

- tea or coffee
- alcohol
- chocolate
- bread or baked treats
- pretzels or chips
- fruity candy, mints, gum
- ice cream

Listen to the Noise

Deliberately eat a noisy food. It could be a few pieces of strong dark chocolate (try the kind made with over 70 percent cocoa) or a shot of espresso or maybe even a bag of flavored chips. Give yourself a window of twenty minutes after consuming it to be quiet and introspective—while reading, driving to work, preparing dinner—and notice the chemical effect in your body and mind. Has your heartbeat risen? Do you feel a surge of adrenaline? A feeling of happiness? Do you feel a buzz in your head? More focused? Jittery? Excited? Note the sensations during the twenty minutes. Then check in on yourself again in an hour to see what's changed. These physical and mental sensations are what I mean by noise. Now that you can hear it from extreme food experiences, start to tune in to it with everything you eat.

CUT THE CRAP
1. REDUCE YOUR SUGAR INTAKE

A sustained level of sugar intake not only make it impossible to lose weight, it may also promote all kinds of ill health, from diabetes and cancer to heart disease. Sugar of any kind causes the blood glucose (blood sugar) to hurtle up in a sugar rush and subsequently dip down, destabilizing your energy and your mood.

Have you ever noticed how, when the subject of sugar comes up, someone always says proudly, "I don't eat any sugar. At all." It's always fun to ask that person what they had for breakfast. They may answer, "Some organic cereal and half a muffin, and some orange-carrot juice." Or ask them what they had for lunch. "Homemade rice and beans." I'm sorry to say the joke is on them. All those things they mentioned are basically sugar bombs that go off soon after they land in the stomach. The fact that they don't indulge in caramels and fudge bars or put heaping spoons of white table sugar in their tea is good, but it's not enough to earn them the right to claim they're sugar free.

The next person may just say no to frosted cupcakes but chug beverages like fruit juice, soda, and flavored iced tea throughout the day. This one's a no-brainer. There's considerable sugar in all of them in the form of natural fructose (in pure fruit juice) or highly processed and detrimental high-fructose corn syrup (in the soda and tea, unless they include an artificial sweetener, which has its own dangers, as we'll see). And what does it mean that the average diet includes plentiful amounts of bread, potatoes, and rice? These things too will rapidly turn to sugar in your blood, which may not be a problem if your metabolism is running fast and efficiently and you can burn it off but will throw off hopes of getting slender if you're slightly overweight.

Once you figure out where sugar lurks in food and you work on eradicating the excess, you give your whole body a break. By *keeping your blood sugar levels low and steady, rather than riding up and down like a roller* coaster, your metabolism can heal and begin to work more efficiently. You stay sensitive to the natural checks and balances of hormones that regulate weight (and keep you protected against diabetes). You avoid some of the serious problems that can occur when elevated blood sugar creates its damaging inflammatory response, such as a suppressed immune system, crucial mineral deficiencies or difficulties in absorbing minerals from foods, and gastrointestinal diseases. Sugar also feeds cancer cells, which multiply more rapidly when it is available, and it has been connected to causing certain cancers, including those of the breast, ovaries, and pancreas. If that's not enough to inspire a scaling back, how about the fact that sugar causes wrinkles and age spots? In much the same way that heated sugar caramelizes in a saucepan, sugar heated up in your body will change form and cause toughening in the collagen of the skin. Want to avoid the leathery look? Cut down the sugar.

TIP Cutting down sugar can help relieve rheumatoid arthritis and vaginal yeast infections.

SOURCES OF SUGAR

Most people know that refined white table sugar is best avoided. But confusion arises about all the other forms that sugar can take. The only real way to decrease your sugar consumption is to refrain from adding sugar to your foods, avoiding the foods that are made with any kind of sugar derivative, and lowering the intake of foods that quickly turn to sugar in the blood.

5 WAYS TO CUT SUGAR CONSUMPTION

1. *Never sweeten your food or beverages with table sugar.* Try the herb stevia, which is incredibly sweet but not a sugar and therefore has no effect on your blood sugar. I use it in smoothies and in drinks. Though it may seem expensive, one purchase will last for ages because a tiny sprinkle packs a powerful punch. If sugar is less refined and comes in the form of brown, cane, turbinado, succinate, maple syrup, or even honey, is that better? I'll make it easy: no, it's not. (Some of the nutrients are still intact, but the negative impact of sugar still far outweighs the positive value of some vitamins.) Your body doesn't say, "That's a nice sugar, I like that." Sure, there's some nutritive value to *uncooked, unfiltered* honey, but most of us put it in tea, which cooks it and turns it to pure sugar.

2. *For baking,* substitute natural sweeteners like xylitol, which sounds like a chemical but is actually red birch bark. (See the Index of Products, at the back of this book, for good brands.)

3. *Pay more attention to the labels.* Sugar lurks in many of the foods we purchase, including condiments and savories.

• Note that one of the most widely used sweeteners in commercial foods comes from corn, which is a very sugary vegetable. If ingredients include such things as corn syrup, fructose, high-fructose corn syrup, cornstarch, dextrose, and maltodextrin, you are eating and drinking sugar. Start looking at ingredient labels and checking for words that end in *-ose* to sniff out the sugar.

• Be suspicious of anything "naturally sweetened." Honey, rice syrup, and cane juice are all sugar. Concentrated fruit juice used as a

37

sweetener is also little more than flavored sugar syrup. Be moderate in use of jams and jellies, or cut them entirely if you can.

- Keep an eye on drinks. The source of most of America's sugar intake today is soda. Try to cut that out entirely, including the diet kind, which has fake chemical sweetener. These are addictive, so be kind to yourself as you are weaning them out of your diet. Beware of sport drinks, energy drinks, vitamin waters, and iced teas. They can be dangerously high in sugar. Note that fruit beverages or fruit cocktails are almost always sweetened with high-fructose corn syrup. Always check the label before you buy.
- Watch out for so-called energy bars and meal replacement bars. They can deliver much more sugar than you realize. Check the carbs and sugar values on the package. Always be a little skeptical of foods that appear to be healthy just because of the name or package design. What counts is the actual stuff inside.

TIP Do not substitute artificial sweetener for real sugar. The chemicals found in saccharin, aspartame, and sucralose can often be worse than the sugar itself. Aspartame, for example, is a chemical that has been linked to neurological disorders, brain tumors, liver problems, and other serious diseases. Using artificial sweeteners can disrupt the body's appetite-regulating system, which is expecting a rise in blood sugar from the sweet food but not getting any evidence that nourishment is happening. It sends messages out to keep eating more and more.

TIP Many products use the word *natural* on the packaging; this is usually meaningless. A "natural" product could be sweetened by sugary fruit (the natural part) and contain additives and preservatives. Evaluate the ingredients for yourself to determine how good it is for you.

4. *Watch your pure fruit juice intake.* Fruits are packed with many valuable nutrients, but they are high in fructose, a form of sugar. Fruit juices have been stripped of the fiber that would have slowed down sugar absorption in the blood, and you're left with a highly sugary liquid. (An eight-ounce glass of pure juice has about eight teaspoons of sugar in it.) In addition, most store-bought juices have been pasteurized, which kills vital enzymes. Some pure fruit juices are still of great value when used in moderation, as they give a powerful vitamin and antioxidant punch (antioxidants are naturally occurring substances that protect cells from the damage that leads to disease and aging). Try splashing a small amount— like a tablespoon—of pure juice of blueberry, pomegranate, and the new "wonder berry," açai, into smoothies. You can also use pure juice moderately to add flavor to water: try mixing unfiltered apple juice with soda water or plain water. Just avoid chugging huge glasses of orange juice or apple when plain water would do.

I'm such a believer in cutting out sugar that I think if you go to a juice or smoothie store and place an order for a smoothie, you're better off eating the fibrous pulp left behind than to drink the juice, which costs five dollars. If that's too harsh, a better alternative is to get a vegetable juice in which green leafy veggies equal or outweigh starchy veggies like carrots and beets.

You'll get major nutrients but minimal sugar. If you do juice your own veggies and fruits, drink the beverage immediately, as many of the beneficial nutrients are lost rapidly upon juicing.

5. *Reduce your intake of grains and starches.* Probably the biggest problem in the modern American diet is the overdependence on foods made from grains. Breads, cereals, crackers, cookies, and cakes as well as pasta and rice have become major staples. Grain products are the biggest section on the official food pyramid—a big mistake since overconsumption of them leads to tremendous weight gain. Second in seriousness: eating too many starches, primarily potatoes. These high-carbohydrate foods, especially the refined grains—watch out for white flour and milled grains—have an effect similar to regular white sugar. Since their energy can't be stored, excess carbs not only turn to fat, they also destabilize your energy and mood in the short term; over time, indulging in them can lead to disease and obesity.

Grains are just another way to say sugar. Your body doesn't differentiate between table sugar and carbohydrates, which become sugar in the blood.Their powerful chemical effect in the body is what makes refined grains and starches so noisy and so hard to self-regulate. They cause a quick rise in blood sugar, which sets off chemical reactions in your body that are designed to counter this sugar rush. The hormone insulin floods out to do damage control, but it rushes out too quickly to defend the body against these extreme ingredients and ends up driving blood-sugar levels too low. This emergency rush of insulin is the reason why many people have hunger pangs a couple of hours after eating high-carb foods and then crave more sugar. It causes the roller-coaster effect—you eat a meal heavy in carbs, feel a fast boost of energy, then later get fatigued and bummed out and ache for a sweet treat. Feed that craving with a candy bar, a wedge of grainy toast, or a caramel latte, and the roller coaster starts up again. It's like a minidrama unfolding as euphoria swings to a funk and back again. Ultimately it can create a condition called insulin resistance, which is a major source of obesity and disease, as well as the common scenario of simply not being able to lose those extra pounds.

TIP I highly recommend reading Ron Rosedale's book *The Rosedale Diet* for a deeper explanation of the connection between insulin resistance and weight issues, particularly if you are struggling with chronic illness or diabetes.

Whole-grain foods turn to sugar more slowly than refined grains and are therefore a much better choice because they won't trigger the extreme roller-coaster reaction; plus, you benefit from the fiber. But the fact is that all grains turn to sugar and elevate the glucose levels in your blood for considerable chunks of time. All grains eaten in excess will therefore cause you to turn their energy into fat. The effects can be serious: if you keep the noise level high by consuming lots of grains, starches, and other sugars, you will become deaf to the hormone signals that want to keep you vital and slim. White is worse. When in doubt, if it's made from white—white flour, white rice, white sugar—make a different choice. Give up buying foods made from white flour. It's devoid of nutrients, and the additives in it can cause vitamin deficiencies.

■ ■ ■

MY RELATIONSHIP TO SUGAR has been interesting, to say the least. In my early teens I was super tall and skinny for my age, and I was constantly hungry. No matter how much I ate, I was never full. On the rare occasions that my family would dine out at a restaurant, I'd be bummed because at a restaurant you can't go for seconds. I'd come home from school and munch on snacks for hours. Endless bowls of Grape-Nuts with orange juice as I watched *One Life to Live* and *General Hospital* with my best friend, or stick after stick of celery with peanut butter. Of course, that incessant hunger is pretty natural when you're shooting up toward five-foot-ten in your early teens. But it troubled me. For one thing, when you're that skinny as a teen and can eat a lot, all the other girls hate you. Even my own sister Margaux hated me. I wish now that their envy hadn't affected me because it indelibly marked food with big red letters that spelled shame.

More difficult was the fact that as the situation in our home got more painful, I turned to food to satisfy more than hunger pangs. I used it to find comfort and solace and to fill a dull ache somewhere below my heart. My mom got sick from cancer and took to her room, my dad retreated more frequently to his beloved fishing river, my older sisters disappeared off to town and teenage trouble, and I ate bread. And more bread. My mother, on her good days, would carefully craft thick loaves of ten-grain bread from my grandmother's recipe, and they were irresistible to me. Straight out of the oven, they seemed to practically glow with warmth, safety, and love. I would eat one slice, then another, carving off thin wedges until much of the loaf was gone. I literally couldn't stop until I felt sick. Sometimes I'd spread the slices with the new "health" food of the early seventies, bright yellow margarine. But I couldn't kid myself. There was nothing nutritious about my habit. Food was my source of love and consequently, when I abused it like this, the source of more shame.

Looking back, I see I was addicted to the crash-and-crave cycle that grains can cause. In addition, when you overeat complex starchy carbs, the neurotransmitter serotonin is released, which is a key chemical in creating a feeling of well-being in the brain. I was so frightened of being addicted to eating like other members of my family had been that throughout my twenties and thirties I cut out all grains and all sugars entirely. I took it all the way because that's what helps me feel most stable.

Salt

The excessive amount of salt in the modern diet contributes not only to high blood pressure in those predisposed to hypertension, but also to taste inflation. If you frequently add salt to your food, ask why. Do you eat a lot of processed and fast food, which typically has high levels of salt and includes preservatives, most of which are sodium based? Has that elevated your tolerance for salt? Or is the food you're cooking lacking in flavor and you're compensating with salt? Use salt sparingly, and look for sea salt, which features beneficial minerals, not regular table salt or iodized salt, which is high in aluminum.

CUT THE CRAP
2. EXAMINE YOUR CAFFEINE HABIT

Caffeine agitates the heart rate and causes the body to release hormones, resulting after prolonged use in a state of adrenal exhaustion.

All too often, you need a caffeine rush because your food is not serving as fuel. Caffeine is often used as the go-to substance when you're flagging, but its benefits are deceptive. It charges up your batteries for a moment but does nothing to give you usable energy. I used caffeine as a crutch for most of my adult life. In my twenties I devised more ways of whipping up zero-calorie, blended coffee drinks than Starbucks could ever dream of. I used it continuously instead of feeding myself real, nourishing foods.

The problem with caffeine is that rather than giving you food energy, it stimulates your adrenal glands to make adrenaline, thus putting you in a fight-or-flight state—the stress response the body goes into in preparing to react to danger. You're amped up and alert, but chances are you're sitting at your desk and neither about to fight nor flee. When that charge wears off shortly thereafter, you're left with the low that comes after the high: you might feel tired, moody, or slightly irritable. If you use caffeine throughout the day, then time and again you're forcing your adrenals to respond as if there's an emergency. It's no wonder that when this becomes a habit it puts great wear and tear on the body. Not to mention you start needing bigger hits to feel as amped as you used to. You lose some

sensitivity to its effects and begin to consume more than a first-time caffeine drinker could ever tolerate. Without a regular intake, you feel withdrawal symptoms, such as powerful headaches. During one notorious episode when I quit coffee cold turkey at the height of my habit, I forgot all my lines on the TV show I was filming, and the crew resorted to holding cue cards saying, "Please have some java!" Coffee had such an effect on my wiring that without it I was turned upside down.

If coffee or tea is something you rely on, you will wean yourself down to minimal amounts during this program in order to quiet the noise in your system. (See "Turning Down the Volume," on page 48.)

Don't forget that many sodas and energy drinks are full of caffeine, and chocolate, especially the dark kind, is a potent source of it as well. If you're not addicted to coffee, you might be addicted to one of these. Follow this program and scale back accordingly.

If you're a committed coffee or black tea drinker, peruse the vast selection of teas in your local health food mart and get inspired by the plethora of interesting green teas and noncaffeinated herbal teas in delicious and satisfying flavors. Online tea retailers carry incredible selections. You can also decaffeinate any tea yourself by pouring in the hot water, steeping for fifteen to twenty seconds, and tossing the water. This removes 80 to 90 percent of the caffeine from leaves. Then pour in more water and steep for several minutes to get your beverage. When purchasing decaffeinated coffee, look for those made with the Swiss water process, which is chemical free.

TREAT YOURSELF: *Rishi teas are my favorite source for fabulous green and herbal teas. A small teapot with an infuser basket is a good purchase; it will ensure you don't oversteep the delicate green leaves, which will give a bitter taste if they're in the water for more than three minutes (certain varieties need even less time). (See the Index of Products, at the end of this book, for all "Treat Yourself" sources.)*

SUPER SUBSTITUTES: Made from a blend of herbs, grains, fruits, and nuts, Teeccino™ is a caffeine-free "herbal coffee" that tastes delicious. I use it for my whey latte (see recipe on page 67), and it's a great stand-in for traditional java when you want to kick the habit. Yerba maté is a potent tea that is quite high in caffeine but can be a good first step away from coffee: it gives a clean, nonjittery lift. Use it to help downgrade your way into the world of teas. (See the Index of Products for recommended sources.)

Since I began treating my body more kindly in my midthirties, I've gone through extended cold-turkey periods when I've not touched a drop of caffeine as well as periods when my green tea habit eked its way up to become nearly a dependency—while I, meanwhile, proudly considered myself a reformed coffee-holic. Today I'm on my guard. I'm the first to say that despite the gentle reputation of tea, be it black tea, green tea, or yerba maté, it is possible to crank up the volume so that you get a real buzz and are totally addicted to it. Anytime I think my green tea is getting out of hand, and anytime symptoms come up in my body that I can't find the source of, I scale back the caffeine. It's my self-imposed checks and balances. But where I used to hold myself to very high standards and force myself to go entirely caffeine free, now I give myself a break to avoid the painful withdrawal symptoms. I scale it back to where I feel neither dependent nor totally bereft: from time to time I limit myself to just one small pot of green tea in the morning, and later in the day I resist the urge for more by making hot water and lemon or herbal tea.

DID YOU KNOW CAFFEINE IS AN INSECTICIDE? It evolved in plants in order to keep bugs away. We're a lot larger than insects, but we're still putting a stimulant into our systems that nature intended to have harsh effects.

Conscious Caffeine Habits

- Instead of relying on coffee in the morning to get you going, eat a healthy breakfast that gives some protein and some fat for a slow and sustained energy boost, and see if that works better.
- Pay attention to your caffeine intake if you are experiencing pain in your joints and muscles. Caffeine can dehydrate the body, and we often drink caffeinated beverages in lieu of water. The combination of its irritating effect and dehydration can cause ill effects in the body and mind. When body pain occurs, notice your caffeine intake.
- Caffeine stays in your system much longer than you may think. If you have trouble sleeping, your first change should be to cut out all caffeine after lunch. Afternoon coffees and teas can affect you even up until bedtime. (And if an evening cup of joe doesn't throw off your sleep patterns, ask yourself: is it a sign that your tolerance is way too high?)

- If you're tired when you wake up in the morning no matter how much you sleep, and you stay sleepy and a bit emotionally unsteady for most of the morning, it could be a sign that your adrenal glands have been maxed out. Though it seems counterintuitive to cut out caffeine when you feel you need the boost most, try cutting it to give your adrenal glands a chance to rebalance.

Get Hydrated

Get up right now and have a tall glass of water.

There is one habit that I'd guess at least three-quarters of the population needs to change. It's the simplest one of all and therefore way too often overlooked. Drink water. We need more of it than we're getting: it's essential for our cells to function in any capacity, for us to metabolize fats, to flush out the wastes. Did you know that dehydration is the cause behind many of your aches, pains, and off-color feelings? Headaches, fatigue, irritability, constipation, dry skin, and that dragging feeling of not being able to get out of bed in the morning all have physiological sources in a dehydrated state. (Not getting enough water also will affect your metabolism so that you put on small amounts of weight.)

What are some more serious cries for help from a thirsty body you should recognize? Pain in the body, like heartburn, rheumatoid joint pain, back pain, and migraine headaches are serious signs that toxic waste has built up in an area and your cells need to drink. If you are chronically dehydrated, far more serious symptoms can show up, from blood pressure and circulatory problems to kidney disease, immune system dysfunction, and digestive disorders.

Chances are you see this advice to drink more water in a magazine from time to time, you briefly up your intake, then after a while you let your levels slide. Maybe you get considerable fluid from teas and nonsweetened, healthy beverages so you imagine it's all the same. But it's not. According to health advocate Dr. Batmanghelidj, who has extensively researched and written about the healing power of water, the body needs a steady supply of "free water," which has no agenda but to hydrate the cells and carry out toxic waste. All other drinks, whether caffeinated, flavored, or enhanced in some way, have some other agenda that gets in the way of this crucial function.

Optimum health is contingent on your supplying yourself with plain water throughout the day and not waiting until you're thirsty: thirst is a sign of dehydration, so by the time you feel it, your body is already under stress. Furthermore, humans lose their ability to perceive thirst as they get older, so if you're always waiting until you've got dry mouth to have a drink, you'll become even more dehydrated.

WHAT: Drink water throughout the day, and try drinking a glass first thing in the morning to get going. (It will also flush stomach acids that accumulate overnight so that if you do have an acidic cup of coffee soon after, you're not creating an even harsher environment.)

HOW MUCH: Some nutritionists advise one gallon a day for every fifty pounds of body weight; others say at least eight tall glasses a day. But the easy way to keep track of your hydration level is to check the color of your urine. It should be light yellow in color—the paler, the better. The darker yellow it is, the more water you need. (Note: some vitamins will make your pee electric yellow, so you'll have to cut them out for a few days to get a good reading.) This should be your default hydration detector all the time: pay attention to what you put out to know what you need to put in.

A tall glass of water can be a quick pick-me-up when you're sleepy and can temporarily quash strong hunger pangs. Try it next time you're longing for a jolt of caffeine or a premeal snack, and see how it shifts your state.

WHERE TO FIND: Having clean, pure water available at all times in your house is a good investment. Tap water almost always contains some chemicals, mainly chlorine and fluoride but also others that contaminate it and slowly take a toxic toll on the body. It is possible to get your water checked, or your town may have information on its water.

Getting home delivery of five-gallon spring water containers (preferably glass bottles, not plastic) is one healthier option; filtration systems are another. The kinds that are affixed under the sink, called reverse-osmosis filters, are the most beneficial. They can be the most cost effective in the long term though require more money up front.

TREAT YOURSELF: *A reverse-osmosis filtration system that fits under your kitchen sink will give you easy access to purified water for drinking and cooking. A quick search online will direct you to many sources.*

CUT THE CRAP
3. REDUCE CHEMICAL ADDITIVES

Artificial preservatives, colors, and flavorings as well as hydrogenated oils and pesticides are unwelcome guests that gate-crash your body and put a strain on your systems of detoxification.

3 Ways to Feel & Look Better Instantly

1. BANISH BAD FATS

WHAT: Trans fats. These are formed when vegetable oils are made into solid form through a chemical process called hydrogenization. They are by far one of the most seriously damaging parts of our diet!

WHERE: Used for many processed foods, especially snack foods, candy bars, and baked goods, and used widely in the fast-food industry. Also found in margarine and buttery spreads. Trans fats are cheap, they lengthen the shelf life of foods, and they keep flavors stable—but at the price of your health.

WHY: The natural vegetable oils have gone through a harsh chemical process in order to be *trans*formed into trans-fatty acids. These acids

Exercise: Archeology Mission

Pull out a few packaged products from your fridge or kitchen cupboard, or look at the packet of the next store-bought food you buy. Look at the ingredient labels. Do you know what all the words on it mean? Do they sound like things you want to have in your body? Consider how much of what you consume you can understand—and suddenly the idea of cooking lentils from scratch can seem pretty appealing.

Lowering your intake of highly processed foods will lower the noise in your system by decreasing the toxic load your body has to process. Anything that contains preservatives, artificial coloring, and artificial flavoring should be vetoed. All these chemical additives are agitating and destructive to body and mind. (It's not surpris-

ing that studies show when you take foods with chemical additives away from kids who have ADD, their behavioral problems improve remarkably.) The engineering that is done to extend the shelf life of foods does not seem to extend our own lives.

Many refined foods have gone through so many processes to transform them from their natural state that they not only end up nutritionally depleted, they also take more energy to break down and expel than they provide. In fact, some nutritionists say that eating foods devoid of the naturally occurring minerals we need will actually contribute to overeating. Our bodies don't want to stop consuming because their essential dietary needs have not been fulfilled.

not only block us from absorbing and using essential fatty acids that we do need, they also disturb the makeup of our cells and are linked to a host of serious diseases, including cancer and diabetes. Trans fats are considered so harmful that consumer advocates have tried to ban the use of this ingredient in the United States—as it is banned in some other countries.

AVOID: Nutritional labels are required to include trans fats. Start checking the ingredients for the word *hydrogenated,* look at the caloric breakdown, and see how many everyday items are full of them. Restaurants, including fast-food joints, are harder to police.

INSTEAD: Use real butter, not margarine, at home; avoid commercially produced snacks, baked goods, and fast food.

It's not just solid trans fats you have to be wary of. The polyunsaturated vegetable oils that are touted to be super healthy, such as safflower, sunflower, canola, and so on, have a downside: they can easily go rancid, which creates damaging free radicals that can harm your cells. And they get damaged by high-heat cooking and further disrupt your cellular function.

One great change you can make in your diet is to switch your fats. Stick with good-quality olive oil (extra virgin is best because it is processed in a gentler way). Buy only "expeller-pressed" or "unrefined" vegetable oils and good-quality butter (organic or, better yet, raw organic if you can find it, full of essential, fat-soluble vitamins and delicious taste). And try a new contender in the health field: coconut oil, which is a healthy saturated fat that is great for high-heat cooking (see recipe section for more). Also try walnut oil and almond oil for dressings and baking. Always store all cooking oils in dark containers so they don't go rancid.

2. CUT CHEMICAL ADDITIVES

WHAT: Synthetic colors, flavors, and preservatives added to processed food to make them more appetizing or more flavorful or to last longer than nature would allow.

WHERE: In many processed foods, from cereal to condiments to ice cream.

WHY: Can build up in your intestines and cross through into your bloodstream, taxing the liver, which must detoxify them. If the liver gets overloaded with toxins from prolonged consumption of these foods, the additives start to circulate in the bloodstream and can lead to problems like skin disorders, weight gain, and possibly autoimmune disorders. In some cases, if you eat a lot of highly refined foods and stimulants, your body starts depleting its own mineral supply. Also factor in the trash and waste that you are adding to landfills from packaged, processed foods. Consuming lots of prepackaged food is not good either for your body or for the environment.

AVOID: Eat meals of whole foods closest to their original state whenever possible (like a home-roasted chicken, not boxed chicken stir-fry). Veto foods that look like nature wouldn't have made them that way, and check the ingredients list for suspicious activity. Harmful nitrates, for example, are added to many lunch meats to make them look pink. Nix those brands.

3. PASS UP THE PESTICIDES

WHAT: Chemicals sprayed on plant-based foods as well as on livestock feeds.

WHERE: Conventionally grown fruits and vegetables; wheat, corn, and other grains and products are made from them. Dairy, eggs, meats, and fish all accumulate pesticides as well.

WHY: Their toxic effect on the body has been linked to cancer and hormonal disruptions, such as reproductive problems in humans, and are especially damaging to an unborn child; the toxic runoff from fields contaminates waters and wildlife.

AVOID: When possible, buy organic or "pesticide-free" produce (which comes from soil that has not received official organic validation but has not been sprayed). Wash all fruit and vegetables thoroughly by immersing in a sink of water with a splash of hydrogen peroxide in it, then rinse in fresh water. This helps to pull the pesticides off the surface in a way that plain water cannot. (Wash even the good stuff: washing also cleans organic produce of any dirt-borne pathogens.)

Fruit and Vegetable Wash, available in liquid form in your supermarket or health mart, is a convenient way to get produce as detoxed as possible. Note that peeling fruits and vegetables will reduce surface contaminants but will also deprive you of nutrients. Vary your intake, wash as best you can, and buy pesticide free whenever possible.

Buy Smart: Lower Your Pesticide Load

- Conventional produce typically most heavily laden with pesticides: apples, grapes, peaches, raspberries, strawberries, cherries, spinach, celery, peppers
- Conventional produce typically least pesticide laden: asparagus, avocado, banana, onion, broccoli, cauliflower, corn, papaya, pineapple, peas

TIP Imported produce is three times as likely to contain illegal pesticide residues. Notice where your berries, fruits, and veggies come from.

GRASS-FED BEEF packs a powerful nutritional punch because it has a higher ratio of important omega-3 fats to the more common omega-6 fats, which most people consume too much of. Likewise, dairy products from grass-fed cows, not cows fed commercial grain, are rich with crucial fat-soluble vitamins. If you can find raw dairy products near you, try them. They not only taste great, they also retain many more nutrients (enzymes, vitamins, and proteins) because they are not pasteurized.

Quick Checklist: Cut Excess Chemicals

1. Avoid canned, sprayed, waxed, genetically modified, or irradiated fruits and vegetables.
2. Limit foods that contain hydrogenated or partially hydrogenated fats and oils.
3. Cut out all sodas as well as desserts or snacks made with artificial sweeteners.
4. Cut out processed meats like luncheon and breakfast meats. They have nitrates that have been linked to cancer, as well as high levels of salt.
5. Avoid most powdered, canned, or boxed soups, sauces, and broth mixes: they often have high MSG levels. Commercial condiments like ketchup often have it too.
6. Buy organic produce whenever possible.

Animal Products:
Lower Your Toxic Load

Shopping for dairy products, eggs, meat, and chicken has become a concern because of pesticides, hormones, and antibiotics, as well as bacteria, that are frequently found at high levels in conventional (nonorganic or wild) animal produce. Purchasing fish is tricky as most fish has high levels of mercury and other toxins. In an ideal world we'd all buy organic all the time. But price and availability render that choice impossible for many. The best you can do is to make organic choices where possible and smart selections elsewhere. It's important to rotate your protein sources to avoid exposure to too many of the same toxins.

■ If your dairy products aren't organic, look for products that are free of recombinant bovine growth hormone (rBGH).

■ If you buy conventional chicken rather than organic, free-range, or cage-free, take off the skin to reduce exposure to toxins that accumulate in the fat.

■ If you buy conventional beef, buy leaner cuts like flank and round steak. Bison, if available, is not only lean, it's often raised without hormones and antibiotics. Never charbroil or grill meat until blackened; this increases your exposure to carcinogens.

■ When possible, buy wild or ocean-caught fish. When buying canned tuna, choose skipjack tuna over albacore tuna, as it has less mercury. Some nutritionists advise eating only fish that has been scientifically proven to have minimal mercury levels; others say the nutritional benefits from fish outweigh the risks. As with every lifestyle choice, you will have to weigh the pros and cons yourself. If you're pregnant, minimize fish intake and research online to find the latest list of safe fish.

■ If you eat a lot of soy-based products or feed them to your kids, look for those marked "GM free." Most soybeans are genetically modified, and the jury is still out on the long-term health effects of these crops.

Exercise: Turning Down the Volume

Which noisy foods do you regularly consume—caffeinated beverages, sodas, energy drinks, sugary snacks, bread products, chips, fast food? Over the four weeks of this program, you will downgrade your intake so that by Week 3 you are eating and drinking none of them. (If you consume only one, focus on that.) Pick two of the three following options—or do all three if it is feasible. Most noisy foods can be cut out immediately without any adverse physical reactions, especially if you substitute something that pleases you, though a strong caffeine habit should be phased out gradually (see "Downgrade Your Caffeine Habit," on the next page). In Week 4 of the program, you will deliberately pick a treat you love and add it back into your food plan in a moderate—but much-appreciated—way, and you will experience how less can be more.

■ **OPTION A:** If caffeine is your noisiest food, in Week 1 you will downgrade it one degree, and in Week 2, downgrade two to three degrees (see chart in "Downgrade Your Caffeine Habit").

■ **OPTION B:** If sugar is your fix (in the form of sodas, treats, sweet snacks, or alcohol), cut as much as you can in Week 1, and continue in Week 2, lowering your grain intake as well if you can.

■ **OPTION C:** If processed food is often on the menu (fast food, chips and snacks, boxed and wrapped products), cut it entirely in Week 1, and work on finding substitutions so that it is easy to avoid in Week 2.

• Notice your physical and emotional reactions to this process. Do you get annoyed at any point in the day or feel a strong craving for your fix, and if so, at what time of day? Do you have a strong physical reaction, like a headache?

• Consider what the reaction means. Does it suggest you may have a dependency on this noisy food, and how does that make you feel? If not having this food has no effect on you at all, ask yourself whether you consume it from habit rather than from real need, and if so, why? What purpose does this food or drink serve in your day?

• When you do add small amounts of caffeine, sugar, or your favorite fix back into your diet, ask yourself if you really want it before you consume it. That way you always consume it because it's a pleasure, not a habit.

Healthier Substitutes

Instead of high-fat, high-sugar treats like ice cream, candy, and cakes, satisfy your sweet tooth with a few pieces of low-fat, natural products like dried fruit, crystallized ginger, or small portions of tart fruit. Fruit ices and sorbets will do in a pinch.

Instead of grainy, sugary snacks or processed-food snacks (cookies, cakes, crackers, cupcakes), try a handful of raw almonds and/or walnuts and some tart fruit like a Granny Smith apple.

Instead of salty chips, nuts, or pretzels, try a small handful of raw or dry-roasted nuts (see Home-Toasted Nuts recipe on page 68).

Downgrade Your Caffeine Habit by Degrees

Caffeine is the hardest habit to kick, but doing so will help you get to a clean slate chemically. If you drink coffee or strong tea consistently, I don't recommend quitting cold turkey. (According to some studies, even one mug a day of coffee can produce withdrawal symptoms when stopped.) Be kind and reasonable in your expectations, and turn down the volume week by week. Get to the point by Week 3 of this program of drinking no caffeine; then you can evaluate during Week 4 if you want it, and you can add back a small amount, which will pack a big punch and taste great. Note that curtailing even a moderate caffeine habit may make you feel unusually tired because you're not getting the kick that you're accustomed to. Stick it out, resist the temptation for a pick-me-up, and know that by cutting the stimulants, you're stripping back the layers to get to the truth of how you really feel.

- *Instead of* three coffees a day, downgrade to two, then one, then decaf coffee, herbal coffee, or decaf tea.
- *Instead of* a large latte, downgrade to medium or small, then decaf latte, then whey latte made with decaf or herbal coffee, or decaf tea.
- *Instead of* regular coffee, downgrade to black tea or yerba maté, then to green tea.
- *Instead of* strong black tea, downgrade to green tea, then decaf or herbal tea.

Instead of a blended frappé drink, try a caffeine-free whey latte (recipe on page 67).

Wild Card: Instead of an energy drink midday or before going out for an evening, try two minutes of Arm Swings (see Exercise section) or the Restorative Pose (see Silence section) to elevate your energy without the aid of stimulants.

SPRING CLEANING EXERCISES

Commit to starting your 30-Day Program with food by physically cleaning the slate and clearing out any clutter both externally—in your kitchen—and, if it feels right to you, internally as well. Building awareness of what types of food work best for you will be easier when you have done a bit of spring cleaning. Here are two ways to expedite the process.

Exercise: Spring Cleaning for Your Fridge

The state of your fridge can cause you to make bad choices. Create the conditions for success by throwing out the old and making room for the new. If you find everything under the sun in your fridge, you'll find it much harder to make good food work for you. You won't eat old pizza, at least not during this 30-Day Program—and certainly not for your revamped breakfast. Toss it. Also get rid of the six drops of Heinz ketchup in the one-gallon jug; the old dressing made from some nasty oil that isn't good for you; the Cheez Whiz; the white bread; the half-eaten pie or cake; and the Cool Whip (it barely qualifies as food). Get rid of anything that isn't a color nature created. Toss any juice; it's just sugar. Take a moment to survey what's in your fridge, and let your instinct tell you what's good and what's bad. Now you're ready to fill your kitchen with the produce that will truly boost your body. By the end of this program, each person's fridge will look slightly different, but all will burst with vital energy—lots of vegetables, lots of natural color, and perishable products that must be eaten fresh.

Exercise: Spring Cleaning for Your Body

In Week 4 you will do a modified, one-day cleanse that is easy and gentle on the system. It gives the body a break from digesting and allows you to press the reset button on yourself. I do a three-day version of this cleanse anytime I need to renew myself or want the feeling of starting fresh in all areas of my life. It is not a harsh fasting cleanse; you stay full and satiated, but the liquid nature of it gives your intestines a break and lets energy go toward healing other parts of the body that may need attention, especially your overactive mind. But even a one-day cleanse will give you benefit: when you introduce different foods back into your diet afterward, your sensitivity to the effect of that food will be much greater.

One-day cleanse: Start your day with a smoothie (on page 66). For lunch and dinner you will eat a broth of pureed vegetables. Steam a mixture of cauliflower, zucchini, broccoli, and spinach, then blend them into a thick puree. Add some sea salt or kelp (dried seaweed) if you can find it; look in the international aisle of your market. Eat this as a hot soup throughout the day, as much or as little as you like. *It is your only food source.*

Although veggies are technically a carb, they are high fiber, nonstarchy carbs, so they don't raise your sugar levels at all.

Drink medium-hot water with lemon throughout the day along with plenty of cool, filtered water. Hot or warm water with lemon is actually a first stage live cleanse. Cool water or room temperature water is better than iced because it doesn't shock the system.

At night take a tablespoon of extra-virgin olive oil before going to bed, and remember to drink water with it.

Remember: no caffeine, no snacks, no bread with your broth.

Everybody does it. Everybody wants to do it every day. But it doesn't always go as planned. Elimination: the taboo subject that is integral to a healthy body and mind. In yoga they say that digestion—the process that happens to your food once it's eaten—is responsible for good health. Any problem eliminating waste matter will affect every part of us, so not talking about it won't do us any favors. It's particularly important for women, as we tend to hold a lot of anxiety in our lower abdominal area, and any stress in our daily life affects our ability to eliminate. Which means that problems with bowel movements are far more common than you realize.

If you are not eliminating waste regularly and efficiently, you will literally feel like crap in your body and your mind. If you are eating plenty of vegetables and fiber, you should excrete up to twelve inches of waste a day, whether in one movement or several separate ones. Any waste that remains uneliminated in your intestines for more than twenty-four hours starts to become toxic. It can create an environment in which peristalsis—the movement of the gut wall to push waste along—is inhibited. If you get off track with bowel movements by eating the wrong kind of diet and you don't try to rectify the situation with better food intake, you are building a situation in which bad leads to worse.

If the waste stays in the colon (the largest part of the intestines) too long, not only do you feel sluggish and bloated and get more constipated, but eventually toxins can seep through the intestinal wall and tax the liver and kidneys, whose job it is to clear the toxins from your bloodstream. The toxins can now also inflame the muscles around your stomach cavity. If you have chronic lower back pain, take note that one possible cause may be waste buildup in your colon. (Getting massages and bodywork may be futile if you don't work on cleansing your internal environment.)

The good news is that if you do suffer from irregular bowel movements, the acts of modifying your diet, exercising, and creating a calm lifestyle in which you're less stressed and have more time for your personal needs will radically improve the situation. Diet is key. As you experiment with cutting out certain foods and adding in others, keep track of what happens in your intestines. Refined foods and processed foods not only lack the fiber to move waste through our system, they contain chemicals that can create that toxic, peristalsis-inhibiting environment. As you play around with your diet in these four weeks, notice the effects on your elimination habits. For example, meat and fish may make some people work more efficiently while slowing others down. Know that nature offers many foods that will help put sluggish systems into high gear. If you can get on track through eating right, your body will be much better off than if you depend on fiber supplements (which are easy to overdo and can cause more constipation) or even natural laxatives. (As for chemical laxatives? Toss them, and add in some vegetables instead.)

Food

Ways to Improve
Your Elimination Immediately

- Drink more water. One of the colon's jobs is to get any water out of food and give it to the body. If enough fluids aren't coming in, your waste is too dry to move easily through the intestines. If you're skimpy with your fluid allowance, doubling your water intake might be necessary to improve your situation. If you use coffee in the morning to promote a bowel movement, now is the time to wean yourself off it. Coffee triggers this action because it is an irritant; the intestines react with a shock rather than because they are naturally ready to move. As with all crutches, you develop a reliance on this stimulant and it gradually loses its efficacy—while you're still flooding your body with caffeine.

TIP Aloe vera juice, available at health food stores, helps with elimination. Try half a glass mixed with a shot of unfiltered apple juice every other morning.

- Lower the load of "sticky foods," such as wheat products, which turn to gluten in the gut, and cheese, which slows down intestinal efficiency.
- Greatly increase your intake of vegetables, particularly cabbage and beets. Dark green leafy vegetables and vegetables with a bitter or spicy taste such as Swiss chard, kale, arugula, watercress, asparagus, and artichoke also help. They add fiber to your diet, plus their bitterness promotes the bile duct to make more bile, which aids in digestion.

TIP Roast several beets in a hot oven, peel when cool, and keep them in the fridge so you can slice into salads daily.

- Use ground flaxseed or flax powder in smoothies or sprinkled on yogurt (see breakfast recipes on pages 64–68). Experiment with adding these high-fiber foods into your diet: beans, peas, and legumes; *moderate* amounts of rough bran cereal and extremely grainy bread products; moderate amounts of dried figs, apricots, and dates (note these are high in sugar, so be careful); berries; broccoli.
- Practice sitting on your heels in Hero's Pose after eating. It aids digestion, and when you sit with one foot crossed over the other, you stimulate pressure points in the feet that encourage overall wellness. Regular practice of Breath of Fire (see Exercise, Quick Fix #3) will also help with digestion.

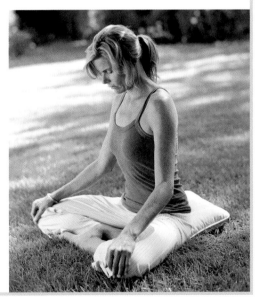

Find Your
Personal Balance

AFTER I LEFT HOME AND BECAME INDEPENDENT, I went through a lot of off-kilter behavior trying to find a way of eating that worked for me. By the time I moved to New York at eighteen to pursue my acting career, I was teaching myself all sorts of interesting ways to rigidly control my food intake. It was a typical actress diet, only I got so interested in the science behind the various food fads at the time, like the ultra-low-fat Pritikin diet, that I always found my own ways of making them more extreme or, as I mistakenly thought, more pure. The food-control issues I'd experienced at home reared up big-time now. Being a young woman on her own in a big city and working in a movie industry that, like today, insisted a woman be skinny added fuel to my self-competitive fire. I subtracted more and more things from my diet that I feared would make me fat and focused on the incredible vitamins and nutrients I surely had to be getting from all the vegetables I consumed. (Not to mention fiber. If there was one thing I was proud of, it was my fiber intake.) Juggling various food philosophies at once, I got rid of all the dairy, much of the protein, and definitely all of the grains. No rice and definitely no bread.

As for fat? Vetoed. In the late seventies and early eighties fat was cast as the absolute nutritional enemy, so I took the news to heart and removed fat entirely from my diet. Animal fats were seen as the worst offenders—they were "saturated" and, the science went, heart destroying, not to mention weight promoting—so I eliminated most animal products from my diet, even the lean ones. At a certain point even fish and eggs left my fridge.

The upshot was that during my twenties I placed so many food restrictions on myself that I could barely eat anything. I basically consumed air-popped popcorn (with no butter or oil), steamed vegetables, and salads and went from eating minimal amounts of tofu to a long period of eating none. I also did a lot of fasting. I'd fast over a weekend because I felt guilty for having fallen off the wagon and eaten a box of organic cereal the week before. This not-so-healthful cocktail was topped off with an endless supply of coffee kickers from morning till night. As we all know by now, coffee is a rapid-fire appetite suppressant. I consumed it in any number of creative ways—blended, ice-frothed "desserts" were my favorite—and it kept me

Food

so jacked up I was convinced I must be doing great because I had energy to spare.

I honestly thought I was one of the cleanest, most enviably healthy people on the block, and yet I was incredibly malnourished. By depriving myself of vital nutrients like fat and protein, I was damaging my metabolism, making it harder for my body to extract the energy and nutrients I needed out of the food I did consume. Without fats, I remained in a state of fatigue—fats are a dense energy source—and I was making it much harder for myself to stay lean, as fat is what helps slow down the quick conversion of carbohydrates to sugar. Lack of fats also meant that my body had trouble manufacturing hormones, and far from being well-stocked with vitamins, I was missing out on crucial fat-soluble vitamins like A, D, K, and E. Without saturated fats, which come from animal products and tropical oils like coconut or palm, I was throwing off many fundamental actions in the body, including the absorption of calcium into the skeleton, immune system function, and proper function of the mood-lifting neurotransmitter, serotonin. (That's why low cholesterol levels have been linked to depression and suicidal tendencies; cholesterol is actually the body's natural healing substance.) Without protein, I was compromising my body's ability to self-repair and, again, stepping on my own foot when it came to regulating my weight. Insufficient protein causes the metabolism to slow down, which makes weight gain more likely.

All this screwing around caught up with me when my thyroid gland got extremely weak. Because I lived on caffeine and no fat and all carbs (i.e., sugar), I was living off my adrenals and cortisal—I was in a constant state of stress by the food or lack of food I ingested. I was forced to hang out the white flag and find a better way to feed. This meant working with a holistic nutritionist, who immediately said I was malnourished and put me on a series of much richer diets, including adding dairy and fats. It was hard to deal with at first; my body reacted by putting on weight, and it pushed every button I had about my self-worth and value. Yet I had to admit, there were major benefits to my body and brain function. With a huge sigh of relief, my body kicked into high gear again. My mind got sharper, my moods stopped swinging between extremes, and all the functions of a smooth-running metabolism, like sweating, getting a period, and staying lean despite eating decent meals, returned.

That said, it took me a few years to find a way of eating that felt totally right. I spent some time following my nutritional guru's advice to the letter despite the fact that the full-fat dairy felt too rich for me and certain aspects of his regime seemed plainly wrong. When I came across something called the Metabolic Typing Diet, however, the loose ends came together. This protocol has been around since the 1950s and basically says that each body needs a different ratio of fats, proteins, and carbs for all its metabolic functions to work correctly. It puts the responsibility on the individual to determine how eating different proportions of these three nutrients affect their physical, mental, and emotional functioning.

I spent some time taking note of how I felt on the healthier diet I was now consuming—complete with more fish, good fats, and nuts and stripped of anything resembling a coffee bean—and then played around with adding and dropping different foods. Do I feel better without all the rich dairy fat? Yes—the noise of dairy makes me feel sluggish, and I immediately put on weight. Do I feel good on red meat? Not as much—but I find myself wanting it in winter. Do I want to put grains back in my diet? No—for my own personal reasons, the memory of how addicting they were makes me want to keep them out. Asking myself these kinds of questions again and again as I ate was how I learned to eat wisely.

Doing this personal investigation allowed me to create the healthy diet that suited me best, and finally I could relax. I knew from experience what worked great and didn't have to explain it to anyone. I became my own expert. I no longer had to have such a vice grip on my diet. As my body healed and strengthened, I grew to new levels of clarity and confidence and learned that I could eat moderate amounts of food that supplied me with good fat, protein, and nonstarchy, vegetable carbs and feel satiated and good about myself afterward. Moreover, I could forget about the calories completely. When I took the panic and punishment out of eating and treated myself more kindly, these healthier habits were able to stick.

The improvement I've seen in my health now that I'm nourished according to my needs is phenomenal. Fueled by all-natural foods close to their original state, in a proportion that works for my body, I find that I never get colds or winter sniffles because with the right biochemical balance, your immune system works far better. True, my body runs so clean that exposure to germs and viruses definitely throws me off, but with half a day of rest and taking a few immune-boosting supplements like shark liver oil and some Chinese herbal teas, I almost always bounce back without falling ill.

So how can you find your own personal balance? If you've already noticed the effects of some of the noisy foods on your diet, you're already on your way.

HOW TO FIND YOUR PERSONAL BALANCE

Most of us grew up hearing clichés such as, "To eat a balanced meal, make sure all the food groups are represented." True, we should include a variety of food sources to get our full complement of nutrients, but as a food philosophy, this statement is too vague. I believe each person must evaluate for herself what types of food work best for her individual chemistry. Humans don't have identical faces or personalities, and neither do they have identical metabolisms—the complex set of chemical reactions that extract energy from food. That's why one person will claim that

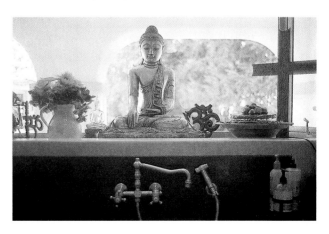

pasta makes her sleepy while the next swears that, on the contrary, a steak slows her down; it's why your neighbor may glow from her strict vegetarian meals but you might feel sickly without some meat and fish.

It doesn't mean that *everything* is open to personal interpretation; certain types of fats, carbs, and proteins are most beneficial and others may be harmful; some power foods are filled with such critical micronutrients (vitamins and minerals) that everyone should consider eating them. But when it comes to the question of how much of each food goes on your plate to help you thrive and which foods to weed out because you can't tolerate them, the choice is yours.

Finding your personal balance of nutrients is the key to operating at optimum. It's also the key to attaining a healthy weight and staying there. Remember, when "what" you eat is right for you, the "how much" take cares of itself. (It's also the reason that all weight-loss diets are a crapshoot. If a diet's rules don't align with your metabolic needs, the chances of getting lasting results from following it are minimal.)

Essentially, what you want to determine is the balance between fat and protein, on one side, and carbs, on the other: Do you need more carbohydrates and less protein and fat to function at your optimum? Do you need more protein and fat and fewer carbohydrates? Or are you somewhere in the middle, needing about even proportions of both?

Eating with your metabolic needs in mind is at the base of my "personal balance" approach to food. It's like picking the right gas from the three choices at the gas pump—

diesel, regular, or premium. Depending on what your particular engine requires, your selection may allow it to run beautifully or will make it sputter and stall. Your personal balance might shift throughout your life, as you can develop different dietary needs at different stages of life, such as during pregnancy or menopause. Once you start becoming sensitive to how your fuel is making you feel, you have the flexibility to make changes forever.

Eating According to Your Metabolic Type

The science behind the metabolic-type approach to food says that no single diet is healthy for everyone. The same nutrient can have different effects in two different people, boosting the health of one body but causing disease in another. What you need is determined by your genes. You get fat and sick if you eat too many of the wrong macronutrients—when you put the wrong fuel in your car. That's why one-size-fits-all diets are not only ineffective, they are also often harmful. Nutritionists who work with these principles will thoroughly explore your metabolic needs to determine with specificity what your metabolic type is. To understand these principles more fully, read the book that is considered the authority on this subject, *The Metabolic Typing Diet* by William Wolcott. One of the biggest advocates of this way of eating today is nutritional expert Dr. Mercola, whose popular Web site, www.mercola.com, is chock-full of information on what to eat and why.

Investigate Your Personal Food Balance

In Week 2 you will begin simply paying attention to the way that your meals affect your energy and moods so that you can understand the macronutrient mix that serves you best. The idea is to understand if you do better on a meal with higher levels of carbohydrates or higher amounts of protein and fat. Whenever possible, ask yourself the following questions after you eat. Try to be really honest with your answers. Remember, we stick to habits not always because they make us feel good but because we want them to make us feel good. The cleaner your diet becomes, the more attuned you will be to what kind of meals fuel you the best.

THE QUESTIONS:

How do you feel in general after you eat? If you feel great most of the time, chances are that your proportions are about right. But if you ever feel sluggish, cranky, or moody or get very hungry or have cravings, chances are that your proportions of macronutrients are slightly off. All that this exercise requires you to do is take notice and ask, "Does this meal work for me or not?"

- After each meal, notice whether you feel satisfied immediately when you're done or whether you are still hungry or you feel stuffed.
- Do you feel a boost of usable energy, or are you suddenly very tired?
- Do you feel good in your body, settled and calm, or are you riled up?

Notice whether your meal was heavy in carbohydrates, heavy in protein and fat, or an even mix of both.

LATER IN THE DAY, NOTICE:

- Do you have cravings for anything, especially sweets?
- Is your mind focused and clear, or do you feel clouded and spacey?
- Do you feel happy, or do you feel down, depressed, cranky, or apathetic?
- Do you have gas, or is your digestion and elimination affected in any noticeable way?
- Do any chronic symptoms or pains feel better or worse?
- If you've eaten the meal close to bedtime, do you sleep soundly, or do you have trouble sleeping?

Anytime you react negatively to a meal, such as having a strong craving for sweets, feeling overly tired, or being hungry before three or four hours have passed, it's a sign that your ratio of proteins, fats, and carbs is not quite right for your needs. Make a different choice next time, and see if the hours after your meal feel different.

Experimenting to find your personal balance shouldn't be a chore; it should be interesting and fun. As you can see, this is not about making strict rules for yourself but about getting more sensitive to what does and does not work for you on a daily basis. It does not mean that if your reaction to one meal is not optimal, you should banish that type of meal from your diet. Knowledge is power, and if you know how your body reacts to certain foods, then you are more empowered to understand why you might feel off balance at times and what you can do to correct it in the future.

Food

A Note on Proteins

As you become more attuned to your body's reaction to food, you might find that lighter proteins fuel you better than richer ones, or vice versa. Lighter proteins include chicken breast, turkey breast, eggs, lean pork, nonfat or low-fat dairy (cheese, milk, yogurt), and fish. Richer proteins include dark chicken, dark turkey, beef, lamb, salmon, beef and chicken liver, and whole-fat dairy (cheese, milk, yogurt).

Take a moment before you order lunch or make dinner to see if you've gone for old favorite carbs (bread, pasta, potatoes) without realizing it. Then make a different choice. It is simpler than you think, and it often comes down to substituting a large amount of fiber-filled vegetables for the bread or potatoes you'd normally have. Go for the salad, not the sandwich, two leafy or chunky veggie sides instead of the carbs. When you're at a restaurant, send the bread basket away. This is an easy and instant way to avoid loading up on sugary grains.

Rethink Your Carb Intake

It's easy to think that carbs simply mean grain and starch products. But did you realize that vegetables are also a carbohydrate source? As I eat almost no grains, veggies are my major carb food at every meal. Because they are packed with fiber, vegetables have a slow and low impact on blood sugar, meaning you get energy without the roller-coaster ride that grains may put you on (particularly if you're sensitive to them). To get energy from vegetables, you can't just have a tablespoon of spinach on your plate. You need to seriously amp up the portion sizes and make them a major component of the meal. Experiment with using vegetables in large quantities in each meal instead of your typical carb source, and see how you feel.

FINE-TUNING
YOUR INTAKE

Apply your observation not just to the major food group but to everything you eat. Listening to your inner wisdom is how you make your own personal diet dos and don'ts and find your way around all the health food "rules" that you may see in magazines and stores. I know that almonds are a great snack choice because they are filled with vitamin E (especially when eaten whole with their skins), yet when I eat too many of them I'm tempted to eat even more, so I limit them to once a week.

Often foods that are touted as super healthy may not work for you, or you may find that you overeat them and then feel out of balance. Many people overdo soy products (such as soy milk and tofu) when trying to improve their diet, and they experience ill effects. If symptoms such as headaches, irritability, itchy skin, or bloating arise, remember to step back and look at your whole diet to see what you can tweak. Play with cutting things out, then adding them back in. Listen to the noise that so-called good foods create, and judge if they work for you. As you learn more about which foods have beneficial effects and which may be harmful, and as you apply your own discretion to whether they work for you, this union of information and instinct will help you build a long-term, wholeful, happy diet you can live with over the long term.

Changing the way you eat might have reverberations among those around you. Other people may suddenly have strong opinions about what you should and shouldn't eat. Family and friends can get pretty weird and almost resentful when you experiment with different combinations of food and new ways of eating. Throughout my life, whenever I've made my choices about how I want to eat and live, there have always been naysayers. "That's wacky!" "Don't be ridiculous; you need meat." "Come on, nobody's allergic to chocolate!" "Everybody can have a little sugar!" "Your kids need milk!" I've always calmly responded, "I don't believe so," and continued with my way. In experimenting with your diet, as with all aspects of this program, you may sometimes have to hold your ground. Decide that this is what you need to do for yourself, and don't let anyone give you grief. Set your boundaries and stick to them.

Choose the Foods That Boost

THINK OF YOURSELF AS AN ARTIST. Selecting food can be like picking paint colors from your palette. You create your plate of dinner or breakfast to please your appetite and your eye. Start with wholesome ingredients and follow your instinct: "What looks good there?" "How many shades of green can I mix in this salad?" An egg over easy, a handful of blueberries, and a few cashews sprinkled atop the berries is pleasant to look at. A piece of grilled fish, two large slices of a ripe and beautiful tomato, and a pile of spinach leaves with a drizzle of balsamic dressing and a few shavings of parmesan is simple, but it makes a lovely-looking plate and your body will love you for it. I like to add unexpected colors—who knew indigo and lavender could show up for supper? When I make my purple cabbage and cauliflower puree, they do. I find true satisfaction in food that is fascinating to the taste buds and pleasing to the eyes and that boosts my energy and mood as well.

The best way to learn what kind of foods will make you look and feel great is to eat them. Fill your fridge with whole foods and make new choices for your meals, and you learn about better nutrition simply by doing it. People often say healthy eating is hard. It's not. I have a very healthy diet, and I know how to make it quickly and smoothly. It is simple and moderate, and its effects are powerful. I focus on including foods that boost in my diet, those ingredients that pack the most nutritional punch possible. It's also often said that healthy eating is boring. Nothing could be farther from the truth! When you focus on buying the freshest, most vibrant ingredients you can find, your meals will burst with color, texture, and flavor.

Creating a healthier, more balanced way of eating is a gradual process. You don't simply start over one day, changing every single thing you eat. You start with one meal, breakfast, and make changes to it, checking to see how you feel. Then you adjust lunch, and you gradually build new eating options. You don't have to commit to an entirely new diet for thirty days. Why not? Because an instant makeover is not what you want; changing everything at once makes it harder for good changes to stick. You're better off gradually introducing new habits that affect the way your cells function so that your metabolism works at its best, which will set you up for optimal health. This is not a cookbook, it's a guidebook: take some of the suggestions that follow, try out my recipes, customize my recipes, or simply let whatever looks good and fresh in your local market inspire you to try something new. Throughout the four weeks of this program, you will be asked to try some new breakfast choices (Week 1), new lunch choices (Week 2), new dinner choices (Week 3), as well as some new snack choices. The intention is build up a repertoire of easy, reliable meals and to learn some nutritional information along the way.

This is microwave-free, TV-dinner-free, take-out-free eating. Planning and shopping smartly are the keys to eating a diet that supports you because if the fresh produce isn't in your fridge, you will rely on take-out meals and convenience products. Both planning and shopping take some discipline. If rushing is your MO, eating *wholeful* foods may require you to go a little more slowly. You do need to eke out a little more time in your schedule to buy fresh ingredients more frequently, and if you spend twenty minutes washing and sorting all your fresh vegetables as soon as you bring them home, your food will be ready to go when it's time to eat. However, after doing a little more prep work up front, the cooking itself comes easily. The recipes I suggest are considerably simpler than those traditional family recipes that might be a staple in your home. The reason? When you use produce that is fresh and flavorful, you can do a lot less to it and get a lot more pleasure.

Personal Balance Essential: When to Eat

There's only one rule for this program. Eat breakfast because eating first thing in the morning will increase your metabolic rate and make you feel boosted in body and mind. If you're underfueled in the morning, the lack of food can tax your body so that it releases stress hormones. As the day goes on, follow your instinct and eat your moderate, healthful meals at the times when you're most hungry. Listening in to when you really need to eat, rather than going on autopilot, helps build sensitivity. But don't eat too late at night. Try to eat three hours before bedtime in order to sleep best.

WHAT TO EAT
Mariel's Pantry Essentials

I use a few key ingredients frequently, and I recommend that you purchase them for the recipes that follow. You can find them at a good health food store or online (see Index of Products for sources). You can start the program right away without them, of course, and eat the dishes that don't use them, but I highly suggest investing in them; they will set you up for success. Six months down the line you might find you have ten or twelve pantry staples you never had before. But for now, these few will do.

■ STEVIA. *This natural sweetener is calorie free and a potent alternative to sugar. Use it to sweeten dishes and drinks, sprinkle on berries, even to make organic whipped cream delicious, if you like dairy. I buy SweetLeaf stevia. If you bake, then xylitol from Kal or The Ultimate Life is another great staple to have.*

■ WHEY PROTEIN POWDER. *Whey, made from milk, is a powerful source of protein, and this powder is superb for smoothies, quick shakes, and desserts. It is important to find a brand that is made with stevia, not fructose, other sugars, or artificial sweetener. Jay Robb vanilla flavor is my favorite kind, especially as it is free of rBGH. Those who are lactose intolerant can often tolerate high-grade whey powders, but if not, egg white protein or soy protein powder can be a substitute.*

■ COCONUT OIL. *Considered by many to be the healthiest oil you can consume, coconut oil is especially good for searing fish and sautéing vegetables as well as for baking since the coconut taste is quite subtle. This superfood is rich in the most beneficial kind of saturated fats, called medium-chain fatty acids, which have antimicrobial properties, are digested easily for quick energy, and boost your immune system. It also helps thyroid problems. Many online health sites sell it; look for cold-pressed or, better yet, virgin coconut oil, and definitely avoid those that have been refined, bleached, or deodorized. It may also be called coconut butter—this is the same thing.*

If you hate even the subtle flavor of coconut, use expeller-pressed olive oil, or try cooking with the clarified butter known as ghee. It is widely used in India and South Asia, and it is a wonderfully aromatic fat with which to cook fish, meats, and vegetables or to drizzle on rice. A small amount goes a long way. A quick Internet search will give you the simple procedure for making it at home, ideally from organic butter.

■ FLAXSEED POWDER. *Flaxseed powder is a good way to enhance your intake of omega-3 fats, which are seriously lacking in the American diet; plus it's a fantastic source of fiber. I love to use it to thicken smoothies; my favorite brand is the ultra-fine-ground Mum's Flax Pro or Flax Probiotic, but you can buy flaxseeds very cheaply from a health mart's bulk section and grind them in a coffee grinder. I also keep flax oil in my fridge, and I use it in several of the recipes that follow as well as for salad dressings.*

- FISH OIL OR COD LIVER OIL. *This sounds scary, but be brave. Used as a dietary supplement, fish oil is the best source of omega-3 fats, which are essential to physical and mental health—better than nuts and flaxseed. Invest in a high-quality brand that is pure and free of heavy metals, such as Carlson's or Nordic Naturals, which have natural nonfishy flavors. Keep a bottle in your fridge, and take one teaspoon a day, or buy capsules that don't need to be refrigerated. If you are avoiding fish due to concerns about toxins, these are a great way to get your essential fishy fats. Many nutritionists consider this a nonnegotiable supplement: everyone needs it.*

- NUTS. *If you try to buy good raw nuts in your local supermarket, you'll likely find a tiny plastic package that is vastly overpriced or nothing but sugared, salted, and roasted nuts. Buy nuts far more cheaply in bulk at a natural foods store or online; almonds, walnuts, hazelnuts, cashews, and pecans should be unsalted and raw or unroasted. If you can find organic ones at a reasonable cost, grab them. It's another way to lower the toxic load.*

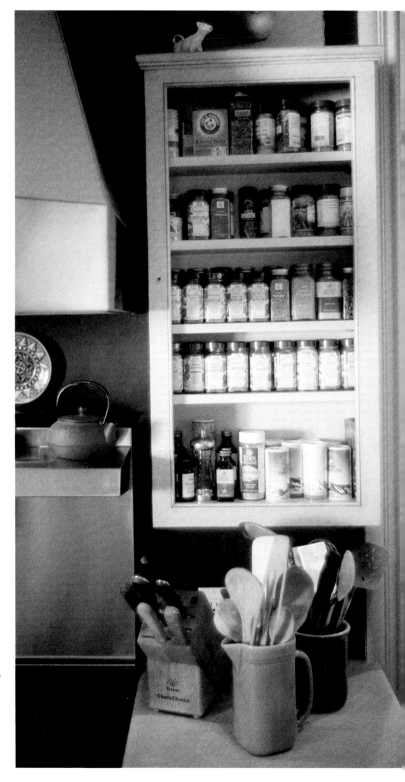

The Best Breakfast

For some reason America decided that sweet food and grain-based food is what should be served for breakfast. But it's not the case in other parts of the world. In Sweden, Japan, or Scotland you might eat fish first thing; in the Alps you'd get cheese and cold cuts; in South India you'd feast on delicious lentil stew. Adjust your breakfast first, and you are more likely to start the day from a place of neutral calm, less likely to ride the roller coaster of sugar highs and lows, and better fueled with protein, good fat, and vegetable-based carbs. For the four weeks of this program, think outside the (cereal) box to make breakfast a bit different. Shelve the typical fare of toast, bagels, muffins, orange juice, jam, honey (and yes, cereal too). Nix anything processed. Instead, create a plate of savory or barely sweet foods that you've made from scratch: soft-boiled or poached eggs served with vegetables; a little good-quality cheese with some avocado; some organic turkey slices and tart fruit; or a smoothie made with minimal sugar. (And no, a healthy smoothie does not contain frozen yogurt!) If you do eat bread, go for the coarsest kind you can find—grainy "peasant bread" rather than shrink-wrapped, refined bread. Invest in organic butter, and cut out the sweet toppings. There are no rules here; if you have salmon left over from dinner, why not try that and see how your energy is later in the day? (PS: Eating salad for breakfast is totally cool by me.)

These four recipes are some of my favorites for a wholesome breakfast. Several share similar ingredients, so once you buy them for this program, you will use them.

Fried Eggs on Greens

2 large eggs
2 cups washed spinach
2 dabs of butter or 2 spritzes of olive oil spray
Salt and pepper to taste

Heat 1 dab of butter or spritz of oil in a skillet over medium heat, then throw in the spinach. If the leaves are not damp enough, throw in a few tablespoons of water and place a lid on the skillet so that the steam wilts the leaves, about 1 minute. Remove leaves with a slotted spoon to avoid excess water, and place them on a plate; cover with a second skillet lid if it's handy to keep them warm. Drain out any water in the skillet, add the second dab of butter or oil spritz, and turn up the heat to high. Crack one egg at a time and let them sizzle around the edges until they're a little golden brown. Put a lid over the eggs for 1 minute so the egg white is cooked through while the yolk is sunny and runny (if runny ain't your thing, leave the lid on for 2 minutes). Lift the eggs out with a spatula and place on the leaves. Season with salt and pepper to taste. Serve with a bowl of raspberries and blueberries or any other vegetables you have on hand.

TIP Commercial ketchup tends to have sugar and preservatives; if you like it with your eggs, try substituting a healthy salsa from Newman's Own or Muir Glen, which have minimal sugar and sodium and no additives.

Mariel's Muesli

1 cup organic plain yogurt (whole milk or
  nonfat) or 1 cup plain kefir
¼ cup mixed chopped raw nuts (any of:
  almonds, walnuts, hazelnuts, brazil nuts)
1 tablespoon currants or dried cranberries
  or a handful of fresh berries
2 tablespoons vanilla flavor whey protein
  powder
1 tablespoon flaxseed powder or
  flaxseed oil

Mix yogurt, whey powder, and flaxseed oil together. Sprinkle nuts and berries on top.

Note: Though my husband loves full-fat dairy, my female body does not process it well. I go nonfat for this recipe and add some fat with the nuts. Experiment and see what kind seems to sit best in your tummy. Always go for plain yogurt, not flavored or diet yogurt, which can be heaped with sugar or fake sweetener.

KEFIR is a high-protein, rich yogurt drink that is full of the live, beneficial bacteria needed for the digestive system to run smoothly. The good bacteria support immune system function and make nutrients in food more available. Everyone can benefit from adding more good bacteria to their diet, and if you have taken antibiotics, consider them essential, as your levels of intestinal bacteria will be greatly diminished. While kefir is one of the best fermented foods for adding good bacteria, other foods such as yogurt containing active cultures (check the ingredients list to make sure), as well as fermented vegetables, like sauerkraut and Korean kimchi, are also beneficial. Kefir can be digested by the lactose intolerant. Look in your grocery store for the plain, unflavored kind as fruity flavors can have a lot of sugar; if you want to get really hippie, you can get a kit to easily make your own at home.

BERRIES of all kind are wonderful additions to your diet. They are loaded not only with important vitamins but also with antioxidant compounds. If you can find wild berries (look in the frozen section), they will pack an even stronger punch since wild foods tend to have greater amounts of trace minerals. As with all fruits, go for fresh or (unsweetened) frozen, not canned.

Superfood substitute: Look for tart, tasty goji berries from the Himalayas, and try using them instead of cranberries or currants. Now available in most health food stores, goji berries are considered one of the healthiest fruits on the planet because of their extremely high antioxidant levels, vitamins, and minerals.

Egg White "Pancake" Dipped in Pureed Fruit

3 or 4 egg whites
1 teaspoon vanilla extract
Dash cinnamon
Olive oil spray or butter
Pick from: ½ papaya, if available, plus ¼
  cup blueberries, raspberries, or blackberries *or* 1 cup frozen unsweetened berries
  (any kind) or peaches
4 raw almonds or a palmful of sliced almonds, organic if possible

Put egg whites in a blender, add vanilla and cinnamon, and whip it up good. Heat a large round skillet, and oil with a small blast of olive oil spray or a dab of butter. Pour the mixture in, and let it cook on fairly high heat. Turn it over when it easily lifts from the side with a spatula. It should be golden colored on both sides. (I like mine a little toasty so I let it get golden brown with a slight crisp.) Puree the fruit you've chosen in a blender, add berries and almonds (toast them under the broiler for a few minutes first if you have time). Blend briefly, and use as a dip for the pancake. It's breakfast heaven.

TIP If using frozen fruit, place it in blender with a few pinches of stevia and some hot water to get the mix moving. This will make enough fruit dip to keep in the fridge for a couple of days.

✴ I'M A HUGE FAN OF WHOLE EGGS. The yolk is an essential part of the nutritional value and a great source of good fat. I do this recipe with egg whites, however, because they are responsible for the light, fluffy, and crispy texture. You can buy egg whites in a box—I like the Eggcology brand—or simply separate your eggs. Cage-free or free-range eggs are a kinder purchase.

✴ OLIVE OIL SPRAY is a great kitchen tool because it squirts very moderate amounts of oil at a time. Remember to look for extra-virgin oil. Spectrum Naturals makes a good one.

The Morning Shake

Note: This may seem a bit wacky, but try it: each ingredient has nutritional value. This is my breakfast at least three times a week. And it is divine!

> 1 scoop vanilla flavor whey protein powder (the scoop comes in the package)
> 1 scoop flaxseed powder
> ¼ cup frozen blueberries
> Water
> Ice
> Hot water (if needed)
> ½ stevia packet (optional). *Add stevia if shake is not sweet enough, though the whey powder will make it quite sweet.*

Put a cup of drinking water and some ice into a blender. Add whey powder, flaxseed powder, and frozen berries. Blend on high. Mixture should be thick and smooth, not icy. If it is too frosty, add a little hot water to soften the texture. Drink in a tall glass, or pour over fresh berries, shredded organic coconut (unsweetened), and a handful of toasted plain almond slices.

T REAT YOURSELF: *A great blender makes whipping up smoothies, soups, and purees a whiz. My Vita-Mix blender can make even the chunkiest vegetables, ice cubes, and frozen fruits silky smooth; I use it daily.*

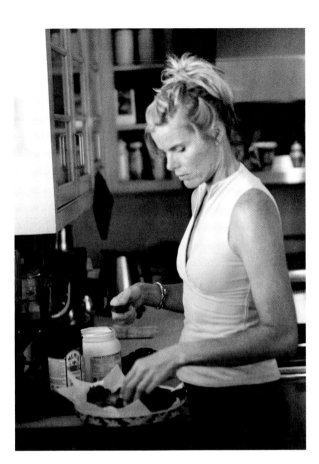

Superfast Smoothie

2 cups almond milk

1 cup frozen or fresh berries

2 tablespoons flaxseed powder or freshly
ground flaxseeds

Throw in blender, give a quick whiz,
and serve.

SUPERFOOD SUBSTITUTE: Hemp
seeds sound highly suspect, but if you
see them, try them! Use them instead of flax
in the Superfast Smoothie.They're nutritional
powerhouses, full of essential fats, vitamin E,
and protein.

Frozen Whey Latte or Cappuccino

1 cup freshly made decaffeinated coffee
or 1 cup Teeccino™ herbal coffee
1 scoop vanilla flavor whey protein powder
Ice

Pour the hot coffee into a blender, add
protein powder and enough ice to fill the
blender at least halfway, and blend. This is a
frozen decaf coffee drink that is actually good
for you and makes a great snack, thanks to the
protein. Naturally sweet—if your whey powder uses stevia—it is far better than the sugar
bombs sold at Starbucks. You'll feel you're
cheating each time you have one.

To make a hot version: If you have a coffee
machine with a milk steamer, it's easy. Put
1 cup of cold water plus whey protein into a
blender and add ice. Blend until foamy, then
pour into stainless steel steamer jug and use
your steamer the way you would steam milk. It
must start cold. Pour this into your cup of coffee or coffee substitute just as with a regular
latte or cappuccino, dolloping foam on the top.

If you don't have a coffee steamer, blend
protein powder with a cup of boiling hot water
until foamy, then add ice, which will make it
extra foamy.

Snacks

Reach for one of these snacks instead of normal sweet, salty, or processed treats:

- One piece of string cheese and half an apple plus 4 raw pecans
- 2 large celery stalks with 1 to 2 tablespoons almond butter
- A small handful of raw nuts, or if you don't digest raw nuts well, *lightly toast them yourself to avoid the bad fats and salt in commercially roasted nuts.*

Home-Toasted Nuts

Take 1 cup sliced almonds, 1 cup pecan halves, and 1 cup cashew pieces and scatter them all over a baking sheet or roasting pan. Roast them at 150 degrees for an hour. If the oven is too hot, the fat in the nuts will turn rancid and give you a stomachache.

For added taste, sprinkle cinnamon on them, a natural metabolism booster. If you like a savory taste, sprinkle Cajun seasoning on them. If the seasoning isn't sticking, spray lightly with olive oil spray after toasting, then sprinkle the flavor.

TIP Nuts make for good snacks but are very "moreish"—meaning you barely notice as you pop them into your mouth. Measure out small portions of nuts in a ramekin, and put the container away so that you eat only as much as you've served.

Trail Mix / Granola

Can be a great snack, dessert, or breakfast with your whey shake or some almond milk.

To the Home-Toasted Nuts recipe, add the following:

½ cup dried cranberries or other dried berries

½ cup pure coconut flakes

1 tablespoon cold-pressed coconut oil

1 tablespoon cinnamon

1 packet stevia or 1 tablespoon xylitol

Spread coconut oil on your hands, and spread it around your bowl of nuts, flaked coconut, and berries, just enough that there is a bit of a coating on everything. Sprinkle cinnamon and stevia or xylitol on top, and mix it into the mixture with your hands.

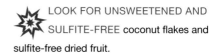 LOOK FOR UNSWEETENED AND SULFITE-FREE coconut flakes and sulfite-free dried fruit.

TIP Except for making salad dressing, I use my hands a lot in food preparation. Of course I wash them a lot as well. They are great for mixing things up, and you connect to the food in a more loving way.

Let's Do Lunch

Lunch can be a challenge. You need things that are quick and easy and keep your energy consistent. It's all too tempting to reach for what's most convenient from a deli or take-out spot (like sandwiches that are all bread and minimal filling) or to wait until you're too starving to make a smart choice. Taking food in to work is great if you find a few more minutes in the morning (and it feels so good to finally put all that Tupperware to use). Let loose your creativity on salads, and have them "your way." Look for the most interesting greens you can find, then throw in whatever vegetables and proteins are freshest and most colorful; if you prepare a little extra fish or chicken or seared tofu the night before, you'll have the makings of a great salad ready to go. If that's too complex, bring your own hard-boiled eggs and add them to a salad bar plate, or simply bring your own dressing so you can control one aspect of the meal. Healthful soups are easy options for work or home; you can even keep miso soup at work if there's a small kitchen available, and customize your own hot soup with leftover fish, chicken, or vegetables that you bring in. Here are four wholeful lunches to get you on track:

The Perfect Wrap

Start with:

 1 small low-carb tortilla

Spread with:

 1 tablespoon pesto (recipe on page 74)
  or 1 teaspoon Dijon mustard

Pile on:

 Half an avocado, sliced

 A handful of grated carrots

 A small handful of grated mozzarella cheese

 A thin slice of turkey, preferably organic or
  nitrite free

Top with:

 Shredded lettuce

 A drizzle of salad dressing of your choice,
  found on pages 70 and 71 (optional)

Note: If you are vegan, sprinkle soy cheese instead of mozzarella, add more avocado, and include a sprinkle of nuts. Use soy products in moderation.

MANY ARE SCARED OF AVOCADOS as they are so full of fat, but when you're diet is clean and free of bad processed fats, you should enjoy moderate amounts of these satisfying and rich fruits when they are in season. Eat them slowly, and notice how filling they are. (They are also delicious in smoothies!)

TIP I recommend low-carb tortillas made by the La Tortilla Factory brand, available in most supermarkets. Buy your sliced turkey from the deli section rather than prepackaged, and look for roasted or naturally smoked meat.

Superior Salad

Start with a bowl of one or more greens:

Lettuce, baby spinach leaves, arugula, watercress, radicchio

Then customize it your way with several of the following:

A sliced hard-boiled egg, pieces of seared fish, grilled chicken, tofu, feta or goat cheese

Cold steamed veggies: cauliflower, broccoli, zucchini, green beans, asparagus

Raw red and yellow peppers

Grilled veggies: eggplant, zucchini, tomatoes

Marinated veggies: artichoke hearts, roasted peppers

Chopped onions

Olives

1 tablespoon currants

A palmful of fresh sprouts

A few crumbled pecans, hemp seed, pumpkin seed, sunflower seeds

TIP You don't need any special equipment to steam vegetables. Fill a medium-sized saucepan with about two inches of water, heat to a boil, and place a metal strainer on the pan with a lid pressed down on the vegetables. Depending on the thickness of the veggies, it will take between 2 and 3 minutes; use a fork to test if they are done enough.

Salad Dressings

Different dressings will give your salads distinctive flavors. Here are a few to try. Make them in bulk, and keep some in the fridge at work to ensure you have the healthiest topping possible for store-bought salads.

Dijon Dressing (with a Twist)

1 tablespoon olive oil or flaxseed oil

Juice of half a lemon

1 tablespoon Dijon mustard

Dash dulse

Dash turmeric

Note: Turmeric is a great antioxidant; use it whenever you can.

Whisk together and drizzle on your salad.

SUPERFOOD SUBSTITUTE: DULSE is a powdered seaweed. Instead of putting sugar into salad dressing, try this unusual ingredient. Then look for other tasty seaweeds to snack on or throw in soups, like toasted nori sheets. Sea vegetables offer the broadest range of minerals of any food, containing virtually all the minerals found in the ocean—the same minerals that are found in human blood—and they are an iodine source, which we need to make the thyroid work well.

Ginger Miso Dip
or Dressing

1 inch grated ginger

1 clove garlic

¼ cup light miso

1 tablespoon apple cider vinegar

2 tablespoons olive oil

½ cup water

Blend until smooth. Add more water as necessary for your desired consistency.

This also works great with your favorite vegetables as a dip.

TIP Miso is a delicious, high-protein paste made by fermenting soybeans, cultured grains, and sea salt, and is used to season soups in Japan. My favorite brand of miso is South River, which is unpasteurized, meaning that good bacteria are available to aid your digestion.

Lemon Tahini Dressing

½ cup tahini

1 lemon, squeezed

1 cup water

2 tablespoons olive oil

¼ teaspoon sea salt

Blend together. Add fresh dill or other herbs for variety.

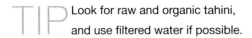 Look for raw and organic tahini, and use filtered water if possible.

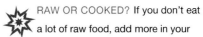 RAW OR COOKED? If you don't eat a lot of raw food, add more in your diet through salads and raw snacks. This will increase the amount of enzymes that are needed to aid in digestion. However, be conscious that we get less efficient at digesting food as we get older, so notice when you have too much of a good thing. Steaming and waterless methods of cooking vegetables are also great, and they preserve vitamins better than rapid boiling.

Easy Gazpacho Soup

SOUP:

4 large fresh tomatoes, preferably Roma

1 fresh garlic clove (or more to taste)

1 teaspoon red pepper flakes

¼ cup olive oil

2 tablespoons fresh cilantro

1 tablespoon fresh parsley

¼ cup onion, minced

¼ teaspoon cumin seeds

¼ teaspoon oregano

Juice of one lime

Salt to taste

GARNISH:

One small cucumber, diced

One small red pepper, diced

One small green bell pepper, diced

Combine the soup ingredients in a blender and puree until smooth. Chop the remaining ingredients and add to tomato mixture. Serve with extra lime and sour cream if desired. Garnish with more cilantro and onions (optional).

If soup is not enough, pair with a low-carb tortilla and a few slices of avocado or some rye crackers.

Heavenly Egg Salad Sandwich

1 large hard-boiled egg

2 tablespoons "real" mayonnaise

Salt and pepper

Paprika

2 thinly sliced pieces of good-quality bread, either grainy and unrefined or flourless, sprouted-grain bread

Mash egg, mayo, and flavorings together in a bowl. Spread egg mixture on bread and put a swipe of Dijon mustard on one slice of bread if you are a mustard fan like me.

TIP Get the most natural mayonnaise you can, one that is organic or additive free, or make your own from olive oil, egg yolk, salt and pepper, and vinegar.

SPROUTED-GRAIN LOAVES have lower impact on blood sugar and more available nutrients than regular loaves. I like Manna from Heaven or Food for Life (red label).

Lemonade

1 green apple

Juice of 1 lemon

1 tablespoon flaxseed powder

1 tablespoon flaxseed oil

½ packet stevia *or* ½ cup blueberries in place of sweetener

¼ teaspoon sea salt

4 cups water

1 cup ice

Blend together in a high-speed blender. Serve chilled or at room temperature.

Dish Up a Great Dinner

Most frequently seen on my evening plate: a piece of seared fish, or occasionally tofu, with a heap of vegetables and salad. It's simple: I buy a nice piece of tuna or salmon, heat up a skillet until it's hot with a spritz of olive oil or dab of coconut oil, then sear the fish so the outside gets lots of flavor, and add salt and pepper. Tuna gets only a quick sear and is eaten while pink in the middle; salmon is cooked on a low heat for longer. Each can get topped with my delicious green-green sauce, found on the next page. Other nights I'll throw some natural or organic meat on the barbecue or broil it: first I sear it hot, then I lower the flame to cook through. Throw together vegetables that burst with freshness—I especially love cauliflower, broccoli, brussels sprouts, or red cabbage or a

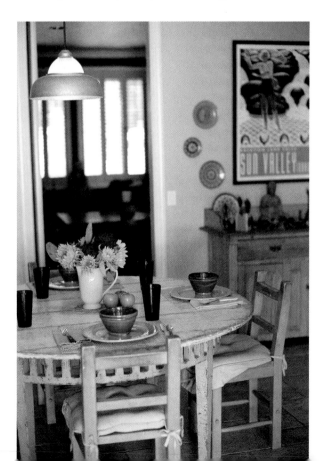

huge side of steamed or raw leafy greens like chard, kale, or collard greens—and it's a most satisfying meal that is quicker than heating a pizza. Below are some of my other favorite homemade dinner specials, which are offered in larger amounts so that you have leftovers for lunch or for another dinner that week.

Green-Green Sauce and Dip

1 large bunch fresh basil (must be fresh)

1 bag baby spinach

1 cup olive oil

½ cup French's mustard

4 kalamata olives and a splash of the juice from the bottle of olives. (It has just the right amount of vinegar to make the dip tart.)

Put everything in blender and blend until smooth. Use for veggies, fish, meat, and chicken and even as a dressing.

Seared Orange-Butter Tofu with Kale or Spinach

1 package organic GM-free tofu, medium to firm

2 tablespoons unsalted butter or coconut oil

Zest and juice of ½ orange or ½ cup fresh orange juice

1 clove garlic

2 tablespoons tamari sauce or Braggs aminos or wheat-free soy sauce

½ packet stevia

⅛ teaspoon grated fresh ginger

⅛ teaspoon pepper

3 cups chopped kale or spinach (add more if the tofu is dominating the dish)

Combine orange juice, tamari or soy sauce, stevia, garlic, and pepper; set aside. In a skillet, heat butter or oil, add tofu steaks, and sauté over high heat for 3 minutes each side, browning them well. Reduce heat to low, and add reserved marinade to the skillet and kale or spinach. Kale takes about 3 minutes to cook and spinach 1 to 2 minutes; they should both maintain a bright green color. Serve with quinoa as instructed per box, 1/3 cup cooked per serving.

KALE—along with cauliflower, Swiss chard, cabbage, bok choy, mustard and turnip greens, arugula, watercress, and brussels sprouts—stands out as an anticancer food. These cruciferous vegetables contain compounds that increase the liver's ability to neutralize potentially toxic substances. Kale and spinach are both high sources of folates, a B vitamin that is essential to cell building and is crucial during pregnancy. Although kale is super nutritious, some think its flavor is too strong; in that case, choose spinach.

QUINOA looks and tastes like a grain but is actually the nutritious seed of a plant related to chard and beets. Quick to cook, satisfying to eat, full of protein, it has a low gluten content and is great for those who are wheat intolerant. Use it as a delicious side dish similar to couscous or rice. Rinse in a fine-mesh strainer with cold water, rubbing gently, before cooking.

Chicken or Salmon Pesto

2 whole, free-range, boneless and skinless
    chicken breasts or 1 salmon filet (8 to 10
    ounces of fresh, wild-caught if possible)
Fresh pesto can often be found in the deli
    section of your grocery store, but you
    can easily make your own and save it
    for several weeks or freeze the extra. If
    you are sensitive to dairy, leave out the
    cheese and simply add salt.
2 large bunches fresh basil
2 cloves garlic
1 cup extra-virgin olive oil
Finely grated fresh Parmesan cheese or
    1 tablespoon sea salt
¼ cup ground pine nuts or walnuts

Preheat oven to 350 degrees.

Put pesto ingredients in food processor or
blender. Blend until smooth or slightly lumpy,
depending on what texture you like. Slather the
chicken breasts or fish in pesto sauce and put
into a casserole dish. Place in oven and cook
chicken breast for around 30 minutes, checking
it after 25 minutes, and then place under your
broiler to brown the top. Cook fish for half the
time, and put under broiler to brown. Use the
extra chicken or fish for lunch the next day.

TIP Limit take-out for the duration of
this program. You can't control
the ingredients in take-out food. Think ahead,
and take any needed dinner ingredients out
of the freezer earlier in the day so that you're
prepared to eat well. Even after a long day you
can put together a better kind of take-out; buy
a supermarket roast chicken, and pair it with a
homemade salad.

POACHING a nice firm white fish in a
vegetable broth filled with fresh broccoli,
cabbage, and sautéed onions, carrots, and celery is a supereasy way to do supper. Use some
white wine, lemon, and dried herbs to make a
French-type dish. Or mix miso paste, soy sauce,
and wasabi powder if you can find it, to make a
delicious Japanese-style fish soup. Or go for a
splash of coconut milk and Thai curry paste from
the supermarket to turn it Thai. Throw chunks
of fish into the broth for just a few minutes, until
translucent flesh has turned opaque. Fresh parsley or cilantro on top add the final touch.

Simple Scampi

¼ cup olive oil
1 onion, peeled and chopped finely
2 cloves garlic
Several leaves fresh tarragon or a dash of
    dried
Dash of salt and pepper
12 medium-sized fresh or frozen (defrosted)
    shrimp

In a small skillet heat olive oil, and sauté
onions and garlic over medium to low heat for
2 to 3 minutes, till they are translucent. Add
salt and pepper, and sauté for 1 minute more;
don't let it brown. Remove from heat and cool.

In a bowl put shrimp with sautéed mixture
and lemon juice. Use your hands to make
sure the shrimp are coated with the marinade.
Again, I think hands make the best tools for
cooking with love. Let this mixture set for 20 to
30 minutes before cooking fully.

Preheat broiler. Line a cookie sheet or
broiler pan with aluminum foil. Place shrimp on
sheet, and put a dollop of the onion mixture on

each shrimp. Broil at high heat until the shrimp is no longer translucent but pink and the topping is brown—around 4 to 5 minutes.

Serve with zucchini "pasta," on the next page.

Serve with zucchini "pasta," on the next page.

T I P Stainless steel cookware is a better bet than aluminum or Teflon, both of which have slightly toxic effects.

Chicken or Turkey Meatballs Marinara

MEATBALLS:

2 tablespoons olive oil

1 large clove fresh minced garlic (or much more to taste)

3 tablespoons minced yellow onion

¼ teaspoon Italian seasoning

1 pound ground chicken or turkey (free-range, hormone-free, or organic if possible)

½ cup whole wheat bread crumbs or almond meal

2 eggs

1 teaspoon sea salt

½ teaspoon ground mixed pepper

½ teaspoon cayenne pepper (optional)

Heat oven to 425 degrees. In a sauté pan, combine the olive oil, minced garlic, onion, salt, and peppers. Cook over low. Heat until the garlic and onions start to caramelize. Add the rest of the seasonings and remove from heat. In a medium-sized bowl, combine the ground meat, eggs, and bread crumbs and mix well. Form into golf-ball-sized rounds and

place on a foil-covered baking sheet with sides of some sort. Place in the oven and cook until the top turns light brown, then turn them over. When the other side is done, the meat should be cooked but can vary according to the size of the meatball. To be sure, take a meat thermometer and test to 165 degrees internal temperature, or split one open and make sure the meat is not pink. Remove and place in the marinara sauce.

MARINARA SAUCE:

3 cloves minced garlic (or much more to taste)

½ yellow onion, minced

¼ cup olive oil

½ cup dry (not sweet) red wine (optional)

¼ cup butter

1 24-ounce can crushed, strained, pureed, or whole Italian tomatoes (organic if possible)

1 small (6-or-7 ounce) can tomato paste

1 teaspoon sea salt

1 teaspoon ground pepper

2 tablespoons fresh oregano or 1 teaspoon dry

2 tablespoons fresh basil or 1 teaspoon dry

1 teaspoon cayenne pepper (optional)

In a large saucepan, combine the olive oil, garlic, and onions. Cook on low heat until they begin to caramelize and turn golden brown. Add the red wine, and simmer on low until the wine reduces volume by half. (If not using wine, go straight to the next step.) Add the remaining ingredients except butter and place into a blender or food processor. Blend until smooth. Return to the saucepan and heat until

Food

a slow boil with the lid on. Add the butter and meatballs and reduce the heat to keep warm.

Note: To make an amazing soup, add 1 cup of cream (organic if possible) to the marinara sauce recipe.

TIP Instead of serving your meatballs with pasta, try this variation. Take 3 zucchinis, and use a vegetable peeler or the long blade of your food processor to make ribbon slices of faux pasta. Steam them in a wide steamer so you don't break the ribbons, and steam until they are tender and slightly floppy yet still colorfully green. Place meatballs and sauce on them, finish with grated parmesan, or serve with marinara sauce alone as a side dish on another night.

Butternut Squash Bisque

4 cups butternut squash, diced medium

2 yellow squash, diced medium

2 medium tomatoes, diced small

½ yellow pepper, diced small

2 sticks celery, diced small

½ medium red onion, diced

¼ cup olive oil

2 tablespoons apple cider vinegar

1 tablespoon each fresh thyme, parsley, and rosemary (finely chopped) or large pinch of a dry blend

½ teaspoon cayenne pepper

1 teaspoon sea salt

Steam vegetables lightly for a few minutes. Blend all together with about 6 cups of water.

Add olive oil and everything listed below it. Whisk all ingredients together and serve warm, not too hot!

Note: This recipe makes at least 6 servings so it can be used for several lunches or dinners, or freeze it in small containers so you have individual servings ready to go.

Sides

Cauliflower "Mock" Mashed Potatoes

1 small cauliflower, broken into pieces

2 tablespoons unsalted butter

1 tablespoon organic cream (optional)

Salt and pepper to taste

Pinch of fresh thyme

Steam cauliflower so that it is soft and falls apart easily, not mushy. Put into your blender or mixer. Add butter and some of the water from the steamer to get things moving. If you want a richer flavor, add a tablespoon of heavy cream and salt and pepper to taste. Mix until well pureed. Garnish with fresh thyme.

Purple Puree

This is my signature side dish: I eat it with many meals to get a huge dose of nutrients, and it is fun and comforting to eat. Use it as a soup or as a dip for anything you like.

1 whole cauliflower, broken into small heads

¼ purple cabbage, shredded

Steam vegetables until soft, not mushy. (If it is too raw, it will have a bitter taste.) Put all of this in your blender (blenders work better than food processors for this, for some unknown reason). Pour the water from your steamed veggies in with your mixture, and blend. Eat this as a healing puree or as a side dish to any protein meal.

■ ■ ■

WITH EVERY DINNER I MAKE, I serve a simple salad. It was the way I was brought up, and it was the way my father was brought up in Paris, so he insisted on it when we were kids. That was one of the few family food patterns that I thought worth preserving as tradition. Salad is a tremendous source of fiber and feels good with your meals. Choose the greens you like—rip up lots of different lettuces if you have a few varieties—and often that's enough. (I love the huge floppy leaves of butter lettuce.) You have the option of a Superior Salad as well, of course, but with a meal I usually find the simpler the better. Wash and dry some greens, make this simple vinaigrette, and it's ready to go.

> 2 tablespoons olive oil
> ½ tablespoon lemon juice
> Salt and pepper

Mix all ingredients together, and if you want more zing, add 1 teaspoon Dijon mustard. Now that's easy!

■ ■ ■

I MAY BE THE MAIN (okay, the only) chef in the house, but I still have to accommodate my family's needs and work within a set of limitations, like the time available and my own willingness to cook. I don't always eat exactly what the others eat because what works for me is different from what my husband needs, and my teenage daughters have their own tastes. So when it comes to pulling together a family dinner, I lay out a few components on different platters—some fish, some vegetables, some rice for those who want it—and let each person make their plate the way they like it. My plate ends up with heaping piles of salad whereas my husband takes more rice and fish. I eat my dessert berries plain; he squirts organic whipped cream all over his. My motto is, provide healthy options, then each to her or his own.

CONSCIOUS CHOICES: SHOPPING AND PREPARING

QUESTION: HOW OFTEN DO YOU SHOP FOR FOOD?

If once a week, consider whether that reflects something about the importance you place on food. Does buying, preparing, and eating food have to be as convenient as possible for you, and if so, why?

TO AID in reinventing your diet, it helps to see your shopping expedition as a creative act. The supermarket might strike you as the most boring place on the planet—a place you rush into and try to get out of as quickly as possible. If so, what does that say about your relationship to food? For the duration of this program, slow down and spend just five minutes more than normal looking at what's on offer. Pick one section of the market and see what you haven't seen before; pick up a new vegetable, smell it, feel it, study the color. Or, if you like bread in your diet, look at the diversity of bread products you'd normally sprint past, and read the labels. Each time you shop, make it a mission to bring home one new food, be it a leafy, green vegetable you haven't used before, a new grain like quinoa or whole-wheat couscous, or dark berries. There is huge value in introducing just one new food each time you shop. Four months down the road, your diet will be very different and more varied than it was before, and it will reflect your tastes and needs, not the dictates of some outside expert.

✷ KNOW WHAT RESTAURANTS near your home or office offer the kind of food that supports you, so you're not wandering in to some random place because you don't know where you're going. It helps to make a list so that you always have a good idea of where to go.

Exercise: Get Fresher

Do you have opportunities to buy more fresh foods, such as fresh vegetables and fish or meat, on the day you want to eat them? On your way home from work, do you pass any vendors that you could stop at? If you can shop more than once a week, you will be more likely to eat fresh food daily. And you become more connected to the food you eat, getting more sensual pleasure out of selecting vibrant, wholesome items and eating them when they're at their best. Make the intention to alter your food-shopping routine for the week.

• If you rarely do an organized shopping trip for groceries, and more often get take-out or pre-made food, your challenge is to hit the grocery store or health food mart with a list and spend a good thirty minutes browsing.

• If you do a bulk shopping trip once a week, make a midweek stop to pick up fresh produce for dinner, selecting something that looks freshest and most appealing.

• If you already visit your local food stores frequently, your challenge is to try out a new source, such as a local farmer's market, and stock up for several days.

Exercise: Buy Two New Foods

Each time you go to the supermarket during this program, make sure your cart includes at least two new wholeful foods that you have never tried before. If you are following the meal guidelines above, this will happen automatically, but if you are familiar with all the foods in the recipes, look a bit further and try a fresh product or wholesome frozen or jarred item that piques your curiosity. PLAN AHEAD. Make a meal list for the week. Out of that, make your shopping list. Being prepared will help you, for example, to not rely on the microwave to defrost your chicken at the last minute. You know in advance what you need each night.

It's time to bring back a sense of simplicity and satisfaction to shopping and eating. In an era when fruit is flown halfway around the world to indulge us in winter, I think it's wiser to honor the course of nature and the seasons as best we can. Notice what local produce is abundant in your stores and markets each season, and choose to cook with it—even if you hadn't planned to use it. When possible, choose foods grown locally. Not only will the "vital stock" of the food (its nutritional value) be much higher if it has been picked closer to ripeness and transported quickly to the sales point, but even if it is not organic, it will have fewer of the "chemical cosmetics" that are applied to veggies to transport them from their place of origin to your supermarket.

As for the expense, plenty of simple whole-food ingredients are very inexpensive, particularly compared to the price of buying premade meals or eating out. Buying bulk cereals, grains, and pulses (peas, beans, and lentils) from your local health food store saves on money and wasteful packaging. If you have a local farmer's market, you'll find great-quality vegetables for competitive prices. Other items, like organic or raw dairy or grass-fed beef, are considerably more expensive than the conventional versions. It's not realistic to expect everything you consume to be top-end product. You will have to make choices and evaluate for yourself which things are worth the extra to you, by tasting them and tuning in to how they make you feel. You might also have moral and ethical considerations to factor in regarding the animal product you choose. Is it worth it to you to spend money on animals that have had a more humane existence? As you factor in different choices, consider food as your health insurance: what you invest now in feeding yourself well, you will get back tenfold in the future from staying boosted and healthy.

Eating with Peace and Moderation

QUESTION: WHICH STATEMENT BEST REFLECTS
YOUR ATTITUDE TOWARD FOOD?

A. I love to eat, and I often find myself thinking about food—to the point where it sometimes causes a problem of overeating or denial.

B. Feeding myself is a time-consuming chore. If nutrition came in capsule form, I'd take it!

C. I can get excited about eating sometimes, but my attitude toward my daily diet is pretty utilitarian.

THE WAY YOU EAT is just as important as what you eat. The act of eating should provide a moment of respite during your day. After all, eating is the most fundamental act of taking care of yourself. While choosing nutritious, whole foods is one aspect of eating well, learning how to treat food with the consideration and respect it deserves—creating a good eating experience, whether alone or with your family—is equally crucial. Only when your attitude toward eating changes can food truly become one of the cornerstones of the balanced life—something that positively affects your life and brings you not just health but also pleasure and peace of mind.

You should be able to eat in such a way that food makes you happy, not anxious, each day and so that you feel satisfied after every meal. If you are rushed, distracted, or fighting yourself over your desires, you won't get as much goodness from your food no matter how well chosen it is.

Good eating is about moderation. Occasionally eating imperfect foods is not the problem; it's overindulging in those foods that's the problem. It's time to shift to the way our predecessors ate: their diets included some sugar, some carbs, and certainly some good fats, but none of it was supplied in the vast amounts available to us today. Plus, their diets usually maintained active, physical lifestyles rather than sedentary ones. In my household the one person who ate moderately was my mother; she had her eggs and toast in the morning; her meat, salad, and baked potato at lunch; her cup of coffee and maybe one cookie or a sliver of pie in the afternoon. It was simple, homemade fare, and she never needed more than the moderate portions she served. Though she had her problems (her alcohol consumption was not quite as limited), she did not use food for emotional purposes; it all seemed so straightforward for her.

That's why the most important message about food is to eat moderately with awareness. It's not enough to simply say, "Eat less and still have your chocolate cake on Friday." You need to get to a neutral territory first. That's why reducing the noisy, addictive bad foods entirely for several weeks is so helpful. It rebalances your chemistry and palette so you eat less and start to discern what's really in your food; meanwhile, adding healthful foods will satisfy your hunger at a deep level. Now you've got a healthy "clean slate" onto which to add a treat here and there as a deliberate choice: it should be something special. Delicious treats are on the planet for a reason—but while they're exciting when eaten occasionally, they're polluting when eaten every day.

Taking some time to investigate not just what you eat but also how and why you eat makes moderation more achievable. Pausing long enough to look inward each time you are hungry can shed light on why you make poor choices. When your new repertoire of foods is combined with self-knowledge and self-acceptance, healthy eating becomes simple, pleasurable, and sustainable.

Eating with Peace: The Ritual of Food

QUESTION: WHAT IS HAPPENING AROUND YOU WHEN YOU EAT?

A. The TV is on (whether I'm watching it or not), or I'm listening to music, or I am reading something, or I'm at my computer.

B. Various family members or roommates drift in and out at different times, sometimes sitting down to join me, other times not.

C. I frequently find myself standing at my kitchen counter eating because I've gotten distracted by something else, like talking on the phone.

D. I'm sitting quietly enjoying a meal with someone I love.

HOW CAN WE GET MUCH GOOD from our food when we treat it like we expect so little from it? In many cultures eating is an important ritual: by preparing and consuming food deliberately and even reverentially, people acknowledge the food before them, bless it, and appreciate the energy it is giving them. Mealtimes become moments to pause, take stock of their lives, and commit to the act of self-care. Instead of being a chore or a drag, eating becomes a daily ritual that can anchor a person more firmly into their life.

That's why it's such a shame that in our modern, fast-paced lives, we've lost track of how we eat. Instead of being a calm and deliberate act, a meal is often squeezed in on the go. Instead of appreciating the food, we often barely notice it as we eat, or we struggle with it, feeling guilty about it or maybe wishing it were something else. Bringing food back into focus is integral to finding balance through eating. For the four weeks you're on the program, you're going to agree to refrain from watching TV, reading, or working while you eat. You're going to put some time into laying the table and presenting your food beautifully, even if you're eating alone. You're even going to do the preparation and cleanup with a more creative and calm perspective. The idea is in small ways to make the act of eating more meaningful.

Bringing this attitude to food makes it hard to overeat and overindulge: you take a moment to decide in advance how much you will consume. You notice how the food is affecting you as you're eating it, and you notice when you're satisfied. The relationship between you and your food grows closer—you know exactly why you're eating instead of confusing the purpose by making food fill emotional needs. Much of the time we consume too much because we're not present.

QUESTION: IF YOU'RE ALMOST SURPRISED WHEN THE FOOD ON YOUR PLATE IS FINISHED, HOW MUCH OF YOUR MEAL DID YOU NOTICE?

If your attention was not there, did you get as much nourishment as you could have?

THE ABCS OF PEACEFUL EATING
A. Put love into your food.

If food is made with care, it changes. Try to plan in advance so you give yourself enough time to prepare the food without rushing. If you plan well, you can go from one food prep activity to the next being aware and conscious of each step, and the act of preparing food becomes more creative and rewarding. As a wife and mom, I can find satisfaction in feeling that I'm doing service for my family—if I take the time to tune in to what I'm doing. The dish doesn't have to be gourmet—it can be the simplest food—but if done with consideration, it carries an energetic message into the meal. It feeds you and your tablemates with more than just nutrients. That's why it pays to avoid the microwave and know in advance what you're going to cook each night.

B. Present meals like they matter.

After cooking, take two extra minutes to lay food beautifully on platters or plates, even if it's just for you or for you plus one other person. I sometimes decorate the platters: a flower grabbed from outside sits next to slices of seared fish, or curls of orange carrot next to slices of tofu. I juxtapose colors and textures and arrange foods in neat ways. It pleases the artist in me to pay attention to how the food looks all together. As my round-the-island family dinners often include separate plates and bowls, it is a good opportunity to make a meal look colorful and appealing or use fun serving utensils. When you put consideration into all these details as you serve a meal, you bring the focus to the moment and make even a daily act more significant.

C. Make mealtime meaningful.

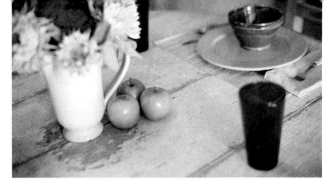

Do you have a dining room table or a kitchen table? It's there because you're supposed to sit at it to eat, whether alone, with friends, or with your family. If you don't have a table dedicated to eating, then might you make a space in your home that is devoted to meals? I spend five minutes to lay the table while the food is cooking. I put out a place setting for each person, including mats and napkins, and I fill a water glass for each person. I put something in the middle of the table: a potted plant or some flowers if I have them. The dogs get locked outside, and the TV in the living room is switched off so we can't hear it. Phone calls do not get answered. Lunchtime, when I'm home alone, is often a time for me to sit and reflect. Dinnertime is a chance to connect with my husband and kids and sometimes with friends. Life rushes by so quickly that if we don't sit around a table, our days could go by with minimal communication. If you're a parent, I believe that you lose track of your kids if you don't once in a while sit down at the table and have those family talks. It may be unrealistic to do it every night, but perhaps one day a week you could alert the kids in advance: "Tonight, guys, we're eating together."

TIP If you're at work and your options are limited, make a small gesture of treating food with respect. Find a place to eat that is well away from your workstation, and go outside if the weather is nice. Leave reading material and cell phones behind. State an affirmation quietly and deliberately as you sit down for your meal: "This is my time for nourishment and calm."

TIP Everyone occasionally eats a store-bought meal at work or at home. Even if it's just a sandwich or sushi in a plastic tray, take two minutes to transfer your meal to proper dishware, and ditch the disposable cutlery and paper napkin that came with it. Use real cutlery, and sit down at a table (note: not your desk) to eat. You won't lose any time, but your experience of your food will be different.

Banned Behavior

1. Eating while talking on cell phone: a common crime among those who eat out or munch lunch on the run. Okay, so you caught up with your girlfriend. But did you even notice what you were eating?
2. Eating while driving: a wrong combination. Bear in mind that some researchers have correlated obesity to driving an automatic. When drivers had to shift gears in a manual transmission car, they didn't have that free hand for eating.
3. Eating while walking around the house: it makes you think you aren't consuming so much or perhaps even that you're burning calories. Sit down and take responsibility for what you eat.

Exercise:
Ritual Dinner

Alter your eating routine so that you start the meal feeling centered, and give your food the attention it deserves. Include at least three of the following elements:

1. **LAY THE TABLE AND PRESENT THE FOOD** in a way that you find beautiful.

2. **SAY A GRACE BEFORE YOU EAT.** One sentence of thankfulness, however you want to phrase it, said aloud or in your mind, brings awareness to the food before you and makes the act of eating intentional.

3. **LIGHT A CANDLE.** If you don't have access to a calm dining area, or if you eat alone and have a tendency to multitask through your meals, lighting a candle will remind you to slow down and be nurtured by your food.

4. **PLAY CALMING MUSIC.** If you are used to some sound in your environment, switch from raucous rock to classical tunes or even some melodic mantras or chanting. Research has shown that subjects overeat when listening to overstimulating music.

5. **BREATHE BEFORE EACH BITE,** or put your fork down. Decide to slow down the pace and focus your attention on each bite. What's the hurry? Notice how each bite tastes and how it makes you feel. Ask yourself, "What feels good about this food?" Swallow and breathe before taking the next bite.

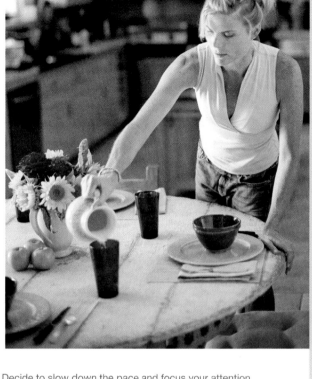

MOVING TOWARD MODERATION

Moderation = a state of panic-free eating. There is no panic when you are moderate in whatever you do. This is especially true with food: if you can keep your intake of whatever you enjoy to a qualified minimum, then you feel a sense of satisfaction, well-being, and calm. If you overdo for the sake of the limited amount of pleasure it will give in the moment, you spend a great deal of time later on feeling guilty and stressed, trying belatedly to make a deal with your overindulgence.

Why, to paraphrase a recent best-selling diet book, do French women stay thin? Because there is no abstinence, but there is no abuse either. They consume small amounts of delicious, high-quality foods in their diet frequently enough that they don't fear of missing out on pleasure. They know that if they only eat a few bites today, it's okay. The good food will be there tomorrow as well.

In order to enjoy a sane and rewarding way of eating, it's important to indulge in the yummiest food on occasion, but only on occasion. Rather than operating from denial and fear, appreciate things that should be savored. The bane of our existence is wanting more. Think what happens when something indulgent becomes a daily habit. It loses its fabulousness, and instead of being thrilled by the experience, you simply want more. The idea is to get away from the addiction—that constant desire or need that can never be fulfilled.

Moderation is a habit that can be cultivated through knowing that you will be happy and satiated by giving yourself what you *need* instead of letting that thing you desire become your master. Whenever you feel you must have a thing, it is almost certainly time to try letting go of that thing, at least for a while. If you love something and can learn to use it moderately, you never have to give it up. You can enjoy chocolate once in a while, that little bit that makes you feel good when you're premenstrual. You can decide that wine is your treat and have one glass at a time or maybe two, but then you make a choice: you say no to the bread or you turn down the dessert and really enjoy that wine because it's your sensual pleasure. Moderation means evaluating your choices for yourself and sticking to them because you know how bad overindulgence makes you feel.

If we can treat ourselves kindly enough to plot out a more moderate path, we can enjoy our food, share it with our families and friends without stressing, and drop a lot of the bad patterns that no longer serve us. Sense pleasures are on the planet to be enjoyed—

if we can enjoy them in moderation, in the spirit of celebration.

THE KEYS TO MODERATE MEALS

The vocabulary of food, especially for women, is so often about eating *less* of some things and *eliminating* others, as if food is the enemy and we are endlessly under siege. Even when we're trying to get healthier instead of lose weight, the emphasis is on deprivation: detoxing, fasting, and ruthlessly cutting out this, that, and the other in order to look and feel better.

Armed with this negative attitude, we are setting ourselves up for instability. I've come to understand that suffering happens in large part because the psyche doesn't understand the concept no. If your thoughts are focused on trying to not eat food, what your mind registers is not the no but simply the tempting idea. By trying to banish food from your mind, you only think more about it. The key instead is to focus on the positive, on the delicious, wholesome foods you can have, and to welcome their abundance by actively seeking out new good things to add to your diet. (As wacky as it sounds, the logic of this clicked for me only when I house-trained my dogs. Constantly warning them "not" to pee inside was useless; they kept doing it. Encouraging them toward the positive by saying, "Go outside," worked like a charm. A strange way to learn how not to crave bagels, but it worked for me.)

Here are the three steps to achieving an empowered and positive state of moderation instead of the negative mind-set of deprivation.

Food

Self-Inquiry

Throughout this section, you've been encouraged again and again to ask questions. Here's why: It's how you stay present and make good choices. When it comes to food, asking yourself questions is the key to staying on track, eating what is right for you, and not overeating. Perhaps you graze at the fridge and can't stop picking at things. From now on, when you find yourself standing at the fridge, about to open it, stop, put your arms by your sides, and take a breath. Ask yourself a series of questions:

1. What am I feeling in my body that makes me want food? Am I feeling true symptoms of hunger?

    If the answer is no, walk away and get busy doing something else. If the answer is yes, ask:

2. Is it possible that these hunger pangs are coming from my emotional mood or current circumstances rather than my body's need for fuel? For example: Am I bored, restless, or blue? Am I seeking procrastination, seeking comfort, or seeking something exciting and new? If you determine one of these things is the case, have a glass of water and turn your attention to the real problem (your bored or blue state) instead of the imagined symptom (hunger).

    If the answer is no, ask yourself:

3. What is my body hungry for right now? What nutrients have I missed in my diet today? Your taste buds may be yelling, "Pop tarts!" but the true answer to this question will more likely be clean protein or an avocado. If the craving for something crappy continues, put your hands on your belly and ask yourself, "Do I really need this fuel today?"

4. If necessary, draw a big question mark and stick it on the fridge to remind you to ask the questions.

Remember to ask these questions at other places too, such as the coffee-shop counter; the deli counter; restaurants; the snack corner at work. If you're out, remember to ask whether the environment is influencing you. For instance, a cozy teahouse on a rainy afternoon may make your mind yearn for chocolate chip cookies while your body isn't that interested in them. Be conscious of where desires come from.

PRACTICE NOT EATING EVERYTHING ON THE PLATE. Leave a few bites, and push the plate away. Save the leftovers if you like, so as not to waste, but from time to time just pause and decide it's okay to stop before you reach the end. Alternatively, use a smaller plate to get accustomed to smaller portions.

Self-Acceptance

If you are so rigid in your eating habits that you can't accommodate unexpected events, your food has gotten the upper hand over you. When situations happen that are outside your control or you get served something that's not exactly what you want, don't stress out. Just give yourself permission to enjoy it. Consider it a feast for your senses, bless the food quietly, and eat some. Fattening or even unhealthy food eaten with love and acceptance won't kill you, as long as it's relatively infrequent. Refuse to eat with stress or negativity, and celebrate the fact that someone has served you food they've made with care.

To enjoy a healthy relationship with food, you support yourself with daily habits that nurture your needs. You find the food that makes your body function properly—

Comfort Food

Why, when we want to be comforted by food, do we so often pick foods that throw our body chemistry off—with sugar or heavy starches—and that later make us feel physically gross or emotionally guilty? If you feel that yearning, it's important to inquire where it comes from; most of the time when we yearn for comfort food, it's not because our body is run down. Often we yearn for warmth or love, not doughnuts. It's a longing for memories of times when we felt good in the past. So the challenge is to pause, ask what you're actually longing for, and see how can you find that satiation, that warmth, in other ways. I find it through meditating or curling up in a chair by the fire and reading. The only times I seek out the soothing effects of food are when I'm under the weather. That's when I listen to my body's signals: usually it is tired and wants some clean, easy, cozy-feeling food that is easy to digest. I find pureed foods like green vegetable soups make me feel comforted, perhaps because they're like baby food.

If you crave comfort food on a regular basis, start using these easy tools to determine whether you are actually hungry. First, drink a glass of water to make sure what you're feeling is not dehydration. Then take a short walk or do twenty-five Arm Swings (see page 100). Now ask yourself if you're still hungry. If yes, make a choice before you reach for the food so that when you run to the kitchen, you have decided that ten cashews and half a pear will be enough (or some cheese if you don't like nuts). Eat this, and wait at least ten minutes before you decide you're still hungry. Allow yourself to find out that this reasonable amount of food has satisfied you. Simply by slowing down and asking questions, you can loosen the grip of your desire enormously.

and then allow for breaks from the norm. The super-rich macaroni and cheese your aunt serves at her house isn't going to throw you off the health track entirely. Just know you can get back to your place of balance tomorrow because you know what to feed yourself and you have a calm approach to food.

Likewise, there will be work or social situations that you're not in control of and you'll just have to take what is offered. So forgive yourself and eat if you need to eat. Doing the tragic lettuce-leaf-and-an-ice-cube thing for lunch might serve a purpose every now and then, but you can't build a lifetime of health on it. If we're holding ourselves to such high standards that one deviation from the rules leads to hours of self-recrimination, we'll never find our footing when it comes to food.

Self-Awareness

A weird thing can happen sometimes while eating. Your food tastes okay, but by the end of the meal you like the food more than when you started and you want another serving. In fact, you can't stop thinking about how badly you want more. The whole process of eating has somehow become more interesting to you because it's over. The truth is, you weren't paying attention at the beginning because you were looking ahead to the end and worrying about how it would be over soon. Practicing being present as you eat, by making meals a ritual and checking in with how you feel before and during the meal, can help you enjoy what you're eating now instead of thinking about the future and wanting more.

Exercise: Add Your Food Treat

By Week 4 of this program, you have adjusted to life without your noisy-food fixes. With this clear mind and quieter body chemistry, pick the treat that you would most love to have back in your diet, and decide upon a reasonable portion of it. Don't double up on treats, like splurging on the bread basket and the wine. Pick one thing, and make it the smartest but most enjoyable choice you can. Choose the day you will eat it, and mark it on your calendar. Get excited for it, and consume it with care instead of on the run. Most important, give yourself permission to love it, and savor every bite or sip! Allow it to be a feast for the senses. Eat your treat *once* this week, and no more.

If your treat is chocolate, make your treat a *small* bar of good-quality, dark chocolate, preferably organic. Not only does dark chocolate have less sugar than milk chocolate, it has far more health-building antioxidants. The finer (and more expensive) the sweet, the more satisfying it will be and the less you will need to consume to get the effect.

If your treat is wine, choose *one glass* of good-quality wine; red wine has beneficial antioxidants, but let personal taste direct your choice.

If your treat is cookies or cakes, there are plenty of varieties made with all-natural ingredients and no trans fats that are still loaded with yummy ingredients. Look in your health food mart.

No matter what your fix is, make conscious choices and upgrade your treats to the best variety you can.

TIP Gather and ground yourself before eating. Sitting at the table before you start to eat, feel your feet grounded into the earth. Place your palms on your thighs. Take a moment and breathe in. Become conscious of yourself in your body. Think about the meal you're going to eat. Visualize how you'll feel at the end. Say to yourself, "I'm rooted, I'm here, I'm in my body, now I can start." Come back to this posture throughout the meal. It keeps you grounded in your physical experience, not drifting into your head, thinking about what else is out there.

■   ■   ■

QUESTION: WHAT WERE FAMILY MEALS LIKE WHEN YOU WERE A KID?

Were they happy or tense? What did you eat—what was considered "good food" in your family?

IF YOU ARE CONFLICTED or unhappy in your approach to food, it pays to look at how you were brought up. We learn to eat from our upbringing, and our attitude toward food is powerfully shaped by how we grew up. Perhaps now is the time to disempower those old memories, beliefs, and habits by peeling back some of the layers and seeing what shaped you. (It also pays to think about what your genetic heritage is and what kind of foods your ethnic group has evolved to eat.)

■   ■   ■

I GREW UP IN A HOUSEHOLD of what would today be called "foodies." There was a lot of extremely good food around, but it was always served up with a dish of anger and resentment on the side. My parents were not happy people, yet neither of them expressed their frustrations or disappointments through talking. The unresolved emotions hung in the air as an emptiness, a lack. There was no hugging and kissing in my house; I can't think of a single time I saw my parents kiss each other. I know my older sisters felt it too because they acted out in their own rebellious ways, getting mixed up with boys and drugs.

Food became the way we communicated or expressed any feelings at all. I'm convinced that the Hemingway genes are coded to indulge in food and drink—and suffer for it too. (When I finally got a chance to visit my grandfather Ernest's former house in Cuba, I was riveted by his handwriting scrawled on the bathroom wall, recording his fluctuating weight day by day: "April 7, 1957: 191 lbs.") In fact, my family pretty much did nothing but talk about food because it was the one thing everyone could get behind. Everyone was arguing and screwed up, but we'd plan meals all the time. It was surreal. We'd eat one meal and then talk about the next: "Oh, we'll have mille-feuille and such-and-such for dessert, and what sauce will we put on top of it? And we'll have a bottle of this wine and a bottle of that wine." And at some point something mean would be said, and my mother would run to her room and eat alone, or worse, a glass of wine would get smashed against the dining room wall in the heat of fury, and the rest of us would end up silently eating our fancy meals

off trays in front of the TV. The atmosphere was charged but devoid of real connection. One of my most vivid memories of my childhood is my dad eating a plate of cheese and crackers for an hour and a half after dinner while he watched television, as if he was trying to fill a void that no food would ever fill.

It wasn't until I was older that I saw how these family patterns had informed my relationship to food. My endless eating of grainy bread as a teen, my obsessive popcorn-and-coffee habit as a twentysomething—I was repeating my dad's habits: I'd starve all day, and love myself all night. It was a cycle, using food as love and then feeling incredibly guilty and hateful about it the next day. Even after I was married and had my daughters, I followed my strict dietary regimes because deep down I was scared to open my heart to love and acceptance of others. My identity was built on being skinny, and my pride came from having control over what I ate. I didn't trust that I had created my own loving family dynamic, different from the one I'd grown up in, a family that could fulfill many of those needs for me. In order to build a healthy and moderate approach to food, I had to understand how my compulsive, purist behaviors were not the sign of admirable discipline I'd always thought they were and had deeper emotional roots.

■   ■   ■

I AM A BIG ADDICT. Even if my addictions are so-called healthy, I make what's good for me bad for me by overdoing it. Whether it's green tea or my healthy breakfast smoothie, I can easily develop a dependency on certain foods or drinks and eat them day in, day out, for months until I develop an intolerance to them—like suddenly getting headaches from the tea. But often I'll keep going with my fix, as if scared that my world depends on my getting it. Not only is it bad on the body to eat an unvaried diet, but this kind of dependency is restrictive and limiting. I had to look at my family conditioning to understand why I tend to use food as such a safety net.

There is no instant solution to emotion-driven eating patterns. Unraveling why you eat the way you do may be a long process. But when you seek the source of your habits, you often find they are rooted in thoughts and memories that need not have a hold on you at all. Allow yourself to release the thoughts and memories, and you begin to release the habits. Of course, most habits want to stick. Your ego wants you to believe you can't feel good without your old behavior. Or your ego will make you fear that despite your good work at changing, you will soon fall off the wagon and your old behavior will come back. I've experienced all these things repeatedly. But I've had to recognize that sometimes the thing that pulls us off balance is a tendency to search for a problem when things are going well. When you feel unsteady and screwy in your head about eating, ask yourself, Am I looking for something to feel bad about? Can I give up always looking for the problem?

IF OTHERS ARE BRINGING TREATS and temptations into the home, making it hard for you to "cut the crap" out of your diet, ask them to take those things away. Claim your right to be supported by the people around you. This is hardly a lot to ask, especially if you are the caretaker of the home.

■ ■ ■

THE ONE THING I'VE ALWAYS WANTED in my life is to clear my bad patterns out so I didn't pass them on to my daughters. As they grew up, I was always completely honest with them about the challenges I'd faced over food, and I tried to teach them all the best habits I could. Though they've had their struggles, like any teenagers, they use food smartly and regulate their own behavior, eating more healthfully than any other teens I've met.

The inspiring thing about modifying your own way of eating is that as you change, your family changes. You don't have to do anything; it's all about example. If you eat right, if you do some conscious breathing and movement, and you change your life, then subtly those around you will change. They won't know why and they won't even ask questions, but they will change. They might also need a major wake-up call to do so, as in the case of my husband, Stephen, whose cancer prompted his shift to the vibrant, whole-foods approach to eating outlined in this chapter. Given my own challenges and hard-won lessons about food, I was rarely prouder than when Stephen got a chance to consult the Dalai Lama's personal physician and the esteemed doctor told him, "Your cancer is asleep. Whoever is telling you what to eat is doing a great job."

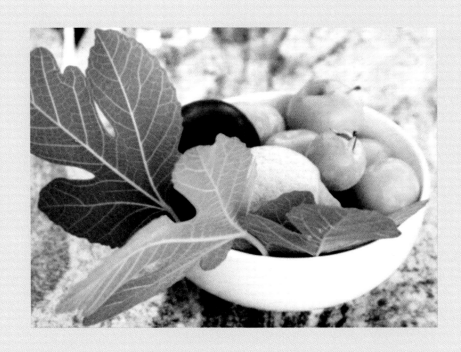

Food

Silence

PART TWO

Exercise

Home

Exercise

QUESTION: THE IDEA OF WORKING OUT EVERY OTHER DAY IS:

    A. Unimaginable. I hardly have time for myself as it is.

    B. Doable. I could find thirty minutes every other day.

    C. Inspirational. I suspect it might make me feel pretty good.

    D. Detestable. I do whatever I can to avoid exercising!

QUESTION: IN ORDER TO QUALIFY AS A REAL WORKOUT,
AN EXERCISE SESSION MUST LEAVE ME:

    A. Winded, pushed to the edge, and covered in sweat.

    B. Conscious of muscles I forgot I had.

    C. Physically renewed and in better spirits than when I started.

    D. Ten pounds lighter—and I want a guarantee on that.

EXERCISE IS A TOOL that everyone needs to know how to use. But it needn't involve extreme sports or endless workouts. It can be a simple yet powerful practice that transforms your state of mind and keeps you well, a time for stripping away some of the excess and turning your attention inward. (Whatever your attitude to exercise may be now, by the end of this program you'll be all about B and C, above.)

▪ ▪ ▪

IF I ADDED UP ALL THE HOURS I've spent working out over my life, it'd be embarrassing. I've owned more stretch leggings than I care to admit and about as many running shoes as Marion Jones. I've done yoga since the days when practitioners wore long, flowy clothes to class and burned patchouli, and over my two decades of practice my heels and palms have worn through countless sticky mats. I've trained at the same level as Olympic competitors in track and field, and left to my own devices, I went through phases of obsessive overexercising, where I jump-roped to excess and watched my skin turn blue.

While sports and yoga have been empowering in my life, they've often threatened to have the opposite effect: to drain me of power. It's just my nature. When I find something that works, I take it to the extreme. In much the way that some people abuse drugs because they want to return again and again to the familiar state where they feel good, I have abused exercise. For years it was my survival tool. As a teen I relied on runner's high to escape the oppressive atmosphere of my home. In my twenties and thirties I became dependent on rigorous workouts to stay skinny and sane.

My tendency when it came to any kind of workout was to click into overdrive—perhaps because at heart I'm a mountain girl whose first instinct when faced with a physical challenge is to do it better and faster than anyone else. My major life lesson when it comes to exercise, just as with food, has been to learn moderation—to stop trying to prove something, to dial down my type-A personality, and to get more benefit from less sweat.

I share this with you because it's important to bust some of the myths about working out. So often when I read books and magazine articles by fitness experts or see them on TV, they look like members of a special breed of superhumans who have a completely uncomplicated, zestfully positive relationship to exercise. They just *love to work out with a huge smile every single day! They use it for good reasons, never screwed-up ones! They never need to rest!* And they definitely *know their bodies are slammin' hot!* My experience in the real world, which includes opening a yoga studio in Idaho and leading workshops around the country, has never matched that image. I'm certainly not that way myself. Nor have I met anyone who's that perfect—not even among advanced yoga practitioners and teachers. I mean, who are we kidding?

Most women I know struggle to some degree with exercise. Motivation can flag on the best of days; even during a great workout that devil can still sit on your shoulder telling you to quit. Insecurities get in the way, making you feel less than the next woman over or that whatever you're doing is not enough to get fit or skinny or sexy. Pride can also cause a few falls—like in yoga class, where the sudden desire for affirmation can lead to doing stupid things that cause injury. I've been guilty as charged on all of the above counts.

Since most of us start with these challenges, isn't it time we approached exercise in a way that doesn't add to the struggle? A way that promotes self-acceptance, not self-criticism, so that no matter how many minutes we move, or how fast or slow, we still get the satisfaction of feeling, "This is good enough"? After many years of using exercise in an extreme fashion, I've found my way back to that middle ground. Today I have an approach to exercise that I can guarantee will make any workout effective, rejuvenating, restorative, or calming, depending on what you need—all with much less effort than you think.

This new, gentler attitude grew as my sensitivity to my physical and mental needs also grew—a shift inspired partly by yoga, partly by meditation, and partly by the simple act of becoming kinder to myself with age. In place of sheer intensity, now I try to exercise with a more subtle quality: *intention.* Instead of forcing a grueling workout no matter how much energy I have (and no matter what the weather's doing), now I check in with myself to ask, "What is perfect for me today?" And rather than worry that I should be signing up for every new workout trend, I know that I get what I need both physically and mentally from my two primary workouts, walking and yoga. They make a simple pair that suits my lifestyle and my personality.

Too often we avoid exercise because of limitations in our lives, especially as women who may have families and personal demands taking up all our time. The good news is that no matter what your limitations of time, terrain, or physical ability, you can learn a powerful way to exercise that takes account of those limitations and still gives you lots of benefit. Exercise should serve your lifestyle and support your needs rather than making you feel like a servant to some rigorous gym or workout schedule. Exercise should fit into your busy life rather than taking it over. And it should be adaptable to changing circumstances. What I love about walking and yoga is that I can do either thing wherever I am. Whether I'm at home or on location for an acting job, all I need is myself, a yoga mat or sneakers, and some comfortable clothing. These two forms of exercise keep me energized, stretched, and balanced. Here, in this segment of the Quickstart 30-Day Program, you will learn to use the same tools.

THE BENEFITS OF EXERCISE

There are lots of great reasons to work out. Your physical body gets conditioned and fit. Your heart is healthier. It helps you keep weight off.

But I prefer to think of this way: exercise is a tool that helps you handle your life.

It's important to see exercise from a whole-person point of view. Exercise affects the body, the mind, and the emotions in equal measure. It lifts your spirits and gives you confidence. (If you're looking for it, exercise can become a spiritual practice too.) It helps you burn through fears and shift from cautious to courageous. When you're feeling boxed in, exercise helps you create some space; it revs you up when you feel dragged down. In short, you need exercise because it plugs you in to your power source.

Without exercise, you compromise your body's ability to function at its best and your mind's ability to focus on what matters. Emotionally, you sabotage your own capacity to *let things go.* And you probably don't look nearly as good as you could.

Notice that the concerns for appearance are last on my list—but not because I deem them unimportant. On the contrary, feeling you look great is one of the best benefits of exercise. The appearance of someone who exercises moderately is always better than someone who doesn't do a lick of it: they have a tighter body; they stand taller, walk more confidently, and radiate a happy, energized glow in their faces. I'm the first to admit that wanting to look better can be a highly motivating force when you're tempted to stay in bed and hit snooze. But vanity shouldn't be the main reason you work out—it's too limited an inspiration, and for most women it can get twisted into self-criticism when what we want to create is a positive relationship to exercise.

My approach is to prioritize internal awareness over superficial concerns. There is simply no need to obsessively focus on external appearances. When you are using your body well, external change happens organically because you're transforming your state on the inside. The first running coach I ever worked with when I was in my late teens called the process "slowly creating the you." He meant that if you zero in on the task at hand, cut out distractions, and cultivate a deep inner focus, then step by step and breath by breath, powerful change will occur both inside and out. Yoga teaches the same lessons. Do your practice with full attention on how your body feels, not how it looks, and you will be working at an intensity that allows your body to carve itself into its best shape. The excess will disappear and the shape will appear. Just as with food, it's not overnight; the change is gradual. But it is far likelier to be permanent because it comes from such deep work.

I've had a much happier relationship to exercise since I stopped doing it exclusively to stay slim and started using it to feel great in my body and mind. Now that I'm in my forties, I'm finally grateful for my body, not critical of it. My body is slender enough and toned enough; it suits the woman I am. The shift to an inner focus is integral to the walking and yoga practices recommended here. I suggest that you constantly check in with yourself and ask, "How do I feel?" and banish all thoughts of "How do I look?" If your ego is running rampant, judging every second how you look, your awareness is going to stay stuck in your head. And who wants to spend more time stuck in their head?

I love exercise because it *un*-sticks everything. Done correctly, it is a powerful way to transform your physical, mental, and emotional state. Warming up the body and loosening the limbs almost always dissolves pain and tension, making way for a new outlook on life. That's why its potential is extraordinary. It gives each person the possibility to shift her state whenever she needs. If you don't already use it as a go-to remedy in times of stress, this program will encourage you to do so.

"Slowly creating the you" means revealing the beautiful body that is already inside of you. It doesn't mean acquiring a size and silhouette that is radically different from the one nature intended you to have. Rather, it's carving away at excess and toning the body shape that is genetically yours. I learned this lesson after years of screwing with myself, and I encourage you to sidestep the suffering. You can't completely alter your body type, your frame, or your natural proclivity to be curvy or straight up and down. But you look and feel your most beautiful when you treat your body kindly, work out according to your own potential, drop the self-critical thoughts, and most important, work on accepting *who you are right now,* as you will in this program.

Exercise

The transformation starts at the physical level. Exercise promotes good respiration and digestion, healthy elimination, effective body repair, and good rest. Even doing a fairly gentle workout like walking will raise your metabolism so that you not only burn food energy better, you draw more nutrients from the things you eat. (It will also make you drink more water, which is always a good thing.) It boosts circulation of the blood, which brings more oxygen to your cells and carries away the waste products. That's why, even if it may sound counterintuitive, exerting yourself can remedy fatigue and make you feel more energized in your daily life. It heats you up so that you sweat out toxins through the skin. It boosts

A Quick Fix

Consider that Americans spend millions of dollars on such things as pharmaceuticals, stimulants, and entertainment to relieve stress and change their mood, yet millions of Americans barely exercise. Commit to trying movement next time you need an instant transformation. Using simple, one- to three-minute exercises during the day can boost your energy, lift your mood, or calm down an anxious mind. These quick-fix exercises are great for spot cleaning: you can use them whenever you need to change your state.

Quick Fix #1:
Wake-Up Twists

Stand with your feet shoulder-distance apart, your knees slightly soft, and your tailbone tucked a little so you feel a powerful center of balance. Shift your feet until you are grounded and steady. Breathe softly through the nose. Begin to loosely swing your arms from left to right about a foot away from your body. Let your trunk and shoulders simply follow the twisting motion. As you gain speed, let the arms go higher, and swing them like a child until the backs of your hands tap the back of the body. (One hand will be at rib level; the other will tap lower down, stimulating the kidneys.) Keep your eyes softly focused on the horizon as your head moves from left to right, and keep breathing softly. Let thoughts go, focus on how different parts of your body feel. This will gently wake up your body and get energy flowing up and down your spine. Do it for one minute.

USE FOR: Waking up in the morning, before a walk, as a break from sitting at your desk.

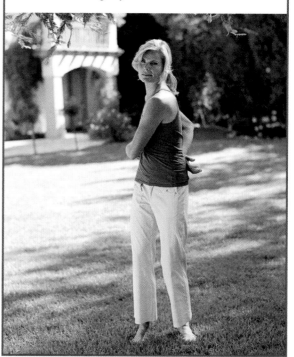

circulation of the lymph fluid, making you more resistant to sickness. Even the fluid between your joints gets pushed around, keeping your joints lubricated. And the deep breathing you do when exercising pushes the diaphragm down so that your internal organs get a massage, which keeps them mobile and healthy.

And a very real physiological effect occurs during this kind of exercise that builds a stress-free internal environment. It's called the "relaxation response." Through steady, deep breathing and calm movements, the heartbeat slows, and respiration and blood pressure decrease. The body seizes this chance to turn on the healing mechanisms.

As the different parts of your body release tension and are cleared of toxins, your mind does so as well. I call it "clearing the cobwebs." You can't see the effect in the way you can see sweat on the skin, but you feel just as light and cleansed afterward. Some feel it as a euphoric high, others as a gentle clearing. For me, it feels like I am processing or digesting my life when I exercise. Things just "come up" as I move and fall into quiet focus: any negative thoughts or old memories are shunted out of their hiding spaces so that I acknowledge them and then let them go. Some people process their lives through journal writing or talking to friends; I do it through moving my body.

This is how exercise becomes a useful tool. It lets you shed the things that no longer serve you. And if you do it right, it teaches you how to be present. Through a combination of steady breathing, repetitive motion, and constantly paying attention to what your body is doing, you train your brain to bring awareness to the present moment and stop dwelling on the past or projecting about the future. Exercising right breaks you out of your thinking patterns and lets you exist in a state of no thought, just being. When you apply a bit of this yogic attitude to whatever exercise you do, physical movement becomes a great way to teach yourself how to be here now.

By the end of a good session of walking or yoga or anything you choose—no matter how gentle or how tough—you can feel like you pressed your own reset button. This will translate to being more grounded, calm, and present in your whole life. When you train the brain to be present in a morning walk or a short stretching session, it's easier to find that feeling doing less active things, like making dinner, tidying the house, and eventually sitting in meditation. If your physical self comes into greater stability and balance, then your psychological and spiritual states will follow.

In the same way that minor changes to diet can create a vast and surprisingly quick improvement to your health, changing your exercise habits a little by adding in a walk where there used to be none, or trying yoga where you used to do the Stairmaster while reading a magazine, will effect considerable positive change in your life. Research has shown that when coupled with a nutritious diet filled with whole foods, the introduction of a daily thirty-minute exercise session caused a significant decrease in subjects' risk of diabetes, cancer, and heart disease in just six weeks.

Quick Fix #2:
Arm Swings

Start with feet shoulder-distance apart, knees soft, arms hanging loosely by your sides. With a slight hop, jump up and swing hands up to shoulder height with bent arms, then swing them down and behind you as you land with bended knees. As you land, roll backward and forward on your heels for momentum, as this stimulates points in your feet that will energize your whole body. Let the arms swing loosely in their shoulder sockets, but don't throw them wildly. As they start to swing forward, hop and bring hands up high again. Repeat the swing-and-hop in a steady rhythm, building up speed until you create a lot of momentum in your arms. Do it for 1 to 3 minutes.

USE IT FOR: Getting your energy going first thing in the morning, to get your body warm before a walk, or in the middle of a yoga practice to add some cardio activity.

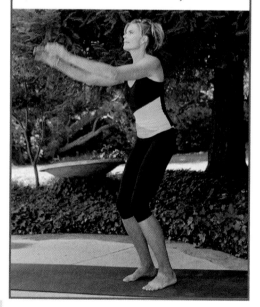

THE 30-DAY APPROACH: EXERCISING WITH INTENTION

QUESTION: THE IDEA OF STARTING A SIMPLE WALKING AND YOGA PROGRAM MAKES ME FEEL:

    A. Anxious that I won't get enough of a workout.
    B. Anxious that I don't have time to fit in exercise.
    C. Curious to try something that doesn't sound too hard.

THIS IS NOT A WORKOUT BOOK. The goal is not to reach peak fitness in a month or to train for competition. Instead, you will learn to use exercise in such a way that it contributes to your balanced life. By focusing on three basic practices—breathing, walking, and a simple yoga routine—you will learn to use exercise in a new way. I call it *exercising with intention.* The goals are to heighten your awareness of what's happening in your body right now, to get powerfully focused in your practice so that you derive more benefit with less time, and to dissolve some of the tension that you may be holding in your body and mind. The four phases of this program will guide you. Step 1, "Turn on the Breath," shows you how to use breath to direct your attention inward. Step 2, "Walk Without Thought," teaches you how to take that awareness to movement. Step 3, "Bring It to the Mat," introduces a yoga practice suitable for beginners and intermediate practitioners. And Step 4, "Set Your Intention," directs you to use a workout to transform the way you feel so that you emerge lighter in mind as well as body.

Learning to exercise with intention may sound weird if you are accustomed to thinking about typical fitness goals like endurance, stamina, and speed. But for the four weeks of this program, agree to let those concerns go. You have the rest of your life to get faster and tougher if that's what you enjoy; for now, you will go slower and more deliberately. It doesn't mean it's easier; exercising with deep awareness is a challenge for the body and mind. But once you begin to develop this more intimate relationship with your body, any kind of exercise you choose to do in the future will become extremely powerful. You can do a sweaty session on a spinning bike, a tranquil ballet class, or an adventure sport like rock climbing, and your experience will be much deeper. (And if you take up golf, you'll be way ahead of the pack.) You'll find that even a three-minute stretch on your living room floor before you go to bed will be more effective at helping you shed the strains of the day.

Don't fall into the trap of writing off things that seem too simple. Your physical body will change during this program. You will find that your ability to walk for a length of time, open your body in a stretch, or even enjoy (or endure) a pose in yoga will improve each time you exercise. It's that inner focus that is most valuable. As that running coach of mine also liked to say, "Exercise will do nothing for you if you're not conscious of what you're doing." Our goal here is to develop that conscious approach, whether you end up walking half a mile at a time or speed-walking for ten.

That's why even if you already do one or more things to keep fit, I encourage you to commit to doing the practices that follow for the entire four-week program. If you are married to your current workout regime, it may be a challenge to lower the intensity to walking and basic yoga for a couple of weeks. Observe if frustration or guilt comes up—and if it does, ask yourself why. If you feel you need to do your regular workout in addition to the practices here, go ahead. But make a commitment to the fact that *this is a different experience.* Shift your attitude from "I must get a fat-burning workout in today" to "I might make more change in my body if I focus on doing it differently."

If your challenge is to get up and start exercising for the first time, then you might have to face other kinds of frustrations and resistances. Don't allow yourself to wonder why you're doing this; just trust that it's worth trying. Simply commit to doing the breathing, walking, and yoga in the program, and make it your task to notice how you feel each time. There are no big goals to meet other than showing up.

I don't expect that you will do the exercises in this book for the rest of your life. Just as with diet, there is no one-size-fits-all way of working out. A sustainable, enjoyable exercise practice is always built to fit individual needs, and each person's preferences will be different depending on her age, body type, and lifestyle. Later on you may upgrade from walking to running or decide to take yoga classes that advance your practice. You may add new sports, such as moderate weightlifting (great for older women especially), or you might try martial arts. This program will be your foundation for any and all of those explorations. It will give you the building blocks of a healthy and happy relationship to exercise, and help you cultivate the right attitude: a graceful acceptance of how much you can do today.

Less Time, More Results

The major obstacle standing between you and an exercise practice may be the belief that you don't have the time. It's understandable, because schedules are jam-packed and there are endless demands on most everyone's time and energy, no matter what their life circumstances. But it's possible to let that belief go because the focus here is on getting more from less.

Having endless amounts of time to exercise can be really fun. But it can also be counterproductive. You can get hazy and unfocused or drift into dreamland as you pedal a stationary bike for fifty minutes. The session can go by without your ever connecting with the experience. When time limits are imposed on you—because of your job, your family, or a low fitness level that leaves you feeling you can't do much at all—picture the limitations as helpful boundaries set there to keep your mind from straying. They fence you in and force you to use the time well. Ten, twenty, or thirty minutes of movement done with a focused mind can feel complete and satisfying and significantly change the way your body feels. Setting reasonable goals, like exercising for a half hour instead of an hour, enables you to fulfill them. (Added benefit: On some days, you'll find that you naturally extend your session without even realizing it—not because it's a requirement but because you're having fun.)

The optimal amount of exercise to do in this program is four thirty-minute sessions a week. I hope that after this program you'll continue exercising and using everything you've learned here. This 30-Day Program will give you the tools you need to help you better understand and maintain your body for the rest of your life.

Though you may start with slightly shorter walks, by Week 3 you will do two thirty-minute walks and two thirty-minute yoga sessions. If you can exercise five or even six days a week, even better. Enjoy an extra walk or yoga practice, or even just a few minutes of Arm Swings, but always rest one day a week. If you have less time available, don't sabotage the mission. Accept that this is what you can reasonably do today, and use the techniques below to be fully committed to the practice. Time spent fretting that a quarter hour isn't good enough, or time spent chafing at all the barriers in your way, is nothing but time lost. The important thing is to keep up the behavior so that exercise becomes a part of your daily life. If time is tight, at least introduce yourself to the yoga mat and do a few Sun Salutations. Once you get quiet inside, you will begin to hear what you need; sometimes just warming up and stretching out is enough while other days your body will crave exertion.

Above all, do some kind of movement every day, including the days that you aren't doing a walk or yoga session. If you have only five minutes for some spinal twists and energy exercises while the kettle's boiling in the morning and five minutes to stretch at night, it's okay—that does not interfere with your day off. Keep focusing on your breathing, and know that these simple things will keep the conversation going between your mind and your body. And if you have type-A tendencies and stress out when you miss a session, remember to allow surprise and be at peace with unexpected changes to your plans.

TIP Whenever the "no time" message tries to derail you from moving your body, refuse to entertain it by reframing it in a proactive and positive way: "I have limited time, and I'm going to use it powerfully."

Create the Conditions for Success

■ **PLAN AHEAD:** Exercise will not happen unless you have cleared time for it. Schedule some time in advance. Tell your partner, kids, or whoever has expectations of you that you will be unavailable for those thirty minutes of the day. When the time comes to start, don't get derailed by other things begging for your attention, like writing e-mails to friends or talking on the phone.

■ **MAKE IT ROUTINE:** When you commit to exercising consistently through the week and make it part of your routine, you avoid having to psych yourself up each time.

Feel Your Body

This modified qigong exercise encourages you to move in a subtle way without expecting anything other than feeling your body in motion. Drop all preconceived ideas of what working out is about, and know that your intention for all your walks and yoga in this program is to connect with your breath, body, and movement. Stand with your legs bent, shoulder-width apart, and hold your hands out in front of your waist. Imagine you have a ball between them. Pull your hands apart as though you are stretching the ball out, then bring them back to their original spherelike shape. It's like you are pulling taffy that's stuck to your hands. Just do this quietly while tuning in to what your breath is doing; see if you can inhale on the outward pulls and exhale on the inward releases. Continue for three minutes. Be conscious of your breath, your weight on your feet, and how you feel when you are done. Then stand with your feet together and your back as straight as possible. Feel the spine elongated and your feet firmly planted on the ground. Arms rest alongside your body; your thighs are engaged (not tightly contracted, but firm and pulling upward). Observe the inner motion of your body and the sound of your breath through your nose.

Exercise

1

Turn On the Breath

WHAT IS THE MOST CRUCIAL CONTRIBUTOR TO LIFE, YET THE ONE TO WHICH WE GIVE THE LEAST ATTENTION?

WHAT BODY-BOOSTING, MIND-CLEARING PRACTICE COULD YOU DO WITHOUT EVEN GETTING UP FROM YOUR CHAIR?

WHAT SINGLE THING, IF DONE WELL, WILL TRANSFORM YOUR EXERCISE PRACTICE?

The answer is breathing.

IF THERE'S ONE THING YOU DO DIFFERENTLY after reading this book, let it be this: breathe more slowly and more deeply. Breathing is the key to intentional exercise. It's how you stop escaping the task and instead commit to it. If you aren't conscious of your breath, you probably aren't conscious of your body. In fact, if you aren't conscious of your breath, you probably aren't conscious of your life. Breathing well is critical to a balanced life—one in which you are present in every moment and go purposefully through your day. That's why before we even start to walk or do yoga, it pays to practice the most elemental exercise of all: inhale, exhale.

■ ■ ■

IF YOU'VE NEVER considered breathing an exercise, think again. With a simple inhale and exhale, we put so many things in our body into motion. In fact, the act of breathing is the most important exercise we do because we simply can't live without it. Food and even water we can survive without for considerable time. But breathing is nonnegotiable. It gives us oxygen, our most essential nutrient, and carries away our wastes and toxins. It both feeds and purifies.

Yet because breathing is an involuntary act—something the body does without our consciously instructing it—we tend to take it for granted. Often we go through an entire day

Oxygen plays a crucial role in all chemical reactions in the body, from releasing cellular energy to fueling our organs. When our blood is saturated with high levels of oxygen, our mind is sharp and our skin is clear and youthful. Consider that when you inhale deeply, you are not only boosting your vitality, you are also cleansing your blood, tissues, and organs. Oxygen not only metabolizes food and refreshes all your cells, it also burns up toxins. You are feeding the brain, which requires more oxygen than any other organ. Studies have shown that over 70 percent of the body's toxins are released through the breath. Every exhalation releases carbon dioxide and relaxes tense muscles. When you breathe well, you stay healthier, have more energy, and can deal with stress better. A full breath will restore a balanced state of mind. When you breathe shallowly and from the chest, you may be contributing to such conditions as anxiety, high blood pressure, nervous disorders, depression, fatigue, sleep disorders, stomach upset, and muscle cramps.

without once paying attention to our breath. We have more important things demanding our attention: the thoughts, worries, and ideas that stream through our minds. But have you ever noticed how when you are stressed, nervous, or concentrating hard, you take short, shallow breaths that inflate only the top part of your chest or are more in your throat than your body? If you're concentrating on reading this paragraph, you might be doing it right now.

Are you?

Breathing in your normal manner, put one hand on your chest and one hand on your belly. As you inhale, notice which hand moves. If the hand on the chest moves, you are chest breathing. Play with your breath so you reverse the situation; can you make the belly hand move gently but keep the chest hand still?

Shallow, rapid chest breathing is the way most people breathe most of the time, whether or not they feel particularly stressed or nervous. Partly it's a learned habit. We lose the natural belly breath we had as infants as soon as we become thinkers who are led by our minds. Soon enough, shallow and fast breaths become standard; the circular belly breath we did in our cribs, where the belly rises and falls without pausing at the inhale or exhale, is totally forgotten. Factor in other concerns that hit during the teenage years, like the vanity that keeps us from letting our tummies stick out, and by adulthood our breath stops higher and higher in our chests.

Partly our poor breathing is an effect of the modern lifestyle. Sedentary work, travel, and leisure habits mean we can get by with subpar breathing. Stress and technology keep us more in our heads than ever before. And some say that since we spend more time than ever indoors, where there are more pollutants and dust than there are out in nature, the body instinctively restricts its inhalations to the bare minimum in order to stay clean. You need to counteract all these tendencies by taking fuller breaths through your nose. When you breathe through your nose, not your mouth, you do have adequate filters to clean the dust out.

To start breathing better in your day, it's important not to force the effort. Your body wants to inhale a satisfying supply of oxygen and get rid of toxins; your job is simply to allow it. Think of it this way: When you slip into the pattern of doing shallow chest breaths, you are unconsciously constricting the natural, full breathing your body would like to do.

Some part of your body is holding tight and not allowing the breathing. Perhaps you are holding your belly in too tightly. Perhaps your back is slumped as you sit or stand, which closes off your chest, or maybe your face is so taut you are not happily allowing each inhale to expand the small facial muscles. Spend a few moments feeling various part of your body as you inhale and exhale to see if you are as open to the breath as you could be.

EXPRESS EXERCISE ## Locate the Breath

For 90 seconds, scan your body as you inhale and exhale in your normal breath. You are looking for places of tension or tightness. Notice the way your scalp feels, and your face, your neck, your shoulders, your chest, your lower back, your belly. If you come across a tight spot, simply ask yourself, "Is this tightness inhibiting my breathing?" Then ask, "Could I let that tightness go?" Let the next breath be your yes.

■ Notice how adjusting your position as you sit may aid the opening of the breath. Is your seated posture slumped, with slightly rounded shoulders? Move your butt to the back of the chair, and place a cushion or rolled towel at the small of the back as you sit up straight, with your spine away from the chair back. This will tip your pelvis forward slightly to promote the natural curve of the back, open the chest area, and let you drop your shoulders back. Lift up your chin so your eyes look at the horizon.

■ As you release tense spots, allow your breath to slow and deepen naturally (you should be breathing through the nose, not the mouth). Notice how air is starting to reach the far corners and forgotten nooks and crannies of your body. Play with making the inhalations deeper to inflate your belly; then play with drawing air up from the belly to expand the rib cage. Small clicking sounds mean that bones are adjusting to the expanded space. Notice if you feel a sense of relief, energy, or even tingling (a sign than oxygen is reaching tissues). Notice if it makes you feel strange to let your belly stick out.

■ Dilate the nostrils on the inhale and see what happens if you let the breath soften your face enough that you smile.

Note: If focusing on your breath makes you anxious or fearful, you will find this exercise easier to do after you have done some of the walking and yoga workouts that follow. These will get you acquainted with the positive power of breath during movement, and it will then be easier to notice your breath when sitting still.

Once you have begun to drop old patterns of constricted breathing, know that there is no one right way of breathing. As we'll see in the third section of the program, Silence, there are types of breathing you can do to produce a calm and introspective state. For now, simply focus on allowing the breath. Remember that exhales are just as important as inhales, and allow them to be luxurious too. Let the smile that comes be the reminder that steady, slow breaths are a gift to your tissues, organs, and muscles.

During the day, play with different speeds and fullness of breath, just out of curiosity. You can do it while sitting at your desk, waiting in line at the bank, or cleaning the kitchen countertops. Whenever you are acutely focused on a task, notice if you have forgotten to breathe. If you find that you are constantly curtailing your breath, try asking yourself, "Why am I not generous to myself?" Consider this idea: accepting the breath is a symbol of accepting life. Allow yourself to have more of it.

TIP The easiest way to remind yourself to breathe throughout the day is the most obvious. Take a piece of paper and make your own personal "Breathe" sign, and stick it where you see it most: above your desk, in the kitchen, or even in sight of your bed. Decorate it with colors and patterns, be as silly and creative as you want, and stick it where you will see it.

TIP Befriend your belly. At various times in the day, place your hands on your belly and breathe softly to feel it rise and fall without constriction. The pleasurable and relaxing state this creates will retrain your brain so that you allow yourself to stop holding your stomach in all the time and get some better breath.

In yoga there is a constant reminder to breathe. Teachers often tell you that if you spent your class motionless yet breathing intently, you'd gain just as much benefit as if you were twisting yourself up like a pretzel. If you simply spent your time breathing, your mind would calm, your body would change, and you'd feel more at ease with the stresses of your life.

I return to breath in everything I do, all day long—whether it's a hard hike or just washing dishes. I tune in to the sound and feel of air rushing through my nose and over my windpipe to draw my attention to the present moment. There is a kind of music in the breath, and when you listen to it you are listening to your body. Breathing consciously is a great way to bring intention to every task. It's like saying, "I am here, I am doing this. There is nowhere else I need to be."

Exercise: Breathe Through Your Morning

Start your day with a large inhale after you turn off your alarm clock and stand up. Hold the inhale for five seconds, then exhale with an audible sound of release. Remember to take the feeling of rest into your standing body. Your challenge this morning is to take a long, deliberate breath before every small task you do, from the moment you awaken until the moment you leave the house. Breathe at the toilet: one deep inhale and exhale. Breathe before you turn on the taps and splash your face with water. Breathe before you take off your nightgown or T-shirt. With these conscious breaths, you are tuning in to your body. When you go into the kitchen, pause at the door and breathe in and out as you observe the newness of the day. As you go about your morning, making coffee or tea or getting food out from the fridge, take a deep breath before each change of action. It will slow your day down very little and improve your efficiency dramatically. If coffee is your thing—that's decaf now, right?—breathe before you grind the beans; breathe before you tip the coffee into the machine; breathe before you fill the water tank, watch it take its liquid course, then breathe one full breath in and out before you turn your machine on. What's next? Go outside and get the paper: open the door, take a full cycle of breath, look at the sky, and feel if it is cool, cold, or temperate. Notice if is there a breeze. Pause to look at something in your yard, or look out your window and notice something natural outside. Take nothing for granted in your life.

The things that you do the most, like taking out the garbage or getting the mail, are the things you want to slow down the most.

Notice how observing the small parts of your life and taking a complete breath before starting a new task will change the way you respond to life's harder challenges: doing your job, parenting, loving your partner— or perhaps trying to love your partner while you feel deep frustration. In yoga class one is sometimes told to let the breath lead your movement rather than moving first and hoping the breath catches up with you. Letting breath lead your movements throughout the day will help you be present in your life as you are living it, connected to the now. Turning this skill toward exercise will make it a much more intense experience.

Quick Fix #3: Energy Breath

This exercise is a great way to start the day. It uses a type of vigorous breathing that in yoga we call "breath of fire," or bellows breath. Note that it may make you dizzy at first, so please start slowly and increase the power and speed of the breath only if you feel comfortable. If you have high blood pressure, are pregnant, or have recently had surgery, do the exercise with regular, calm nose breaths instead.

Sit cross-legged on a cushion with your hands on the ankles. Breathe a few long breaths through the nose, then inhale to an expanded belly, and forcefully exhale through the nose. Let the inhale come in normally, and exhale forcefully again. Repeat and pick up speed. The navel will move energetically in and out in a rhythm, and the sound of the breath will be quite loud, like a pair of bellows. This breath alone is very energizing.

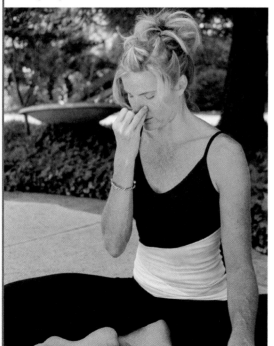

If you feel good, now add the flex. On the inhale, look up and stick your chest out. On the exhale, tuck the chin and curl the back so you are staring at your belly button. Repeat the motion and increase your speed as you feel more comfortable, working up to a vigorous flex-curl rhythm. This exercise will make you energized and ready to go; it cleanses impurities from the nasal passage and lungs, detoxes the blood, and massages your abdominal organs. Research has also shown that three minutes of doing this motion changes the brain waves to a calmer pattern. Do it for thirty seconds to one minute.

USE FOR: Energizing first thing in the morning, or as a pick-me-up later in the day.

Better Body Awareness

Are you treating your body kindly even when you are doing nothing at all? When you repeat poor habits on a day-in, day-out basis, your body's structure eventually changes by adapting to the bad pose, causing pain and misalignment. In addition to bringing awareness to your breath, bringing awareness to your habitual body postures as you sit and stand throughout the day is one of the easiest ways to stay balanced. Watch out for these mistakes.

1. Problem: Poor ergonomics at your desk, including a chair that doesn't support your back. Solution: Use an office chair with elbow supports; add a lumbar-back support cushion. Sit squarely in front of your computer. Knees should be at a right angle to the floor; consider a footrest to elevate feet. Your screen should be at eye level. If you use a laptop, raise it on a stand or dock, and use a separate keyboard and mouse. Keep forearms parallel to floor as you write.

TIP A large-sized Swiss ball (inflatable exercise ball) makes a good chair substitute because it encourages this posture while making you engage your abdominals and support your own back, thereby building strength as you sit. Make sure it is strong enough to withstand puncture by staples or sharp objects on your office floor.

TREAT YOURSELF: *The pricey but superb Swopper stool takes the Swiss-ball idea to the most sophisticated extreme (see Index of Products).*

2. Problem: Long stretches of typing without standing up and stretching the shoulders and wrists. Solution: Every twenty minutes, stand up, stretch arms to your sides, then pull them back by squeezing the shoulder blades. Flex wrists backward as you do so. Lift and drop your shoulders ten times. Breathe.

    If you work on a laptop, use a separate desktop mouse so that your hand is not constantly curled over your touchpad, a habit that is often the source of hand, wrist, forearm, and even shoulder pain.

3. Problem: Cradling the phone between chin and shoulder will shorten muscles on one side of the neck and overstretch those on the other, eventually causing chronic pain. Solution: Get a hands-free headset.

4. Problem: Walking in high heels throws you out of your natural posture and forces the muscles to work hard to hold you upright. Tension headaches, lower back pain, and nagging pains or aches in your muscles and joints are symptoms of high-heel overkill. Solution: Save the heels for special occasions, and use the yoga stretches here to loosen up.

Exercise: Sit-Stand Spot Check

If you work at a desk, drive, or talk on the phone a lot, notice your habits today and see if you can make adjustments to improve them. Your workplace may have access to an expert who can check your desk setup for you. Put a picture above your desk to remind you to stretch and move.

T REAT YOURSELF: *I'm a firm believer in the preventive and healing power of bodywork. I have learned that when my spine is out of alignment, my moods, my energy, and my immune system all suffer—sometimes to an extreme—because the function of the nerves and the cerebrospinal fluid are compromised. I frequently work with a chiropractor to put my structure back in balance, and it improves every part of my functioning. You may find massage helps you to work out the kinks and lift your spirits. These treatments are not cheap, but they are deeply worthwhile additions to your tool kit. Always get personal recommendations for a bodywork practitioner if possible, and talk to the person before starting to make sure you feel comfortable.*

PRELUDE TO EXERCISE: HARDER DOES NOT MEAN BETTER

I got hardwired to perform grueling exercise when I trained for the role of an Olympic hopeful pentathlete in the film *Personal Best* at the age of seventeen. After I'd experienced track-and-field training like a professional athlete, the discipline and, perhaps more important, the addiction to that kind of adrenaline high were firmly established in my body and strongly engraved in my brain. Pushing to the edge, every session, was my approach to exercise. You weren't succeeding unless you were doing a lot—or too much. It played into all of my competitive, perfectionist, and compulsive tendencies.

For the next ten years, pushing my body to an extreme of strength and fitness almost every single day was my way of imposing order and control in a life where much felt unsettled: my career as a young actress, my feelings about my body and food, my fears about my family and its dark legacy. Hard exercise became a way to escape those fears. I'd run and train hard, propelled by sheer willpower most of the time, never slowing down to a walk for fear that I'd not be able to run again.

Even after I was married and a new mom to my first daughter, Dree, I was still in the habit of thinking more is better. In our small New York City apartment, I found a new outlet for my obsession: jump-roping. I didn't jump for just twenty minutes, I jumped for an hour, and sometimes two. Plus I would walk miles and miles around Manhattan instead of taking cabs or the subway, trying to get more and more exercise every day. Often Stephen would return home from work and find me skipping rope madly with a dull and distant expression on my face. I'd gone from hot and sweaty to cold and clammy to the touch. It was freaky. Although it was technically a great workout and I was in very good shape, I was also very tired most of the time. And I had so much anxiety about the subject—always a little nervous if I hadn't done something. I was never overweight, but in order to attain "thin" as defined by the entertainment industry, I had to struggle a lot, especially as I was staying slim without the help of diet drugs, which were huge at the time.

In combination with my extreme low-fat, low-protein diets, my adrenaline-junkie habit weakened my resistance to illness. If there was even a slight change in the weather, like rain or a cold snap, I'd be fighting a sore throat, and if I couldn't fight it with my natural remedies, it would take me down for the count. I would make ridiculous demands on myself: "If I did an hour and twenty-five minutes today, I'll do an hour and thirty tomorrow." And on and on, so that by the end of the month I was doing a crazy amount, and then I'd get sick to recover. I went for years without giving myself a day off. Seven days a week, two to three hours a day of hard work, until my body would finally say, "You are such a jerk, I'm going to get sick so that you have to stop because you won't

slow down, and I can't keep up!" My body was wise: a cold or flu was a last-chance way for it to rest because I was unwilling to listen and slow down. It was my way of feeling in control, but that very need for control was controlling me. My sense of well-being and my health were always at risk. So who was really in control? Certainly not me. It seems obvious to me now, but it wasn't at the time. Body issues are about the desire to control something—anything!—in a life that is always changing. The irony is that you can't control anything, so why not give up trying to control your body? When you give up the compulsions, the body finds its natural place, the weight and comfort level that suit it best. The mind and its anxiety, as I found out, create more problems than does any actual weight gain or loss.

■   ■   ■

MODERN-DAY EXERCISE HABITS tend to fall into extremes. The majority of people are either underexercisers or overexercisers, and neither side is finding a moderate middle ground where exercise is helping, not hindering them. A lot of misinformation is out there. For one thing, it's been ingrained in us for years that pain equals gain and that simply by doing a harder, more exhausting workout, we will be more fit. That is not the case. Similarly, like fad diets and food trends, new exercise trends come along at a steady clip, always promising better and faster results. Exercise, the thing that is supposed to provide relief and fun, can sometimes seem like one more thing to keep

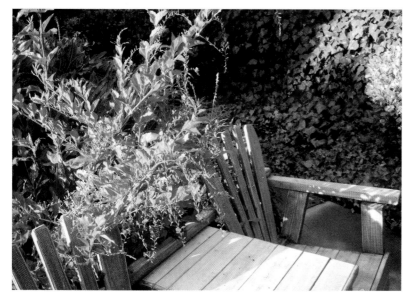

Sickness and injury, as well as reduced endurance and lack of strength, will be far more likely. Overtraining can also trigger emotional responses like irritability, anxiety, and sensitivity to criticism—all things you might, ironically, decide are caused by not working out enough. New mothers who take on hard exercise too quickly can develop postnatal depression.

up with. For the purpose of this program, you're going to slow down, tune out all those external messages for a few weeks, and tune in to a more reliable source of information: yourself.

There's a real danger in the more-is-more approach. Did you know that intense cardio activities actually stress the body? They cause a catabolic reaction, meaning they destroy tissue. The body goes into alert mode and urgently looks for energy. If it doesn't find it immediately from food, the energy will get drawn from the most easily available sources like muscles and organs (rather than the harder-to-get fat deposits). If your life already has its share of stress, including a mediocre diet and too little sleep, or if your health is compromised in any way, this new set of stresses will tip you way off balance.

If, by contrast, you are nourished, rested, and calm to begin with, the stress from intense cardio workouts might be easier to absorb and you might love them. But it's wise to be conscious that you may unwittingly be adding more stress to your life by doing the very thing you're hoping will help destress you. The endorphin rush that comes with high cardio can feel great, but did you realize it's also a sign that you have just pushed your body into emergency fight-or-flight mode? When you are in that state, all nonurgent bodily functions get shut down, like digestion and reproductive functions. That's why chronic overexercising can throw off the entire balance of your body.

Walk Without Thought

TODAY MORE THAN EVER, exercise takes place with so much distraction, you can almost forget you're doing it. Sound and stimulation come from all angles: among runners, bikers, and hikers, MP3 players are ubiquitous, with cell phones a close second. In the gym there are banks of TV monitors playing headline news, pop videos, and talk shows side by side (not to mention scores of other bodies to stare at). And who isn't guilty of trying to read a magazine on the elliptical machine?

All these things serve to pull our focus away from the task at hand. They keep us in a state where we are led by our heads and only half-aware of our bodies. The results are mediocre: you see people doing the same run or workout for years, and they always look the same. They're doing everything they can to escape the task instead of focusing in and getting real benefits. You might think it's easier to work out when you've got the latest episode of *The Real World* to entertain you. But doing two things at once leads to only one end: distraction. It means you get to the end of a forty-minute ride on a stationary bike and realize you didn't notice any of it, and neither do you feel especially rejuvenated. Whether it comes from banks of TV monitors, your wandering thoughts, or even a workout partner who just won't shut up, distraction is destructive.

Exercising with intention is the remedy. It is how you stay present in your process no matter what type of workout you are doing. It is how you harness your mind so that you constantly come back to where you are, right now. It is how you get more from less so that by moving your body, you get a truly refreshing break. It comes down to using three simple techniques:

1. Move in concert with your breath.
2. Sense the moment.
3. Check in with yourself by asking questions.

WALKING: A PRIMER

WHAT: Thirty-minute, brisk-paced walks are what we are aiming for in this component of the program. (You'll start with twenty minutes, but if you have more time, keep going.) You will want to vary the intensity of your walk depending on your energy level from day to day. If you feel quite fit already, adding speed and hills if possible will be important.

WHERE: Consider what routes you have available in your immediate environs. Are there walking trails in your town? Is there a park with trails or a running track? Is there a hilly, residential neighborhood nearby? Perhaps your most accessible resource is a mall. That's okay too: just pick a time when it is quiet so that you can walk quickly (and leave the credit cards at home). Do you have time to drive to nature trails, perhaps for a longer walk, on the weekend? Do some research online, and you may find that local walking and running groups have mapped out circuits in your town. If you live in a big city, walking on urban streets requires heightened awareness to traffic and pedestrians but can still be a vigorous and stimulating exercise. Take a few minutes to map out routes that will lead you down streets you like. Walking indoors on a running track is a fine substitute. Using a gym treadmill can be a good option, particularly in winter or at night or if there are no hills near you and you want to increase the challenge. Follow some of the advice on the next few pages to tune out gym noise and tune in to yourself.

WHEN: Any time of day works for walking. Try to let yourself experience different times to see what suits you best. You may find an early morning walk starts your day with a boost or that early evening is a particularly pleasant time to be out in your neighborhood. If you get a full hour for lunch, try using half of it for a fast hike and half of it to eat afterward. Don't let inclement weather be an excuse not to walk. Unless it's raining hard, walking in all kinds of weather lets you feel nature most fully. Dress in layers, adjust your footwear if necessary, and embrace the day whether it's gray, blue, or even white with snow.

WHAT TO WEAR: Comfortable loose clothing, with layers for cold or wet weather. Either walking sneakers or true running shoes. (I like the latter because they allow you to move at a fast pace and break into a jog if you feel like it.) It is advisable to replace running sneakers every five hundred miles for best support. In snowy weather, outdoor boots will do fine.

TREAT YOURSELF: *I frequently wear Masai Barefoot Technology sneakers, which are designed to mimic the natural rolling gait of bare feet on the earth. This counteracts the compression that happens to your joints when you sit a lot. The spine realigns, muscles get toned, and your posture improves (see Index of Products).*

SAFETY ISSUES: Walk smart. When possible, stick to daylight hours. At night, if the area is safe, be sure to wear reflective strips on your clothes and an LED wristband or headlamp. (If walking outdoors doesn't feel safe for pedestrians, consider using a treadmill indoors.) If you're concerned about safety, pair up with a walking partner and agree to hike together in silence during the program.

WALKING POSTURE: Keep your chin parallel to the ground, your back straight, and your shoulders and arms loose and relaxed. Avoid leaning back or sitting back on your hips. Tuck your hips slightly forward to avoid arching your back, and pull in your abdominals so that your core is firm. Let your head be still as you walk with eyes softly focused twenty feet into the distance. The length of your stride should be long but not uncomfortable. As you pick up your pace, use your arms powerfully to propel yourself forward. At slower paces, let them swing naturally. Breathe.

WARM UP: Try doing at least two minutes of Arm Swings (on page 154) before you start, along with any of the Quick Fixes in this segment that you like. Take a few minutes to loosen up a body that may have been inactive for hours. Shrug your shoulders, roll your head and neck, step wide and bend your knees to the sides. Do whatever feels good: the point is to say hello to your body. Next, set your intention (Step 4). Then go.

COOL DOWN: If you have pushed your muscles hard, particularly on steep hills, take a few minutes to stretch at the end. The yoga poses Reclined One-Leg Stretch, Seated Forward Bend, and Standing Forward Bend are good for this.

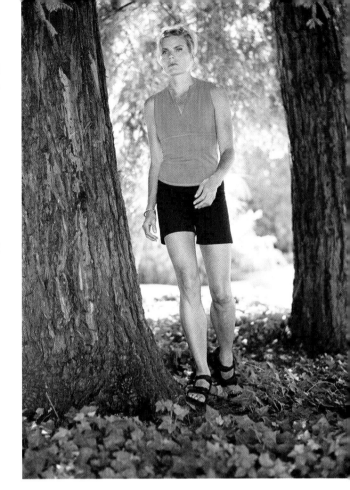

PREREQUISITE FOR ALL WALKS:
Turn off the noise. For the four weeks of this program, check your music players, cell phones, and other communication devices at the door. (If you absolutely need to carry your cell phone, put it on vibrate and answer only urgent calls.) In the future you may find music helpful to get into your groove if you're walking in a busy gym, but for now you want to hear the sound of your breath. Walking with music outdoors, however, has the effect of canceling out the subtle sounds of the world around you and cocooning you from nature. It is also less safe in an urban environment. I advise against it.

Exercise

115

QUESTION: IF YOU INSULATE YOUR-
SELF WITH MUSIC WHEN YOU WALK
OR RUN, IS IT BECAUSE YOU FEEL
UNCOMFORTABLE OR ANXIOUS
HEARING YOUR HEARTBEAT AND
YOUR BREATH?

If so, you're not alone. But hearing your heartbeat is a reminder that you are alive! It's a good thing; it can't hurt you. So resist the temptation to hide under the veil of music and not feel your body doing what it is supposed to do.

CONSIDER HOW ELSE you can make the walking experience more pure. For instance, if you walk your dogs and they require your attention, you may need to have them leashed in order to keep your focus. Tuck keys away in your pocket. Try to avoid bringing clothes that will get tied around your waist. Streamlined and silent is what you're after.

For the first two weeks of the program, you will take twenty-minute walks, minimum, and you will practice one of the following techniques during each walk. For the final two weeks you will integrate them all and focus on increasing the length of the walk to at least thirty minutes, upping the intensity and challenge. In Weeks 3 and 4, please try to push yourself so that you are working up a sweat and breathing hard.

Technique 1: Breathe in concert with your movement.

Try to synchronize your breath with your steps. For at least fifteen minutes of the walk, practice inhaling for three steps then exhaling for three steps. Try to inhale through your nose and see how that feels. In challenging terrain, like steep hills, you will likely need to breathe through your mouth, but experiment and see how breathing through your nose creates a more introspective state. By the end of the week, increase the breath so you inhale for four steps and then exhale for four steps. If you have strong lungs and feel comfortable increasing the steps per breath, do so. The length of the inhale should match the length of the exhale so that you find balance in the cycle.

Let repetition keep you present

Doing a repetitious movement like walking is the way to practice ritual in your movement. That's why repetition keeps you present: it turns any physical activity into a moving meditation. Find the rhythm of your steps, and let your mind follow that rhythm instead of thinking actively. Imagine your steps are windshield wipers clearing the dirt and gunk off your life. Let the repetition bring you to a calm and quiet state of mind. From there you can notice what's going on both inside you and in the world around you, without spiraling off into complex conversations with yourself.

The way you exercise is a good model of how you behave in general. If you're distracted while you exercise, chances are you also check cell phone messages while you drive, write e-mails while you talk on the phone, and so on. Use exercise as a way to learn focused awareness for the rest of life. If you can focus on the process even when it seems boring to you, you are well set up for life. Because, let's be honest, life is sometimes boring. Are you going to try to escape it, or will you be there and hope to catch a moment of beauty?

TIP After you have learned the *Ujjayi* breath (page 125) in your yoga practice, use it while walking to create an audible sound that captures your wandering mind.

TIP After you have learned the *Ujjayi* breath (page 125) in your yoga practice, use it while walking to create an audible sound that captures your wandering mind.

Technique 2: Sense the moment.

I firmly believe that when you learn to observe the external, you become better at observing the internal. When you focus on simply noticing things without judging or analyzing them, you quiet the mind and get in touch with the process. This technique develops that skill of observing. It works best when you are outdoors and will be most fun if you are in a park or in a somewhat natural setting. Now that you are breathing well as you walk, turn your attention outward so that you are quietly observing the world that you are passing through. Drop your internal dialogue, and let your senses pick up information without necessarily commenting on it. Observe the colors and patterns of nature, smell the scents that waft by, feel the change of air temperature against the skin. Give yourself half of your walk to simply notice. Don't comment; don't go off into thoughts about what you see. Feel what you feel.

It's easier to get into this calm state of mind when you've got nature to play with because it automatically gives you a different sensibility. You are stimulated and soothed by the physical world, and your ability to feel the breeze and feel your breath is heightened. Walking outdoors builds sensitivity, so do it when you can. (Plus, in nature there's no mirror and no one beside you to compare yourself with.)

I am clearly a mountain girl. On sunny bright days here in California, if I can get into the hills I am like a wild animal, free and happy. As I walk I let my animal senses notice everything; by the time I return I feel thrilled and refreshed in so many ways.

Alternative: Walking at the gym.

If you are walking inside on a treadmill, don't try to notice the external environment because it will be too hectic. Instead, focus your eyes on a fixed point on the wall ahead of you. Sense the moment by tuning in deeply to what is happening in your body—the feel of sweat on your skin, the sensation in different muscles as they get warm. Notice if you are overworking one side of the body, and how your feet feel as they hit the treadmill. Notice how your arms are moving and if your hands are clenched. Are you smiling or grimacing in concentration? Notice how often you break focus by looking up at the TV monitors around you or at the other people in the gym. Then bring your attention back to your own body. *If you are moving at a slow enough pace that feels safe,* close your eyes for some moments. Draw your attention powerfully inward, and scan your body with your senses. Hear the rhythm of your feet hitting rubber and the sound of the machine.

TIP Closing your eyes any time you use a *stationary exercise machine* like a Stairmaster, bike, or elliptical machine is a guaranteed way to up the intensity of your experience. From here on, any time you use one of these machines, close your eyes, ignore the gym noise around you, and feel what a difference this focus makes.

Exercise

117

Technique 3: Ask questions.

They say good listeners ask questions. In exercise, asking questions is one way to keep yourself present in the process. Wean yourself off using your stopwatch or treadmill timer to know how you're doing (and if you're in the gym, don't use your reflection to tell you if you're doing okay). You know how you're doing because you can feel how you're doing!

At the beginning and end of the walk, ask yourself how you feel and what feels different. Plus, at various moments in the walk, ask yourself: *"What feels good in my body right now?"* Let the answer come by simply noticing what feels good, without analyzing or asking why or how you feel that way. Let your body speak to you, and bypass the mind. This is how you build your physical intelligence: you pick up valuable information that comes from a place deeper than your ego.

Doing this helps you find beauty in things that otherwise you might be resenting or struggling with or that you might simply miss. It automatically creates a kinder and more intimate relationship with your body. So often, our comments to ourselves when we're exercising are negative: "This hurts! Ugh, when is this going to end?" Asking questions about what feels good spins your whole experience toward the positive. You will do it in yoga, and you might notice that a challenging forward bend is opening up your lower back and it feels great. Or you may realize that even though a balancing pose is hard, your breath just got a lot deeper and smoother. Often the act of asking the question will make you smile. Something somewhere in your body does feel better.

BONUS: After you have discovered a positive answer to this positive question, add another question that continues this new kindness to your body: "Can I accept myself as I am right now?" See what answer pops up. If a flood of negative thoughts arises, that's okay. Keep asking the question each time you feel good in your body during a workout, and see how your answers might change.

Add more walking to your daily life.

1. Park your car in the far side of the parking lot from your destination or farther down the street than normal. When shopping, load your car, and then take the cart all the way back to the front door of the market.
2. Take the stairs, not the elevator.
3. Suggest holding casual meetings with workmates while walking rather than sitting inside.
4. Try to shop in areas where small businesses are clustered together so that you can complete multiple errands by foot rather than driving from store to store.

EXPRESS EXERCISE

Take More Steps

Make it your week for walking more, and commit to adding in a few hundred meters here and there during your most ordinary errands and duties. If you spend a lot of time in your car, you may want to put a reminder sticker where you can see it saying "Walk!" so that you park farther away than normal and start these new habits.

Quick Fix #4: Squats

Simple squatting is great for encouraging digestion and elimination. It's how humans have hung out for eons, but since we became dependent on chairs, we rarely sit this way anymore. The squat is part of the yoga sequence that follows, but you can do it anytime as it increases flexibility in the lower part of your body, strengthens major muscle groups, and most important, stimulates blood flow to abdominal organs and gives intestines a good massage. Start with feet shoulder-distance apart, toes facing forward. Bend the knees as if you want to place your butt on the floor, but try to keep feet flat. Shift feet wider if you need to, or place a rolled up towel or two under your heels. (If you have knee problems, you may prefer to do Chair Pose for a few breaths.) Placing hands in prayer position at your heart and pushing elbows into insides of knees helps with stability. Most people will have difficulty getting their heels flat; just hang out on the ball of your foot, and try placing a folded blanket under the heels until your flexibility increases. Fix your eyes on a point on the wall if balance is tricky. Do it for thirty seconds to one minute.

USE IT: A way to condition and boost your body while you do anything at home—even watching TV. It's also an antidote to lower back pain during your period. Good for a cool-down after a vigorous hike.

If you can, do a series of squat-to-standing motions, moving slowly up and down. Exhale on the way down, inhale on the way up. This will give the intestines some movement. Do as many as you can, whether it's ten, twenty, or more at a time.

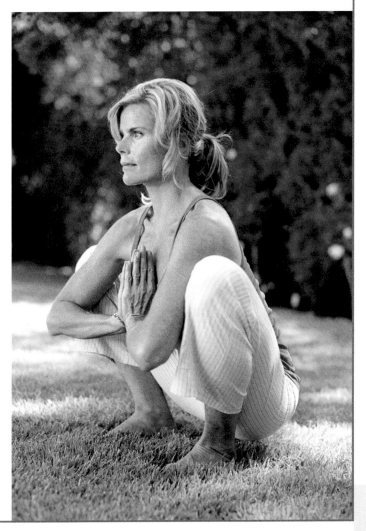

Exercise

119

Bring It to the Mat

YOGA BY ITS VERY NATURE is a practice of balance. The form of yoga you will begin learning here is called hatha yoga; the name combines the Sanskrit words *ha,* meaning sun, and *tha,* meaning moon. Just like the breath creates a balanced cycle of in and out, the postures in yoga create balance of opposing energies. You bend and then you stretch; you expand and then you contract; you move and then you sit still; you twist to one side and then twist to the other. The purpose of hatha yoga is to open up the body to receive vital energy and to bring harmony to the body, mind, and spirit. How could you not feel more at peace after taking some time out of your busy life to do it?

What I love about yoga is that it puts you into a natural state with yourself; inside your body you create the same sensations that you feel when you are moving in nature. Heat comes up from deep in your core; a breeze crosses your skin as you flow into postures. Sometimes I tingle throughout my whole body after a backbend. The feeling reminds me of being on top of a mountain.

In essence, that's how simple yoga can be. It offers you a chance to let your facade drop and to feel real. With each stretch, your protective armor dissolves and you get a chance to soften. With each bend, you reconnect to your own power, and any negative, self-critical thoughts lose their hold. When you do the yoga poses, you develop an intimate rela-tionship with your own body: you become aware of muscles you didn't know you had, aware of how much longer, looser, and taller you can feel, and aware that the body is amazing, able to move in ways you didn't think possible. All this matters because awareness of your body is the first step to acceptance of your body—and what woman doesn't need more of that?

Think of the word *intimacy* as you do the yoga practice here. It may be strange to think about intimacy in relation to yourself. We more often put energy into seeking intimacy with others, by winning people as friends or as lovers. But what about trying to be a friend to yourself? As you move and breathe through some challenging positions, the most im-portant thing you can do is lose any idea of dominating or forcing your body and instead use all three techniques you learned in the Walking component of this chapter. Breathe in concert with your movements; observe what's happening in your body; and ask yourself with kindness, "What feels good about this pose?" When you do yoga with this attitude of curiosity and acceptance, you create a kinder feeling toward yourself. It's like becoming intimate with a friend: knowing that person better increases your compassion toward them.

A yoga teacher I know tells his students that when they are in a pose, they should breathe, quiet their minds, and "Go inward like a turtle going into its shell." Remember that turtle as you move slowly and deliberately through this yoga sequence: imagine her or him ducking out of the busy world to find reprieve within. If you are able to find a moment of stillness even while you are in motion, your yoga practice will evolve from physical stretching and strengthening alone to a harmonious practice in which body, mind, and emotions find relief and release.

Yoga is also one of the best physical therapies you can provide for your body. All the systems are in some way boosted—your muscular, skeletal, circulatory, lymphatic, and respiratory systems as well as your endocrine (hormone-producing) and nervous systems.

I have a secret. I spent most of my years in a yoga class waiting for it to be over. I liked going to class and accomplishing hard poses, and even egotistically I liked when I was watched—even though I pretended I didn't—but underneath I was uncomfortable. I wasn't doing it for me. I was doing it because I wanted to be loved and I wanted approval.

Mostly I wanted my own approval, but of course I couldn't get that because I wasn't doing yoga for the right reasons. At some point I woke up and realized that other people don't care about my path, even if they clap after I demonstrate a really hard pose to the class. Each person is on his or her own path. The motivation has to come from the desire simply to feel great and have fun. These days, if someone in a class does a pose I can't do, instead of being envious and feeling inadequate, I think, "Oh, that is so cool! I bet it feels good. I really want to learn how to do it this year—for me, not for anyone else." And if I don't learn, who cares? I'm enjoying the journey. We look to comparisons to get our sense of surety, but it's so much better to find assurance within. If you get over your need for acknowledgment, true beauty shows.

YOGA: A PRIMER

Chances are you've noticed how fashionable yoga has become. Perhaps you've also come across people who bring a competitive vibe to it as they compare notes on what teacher or studio is better and what postures they can do. None of that really matters. Your practice can start in your living room, with no fancy accoutrements or pricey classes necessary.

The joy of yoga is that it is both democratic and modifiable. Your size, age, and strength levels are irrelevant because the poses can be done with the level of intensity that suits you. Your practice can be adapted to your own limitations of time and space. I've done yoga in hotel rooms, friends' gardens, and, as I mentioned, cramped RVs with minimal clearance overhead. As long as you have room enough to extend arms and legs in all directions, you have room to do a practice. By the end of this program you'll know enough basic postures that you can begin to plug them together in your own special way. You may still consider yourself a beginner, but in fact you are well on your way—because you will have a yoga practice of your own, without a teacher standing over you.

Today, I do 75 percent of my yoga at home, with group classes accounting for the rest. I think of my yoga mat as an anchor in my life, something that's always there for me when I want to move my body or shift my state. All I have to do is show up. Let yoga be your private practice, something that makes you feel great but that you don't have to share with anyone. Do what you need to make your session a sacred time, whether it's turning off phones, placing a vibrant plant or flowers within eyesight, or simply shutting the door.

WHAT: Try to do the complete yoga practice that follows at least twice a week. Doing the whole practice at a moderate pace will take about thirty minutes. If time is tight, simply do as much as you can, always including at least two minutes of the final resting pose at the end. If time allows you to combine a walk with yoga, do it. Bringing your warmed-up body to the mat is especially rewarding.

TIP If you find yourself with five minutes or less, try this: do a few poses to warm and move your body, or some Arm Swings or small jumps that focus on a soft landing, then sit cross-legged, breathing your yoga breath, and run through the yoga sequence in your mind. It will help imprint on your memory how one pose flows into the next.

WHERE: Experiment with different spots in your house until you find one that works for you. It should be relatively clutter free, out of sight of anything immediately connected to work or household duties (for example, a desk overflowing with office papers and bills). Practice in natural sunlight and with some fresh air if possible. Set a boundary with housemates or family (or pets) so that you are undisturbed for your session. You may want to do your practice near to the sacred space that you will create, which is explained in the Home section of the book.

WHEN: An early morning practice can set you up wonderfully for the day. You may be stiff at first, so warm up slowly. A hot shower before your exercise will help. Morning is a natural time to do Sun Salutations, which celebrate the energy of the sun. If you want a more vigorous practice, add more salutations as well as extra Plank and Push-Up poses. Or slow down your Sun Salutations so that you hold each pose for several breath cycles, which will build strength and stamina. Evening lends itself to a more relaxing and restorative practice. Spending extra time in Seated Forward Bend, which calms the nervous system, the reclined poses, and final Relaxation Pose will help you wind down from the day.

WHAT TO WEAR: Comfortable leggings or shorts and tank tops or fitted T-shirts. Anything that hangs too loosely on the body will bunch up and get in your way. Feet should be bare. You can do all these poses without a yoga mat, on carpet or a wooden floor. But a mat will give you far more traction and enable you to get deeper into your poses. Simple sticky mats are absolutely fine; thicker, firmer yoga mats provide extra cushioning for extra cost.

TIP As with the walking sessions, I highly recommend doing this practice mainly in silence for the first few weeks in order to hear your breath (note that Week 2 will throw in a surprise sound element). But if there is a lot of noise in your home, playing either some soft ambient music or mellow classical music during the session can help to create a private space. Do not use music with lyrics or a thumping beat.

HOW TO BREATHE: Through the nose, with long and smooth inhales and exhales. Let the breath lead each movement, as if the rush of air in and out of the lungs is powering the motion. As you get familiar with the poses, start to inhale on moves that open the body and exhale on moves that fold the body or that connect opening postures.

EYES OPEN OR CLOSED: Begin the first Mountain Pose with eyes closed to check in with your breath and body. End with your eyes closed in Relaxation Pose. In between, keep eyes open and softly focused on a horizon point in the distance. When it feels right, you can play with closing your eyes to draw your attention inward, but vigorous standing poses like Warrior I require that you use your sightline as an anchor.

SAFETY ISSUES: It's often said in a yoga class, "This is your process, not anybody else's." You go at the pace that instinctively feels right, and you find your own edge in each pose. Your edge is the point at which you are challenged but not pained. A rule of thumb is to go as far in each movement as you can comfortably breathe; if you find yourself straining to breathe or holding your breath tensely, you are trying too hard and should back off. I still try to challenge my comfort zone because when things get too rote and easy, my mind gets lazy and I lose my ability to be present. But I still remember that yoga is a balance between effort and surrender. Sometimes simply breathing beautifully and doing half the practice while resting for the other half can be a transformative experience.

For the first two weeks of the program you will simply do the whole yoga practice and familiarize yourself with the poses. In Week 3, play with adding an audible breath, and in Week 4, get creative with the sequence. Before each session you will set an intention, even if it's as simple as, "I want to learn the poses so I don't have to look at the book for each one." At the end you will check in to see if you have achieved some of that intention. (See Step 4 for details.)

Find Your Center

Don't underestimate the power of standing still. The first pose in the sequence, Mountain Pose, is in many ways the most important because with it you are discovering how to be grounded and balanced in everything you do. In Mountain Pose you can clearly gauge the quality of your breath and the intensity of your mind. Before you begin the sequence, play with finding the placement in Mountain Pose that feels appropriate to you. Just as there will be a landslide on the mountain if it's weighted too heavily on one side, gravity will pull your Mountain Pose down if you're not standing straight. Go stand sideways next to a mirror, and look at your reflection to see if you are centered. Most of us fall forward because we are afraid of what's behind us; we don't want to revisit our history. (That's why back-bends can be intimi-dating—psychologi-cally we feel, "I'm never going back to where I came from." If that comes up for you during this sequence, acknowl-edge that resistance, then try to move your body past it and just play with how it feels to do the first backbend,

Bridge Pose.) Shift on your feet to find the posture in which you are standing straight and tall, and know that to be truly in your center, you will always be slightly in motion. If you are a little bit in back, a little bit forward, then you've found your center.

Bring that sense of grounding and fluidity to every pose in yoga. Remember, balance is not static. The world is moving, and you have to move with it. Have the lightness and spontaneity to allow yourself to move with the ebb and flow of the earth even when you're supposedly standing still. And if that means you sometimes fall over, look silly, and are less than perfect, welcome those things! Falling down is how you build yourself up. Now you're ready to begin.

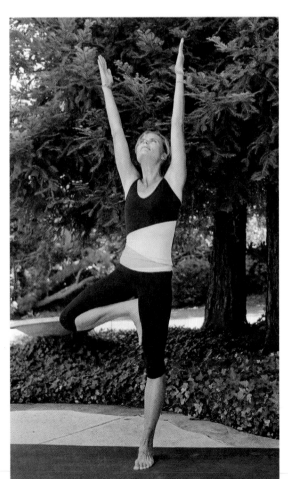

TIP Try to find a bit of mountain not just in every yoga pose, but also in different parts of your day. You can do Mountain Pose while brush-ing your teeth at the sink or waiting for the bus. Breathe, be quiet in your mind, and sway a bit as you sink your feet into the earth and let your body find its natural balance. Yoga becomes easier as your body memo-rizes the poses.

As I became less fixated on performing heroic yoga feats that proved my strength and endurance, I began to receive the full benefits of yoga. Instead of looking at my body as this separate "thing" I could use to prove myself, I began to hear the subtler messages it was sending me. Yoga is all about how to listen to your body. You turn your attention inward and ask, "What's going on here? How do I feel in this posture? You know what, I'm going to bend my knees because otherwise this pose doesn't feel comfortable. Maybe I'll take a little of the bend out." Through slowing down, breathing with intention, and checking in with myself throughout the practice, I became my body's caretaker, not its drill sergeant. Fueled with this new attitude of kindness, I began to accept and love my body for the first time.

YOGA PRACTICE

KEEP IT FUN. Add surprise by throwing on some funky music for five minutes in the middle and dance as wildly and expressively as you like, then turn off the sound and bring that joy and spontaneity back to your mat for the rest of the practice. Lose any preconception that you're supposed to move in a certain way for yoga and that you're doing it wrong if you're not absolutely serious about it. If you bring the freedom of dancing to your yoga and explore the poses in a fluid and lucid way, you will bring fun to your mat and lose any perfectionist tendencies.

UJJAYI BREATHING. *Ujjayi* breathing is a type of audible breath that yogis use to both energize and relax themselves as they practice. The sound that it makes is mesmerizing; it can be a great help in drawing your awareness inward and dropping distraction. Practice it first by sitting on the floor cross-legged. As you breathe through the nose with your mouth closed, gently constrict the opening of the throat so that you create a slight resistance to the passage of air. Your breath will sound like Darth Vader's, just softer and less scary. Focus at first on bringing the sound to the exhales, as this half of the breath is easier. Can you make them sound like ocean waves going out from shore? Then try to inhale with the slightly closed throat. Don't try too hard; it should be gentle and pleasing to do. Bring this breathing to a few poses like Volcano and Downward-Facing Dog, and see if it helps you focus. What if you let this sound be your music for your entire practice?

FREEDOM YOGA. After you have memorized a basic series of yoga poses and can flow between them with a steady and powerful breath, you get the chance to play. This may be in the fourth week of the program, or it may be later. Don't think you have to do them in the same order, for the same amount of time, every practice. Break from the script and start writing your own story. If you feel like doing one pose four times over and dropping the next, play with that. Be curious about how you can mix and match the poses, and don't be overly obsessed with following a formula. Full disclosure: I also occasionally do my yoga routine in front of *Sex and the City* reruns. There are days, after all, when a girl just doesn't want to go that deep.

Exercise

125

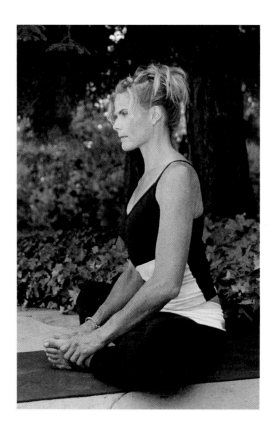

Another day you might add music, dance, and spontaneous movement to your yoga practice. When you let yourself experience exercise in an artful way that expresses something of who you are, it becomes a rich and rewarding part of life.

TIP If you feel you screwed up, ate a bad meal or binged, or didn't walk or be silent or do a small yoga practice, all is not lost. First, there is no screwing up. You are always one meal, one silent five minutes, one short walk, or a few poses away from getting back to feeling great about everything. Give yourself a break. Weirdness happens. Life is full of curve balls, and that's the beauty of it. You then say, "Hey, I just had a Krispy Kreme moment, and now I move on." So what? Even if it was not "treat day," make today your treat day and be done with it. Always give yourself love and permission to have gone a little astray, and then, by being kind to yourself, you are already back on the beam. You don't have to wait till tomorrow or the new moon to begin again.

I've recently come to see all exercise as art. The way you do it can be the way you express yourself. One day you might hike with assertive steps as if you're sculpting a giant sculpture; the next day you do yoga in a very subtle way, as if painting the air with delicate brushstrokes.

Set Your Intention

BY BREATHING CONSCIOUSLY, walking with new awareness, and developing the yoga skill of active body and quiet mind, you are developing a different way of exercising. If you ever had the habit of working out on autopilot, that button is now beginning to get switched off. You are becoming more present in the process, and you feel more in harmony with the changes that occur in your body and mind during a workout.

But there is a final, very simple, part of the plan. In order to exercise with intention, you must literally set an intention for every walking session or yoga practice you do. Simply take one moment before you start moving to gather your energy and state softly for yourself what you want to get out of the next thirty minutes. One simple statement is all it takes.

The intention may be quite pragmatic: to finish a thirty-minute walk at a good clip or to get through the entire yoga program without getting distracted. It may be physical: to relieve sore spots in your body after a long day at a desk, or maybe to feel lean and strong and tall after driving all day. Perhaps it's to get a bit better looking; that's fine too. Your body does change when you visualize what you want and set an intention before and during your practice. As you move farther along, your intention may become more personal or emotional. It will be a reflection of how you are feeling that day and how you would like to feel after you're done.

First, notice your state before you start. "Am I feeling jittery? Sluggish? Moody? Too wired to go to bed?" Then you visualize how the next half hour can help you shift the state, and you audibly speak what you intend to change. If there are people around and you feel silly, say it to yourself, but know that saying an intention aloud and in a tone of voice that expresses what you want to achieve—energized, soothed, relieved, and so on—is important because it commits you to the idea.

Once you have stated your intention, just get moving, and practice the three techniques in both walking and yoga. *One, breathe in concert with your movement; two, sense the moment and notice what comes up in your body; and three, every so often ask yourself, "What feels good?"* Let the intention echo as you move so that occasionally it floats across your mind, but let go of wordy thoughts and concerns about it. When you're finished, remember to take a moment to check in and see if your feelings and physical energy have

Exercise

127

shifted. Has your intention manifested? There is no success or failure on this count, simply observation. If you don't feel the way you wanted to after working out, do you have time to continue for a little longer?

Some examples of intentions include:

- I intend to bend and stretch until I get space in my spine and all through my body.
- I intend to get my heart rate up, sweat like crazy, and smile.
- I intend to get outside and enjoy this beautiful day after being stuck inside for hours.
- I intend to clear my mind so I can think more sharply.
- I intend to work my body toward my goal of being trimmer and healthier.
- I intend to get rid of this apathy and find my optimism.
- I intend to dissolve this anger at my partner/friend/colleague/self.
- I intend to do some quiet, slow exercise to wind down tonight.
- I intend to take half an hour for myself and emerge enthusiastic about all my responsibilities.
- I intend to move and enjoy it, and to trust that my body will feel and look its best because of it.

Setting an intention not only helps you engage in the walk or yoga session with greater effectiveness, it also makes exercise emotionally transformative. It helps guide you from one state to another because you've declared the purpose and set out on the journey. This is how you use exercise to "clear the cobwebs" when you've had a difficult day, have accumulated stress, or are in a rut. Physical activity can be a powerful way to create space in your mind and heart. If your mind is clouded or if negative emotions are pulling you off balance, use a workout as a tool to clean the slate and feel new. No matter what type or intensity of exercise you do, you always feel different at the end of a workout than you did at the beginning.

The beauty of life is that things always shift. A bad day, an uncomfortable mood, or negative thoughts always move on. It may take a few hours, or it may take a few days, but it is a fundamental law of nature: everything changes. Exercise speeds up the transformation. You plug in to your own power, turn up the heat in yourself, and just as in cooking, you burn off some steam.

Explore using walking and yoga to shift your state anytime you feel less than your best. For example, a gentle yoga session can be nurturing when you feel fragile and lonely. A vigorous hike can get you fired up to focus on work when you've lost your enthusiasm. When you set an intention and consider, *"How will the next thirty minutes benefit me?"* you are treating yourself with the kindness that I believe must be at the core of all these balanced-life practices. Whether you eat well, exercise, or make a lovely home environment, you do them not simply to stay in shape or look better to the outside world, but as an act of loving-kindness to yourself. When you set your intention during exercise, you are committing to staying well and dispersing stress before it can make you run down or sick. It's critical to remember that the time you devote to exercise benefits you and everyone else around you—because if you don't take care of your own internal world, then you're no good for anybody else.

I intend to accept myself as I am.

The more you use your body, the more you come to accept and love your body. The more intimate you become with your body's strengths and weaknesses, clicks and creaks, tight spots and loose spots, the kinder you become toward it. Women spend an inordinate amount of time mentally beating up their own bodies; they repeat the same mean thoughts about their size or shape a million times over and criticize themselves more viciously than they'd ever criticize a friend or daughter. They yell at themselves for failing, even though they know from experience that yelling is the worst way to create change: if you do it to your kids, they retreat in anger and hurt. Your body is the same—it will tighten up and create pain or sickness because you are at odds with it. I know it because I've done it.

Sometimes exercise can bring up resistance if you're in the negative state of focusing on everything that's wrong with your body. *"I don't have a skinny 'yoga body'; I'm heavier than everyone else on the walking trail; I look huge in these track pants."* Yet the act of doing exercise burns through that resistance. You might start a workout feeling self-conscious or even self-loathing, but by the end a transformation has occurred. It happens in yoga all the time—you walk into a studio all concerned about how you look in your outfit and checking out who has a better body, and ten minutes into it, you're sweating, your hair's a mess, and you don't care at all. You've reconnected to your physical self and gotten out of your mind, you've experienced *how good you can feel in the body that you have,* and you are thankful for all it can do. (And you realize that there is no such thing as one kind of "yoga body" after all.)

That is how you work toward acceptance; you begin to base your self-worth on the strength, confidence, and assurance you feel in your physical body rather than basing it on phantom ideas about yourself that flit through your head. Physical exercise is so valuable because it allows you to let go of some stuff that wasn't really there in the first place.

The challenge to accept and love my own body never quite goes away. I'll admit that having two gorgeous, tall, skinny teenage daughters messed with my head until I acknowledged that my envy was ridiculous—how crazy would a woman of my age look with their tiny frames?—and until I learned to love that it was their time in the sun, their time to be hot young things who turn heads in restaurants. Getting older in the entertainment industry definitely brings any doubts and fears right up to the surface: it's almost not permitted to look a day over thirty. When self-critical thoughts come up, I know now that there are two choices: I can sit and stew over them—I call it feeding the serpent, that ugly part that lives inside and stays alive only if I choose to feed it—or I can take it to my yoga mat or go on a fast walk with my dogs and reconnect with all that is amazing about a body that can move in graceful ways, hold itself in beautiful postures, and feel utterly new over and over again. I may still have qualms about certain bits of myself—I won't pretend otherwise—but I accept that this is me and I am able to love who I am.

That's why if you find yourself beating up on your body, set the intention for some of your sessions to simply be kind and be a friend to yourself. It's not about suddenly pretending you love your size and shape and would never want to change it. Rather, it's about gracefully accepting where you are, right now, in your body. It's acknowledging that you arrived at this size or shape through some choices that served you at the time, but you know that you don't have to stay there. You can set your intention to become healthier and trimmer, and reveal the best body that is already there inside you.

Much of my own personal journey has been about learning how to stop causing my own suffering and simply practice graceful acceptance about who I am, how I look, what I can and cannot do. And my yoga and exercise practice has been an anchor throughout. Accepting who you are will heal you in so many ways. And it does reverberate to others. As a mother, you're a better example to your kids if you heal yourself and love yourself. You teach them wonderful self-esteem as they grow if you have a healthy, kind *sense* of your own self.

Bonus: Shedding the Schlock

Sometimes your intention to clear out a bad mood and change the way you feel brings up a powerful emotional response. It may take you by surprise—a hike unleashes a torrent of tears or a yoga practice elicits a flush of anger, sadness, or pain. All these things are healthy because moving your body can move some of the schlock that you're holding onto and push it out of hiding. In that way exercise can help you safely process and release things that are on your mind. Insight is one of the best by-products of exercising with intention. It's that windshield-wiper effect: when you fall into a rhythm and drop some of the everyday chatter from your mind, physical activity becomes something of a moving meditation. Without consciously thinking about a problem, something comes up, and you can notice it and go, "How bizarre that I feel that right now."

Sometimes the simple act of sweating and burning through the heaviness is enough. You feel lighter and freer when you're done. Other times feelings come up that are complex and confusing. If you turn toward them and ask some questions, you gain insight into your-self. Ask, "Why are these feelings coming up? Where is their source?" That is how exercise can become an investigation. It can be part of your healing and your self-analysis. You can do some powerful work observing how your history—your family, your past, and your

Releasing the Resistance

Exercise affords a great opportunity for exploring your own psychology. Whenever you are in a state of emotional upheaval or distress, take it on a hike and let yourself feel the emotions as you move. Ask yourself, "Where is this feeling located in my physical body?" Maybe it's the solar plexus, the throat, the shoulders. Then consciously breathe into this tightness. Ask yourself what emotion is coming up—despera-tion, fear, sadness, and so on. Ask if you can accept that this emotion exists. And then ask if you can let it go. As simple as this is, it is the basis of the "releasing" technique that I use any time I feel emotionally off balance.

Perhaps you are not experiencing emotional upheaval, but you find that you feel resistance toward exercise, and each time you are scheduled to work out, you'd prefer not to. Notice that resistance, and ask where in your body it sits. Then ask yourself why that resistance is there—and is it really yours, or is it simply a projection? Did someone once tell you that you were no good at exercise, or have you been telling that to yourself? Perhaps there was a moment in your past when someone made you feel unfit, awkward, or undeserving. On a vigorous hike, the memories often start to percolate up like bubbles to the top of a pan of hot water. If you can, locate the point that is causing your current resistance, and see it as the powerless memory that it is. Ask yourself if you can let it go.

training—inform who you are and why you make some of the choices you make in your life.

I like to ask questions that help me find the trigger points of bad feelings. We all have those stories from our past—a first boyfriend, a teacher, or a parent who said something silly or meaningless about our abilities, looks, or potential that went deep into

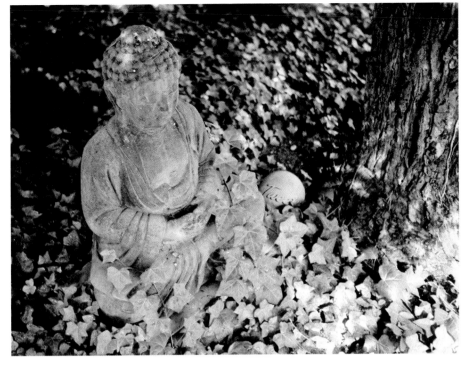

our psyche and became our truth. If you can peel back the onion a little, you often find that these ancient moments are still resonating inside. When I'm power-walking, if I'm emotional about something, I roll the mental tape back and run through my life. I ask, "Where does this feeling come from?" Suddenly, I remember something from way back. "Oh, my god, that awful teacher who said I didn't deserve extra homework time even though my mom was going through chemo, and if I couldn't keep up with the class I was obviously worthless and stupid—wow, she totally messed me up!" If it makes me angry, I visualize a new ending to the story, like throwing

a pie in her face, and then just let that old story go. It's amazing how you can be moving physically while experiencing all kinds of messy emotions rushing around your body. And suddenly a moment of clarity comes out of nowhere and you go, "Aha! I recognize this as a trigger point for my withholding love and approval from myself."

TIP To learn more about releasing emotions that are stuck or that are holding you back, I highly recommend the book that has been invaluable to me, *The Sedona Method,* by Jack Canfield and Hale Dwoskin.

Exercise

131

■ ■ ■

YESTERDAY ON MY WALK, it was hot and I was agitated. I was so antsy that while walking I just felt like pushing into my breath and challenging my body with speed. The exercise was intense, yet I wanted to push up the hills even harder and feel the struggle. I became fascinated with my weird state. I couldn't figure out why I felt so crazily emotional: I thought perhaps the relentless heat on my face was bullying me and I was simply trying to bully it back, acting as though it made no difference to me: I'm tough, I can overcome any kind of weather! All I knew was that I felt like crying, but I wasn't interested in why. I just wanted to power through to feel better through sweat and physical exertion.

It's a familiar state to me: I've used a hard, tough hike to pound out many a difficult and emotional time. The day my mother died, almost twenty years ago, I went out for a long hike—at least nine miles. After over fifteen years of thinking she was going to die of cancer, when she finally did pass I was confused by how little I cried. My emotions were caught inside my head and hiding deep in my gut— and yet I felt a strong agitation, a need to push my legs and body toward a summit to free me from the pain of feelings that were stuck. The only thing I could feel was physical: the feel of

breath in my lungs, pushed by frustration, hurting my throat; the searing heat in my thighs.

It hurt then, and it hurt yesterday but for different reasons. With my mother's death I knew what emotions I wanted to have but couldn't find them. Yesterday I was full of emotions that I didn't understand. Some days are like that, and you just have to surrender to them. By the end of my hike, pushing into that uncomfortable physical place had served me well. I was very alive. I felt motivated and focused, alone with myself: no deep introspection, no extracurricular thoughts. The hike had mimicked the day of my mom's death in that the heat was a constant, a sun with no wind, a dry stillness that matched my mood: dead, itchy, wanting something and not knowing how to get there. Yesterday I was curious only to get past the push. I made it to the top of the hill. I had no mantra or releasing exercise I could settle on, so I watched myself in my discomfort, and like everything in life I knew it would pass as I hit the top of the hill. The top is a place for stopping and feeling how you feel. A place to go into a gentle Mountain Pose, to examine your body, the pulsing of your heart, the racing of the blood, and the feeling of a face flushed with heat.

At the beginning of my hike I had been longing for the quality of calm I get through my yoga practice. Instead, by burning through my agitation and antsiness, I received a different quality of self-understanding. I was watching a different me. I was present. The day had been productive.

I do this anytime I am caught up in negative feelings about my past, my future, my body, my age, my looks—whatever is getting me in a tizzy. We can allow our feelings to emerge by breathing deeply like we do during a hard climb or a strenuous practice or any exercise that forces us out of our head. Sometimes we examine emotions through gentleness and calm; sometimes we need to bypass examination and just burn a hole through the lies we have told ourselves by using pure exertion.

Quick Fix #5: Sausage Rolls

This is good for grounding yourself in your body when you have been in your head all day. Do it at the end of the day. (It feels great after a shower or bath has warmed your body.) It is best done on a carpet or area rug. If you don't have either, try it on your bed. Lie down flat on your back with your arms over your head

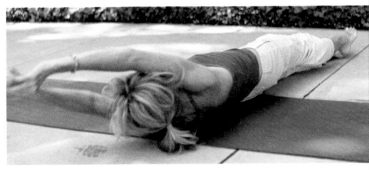

and your legs straight. Roll your entire body over two complete times to the right, like a sausage rolling across the floor, then immediately two times to the left, and repeat both ways for two minutes. Be floppy, be loose, feel your back and abdominal muscles getting a massage as they roll across the floor. After 2 minutes, whether you end up on your back or front, lie there and breathe and notice the space between your body and the floor for at least 1 minute. You will find it rejuvenating and mentally cleansing. It makes me smile, and my back loves it.

Exercise

YOGA SEQUENCE

1. Mountain Pose

—Stand with feet together at the front of the mat, toes spread wide. Your arms rest gently at your sides, palms facing forward. Your shoulders are pulled back and down, away from the ears. Press your feet firmly into the ground, firming your legs and lifting your kneecaps.

—As you inhale, draw energy up through your core, and let it travel up through the spine to the top of your head. Take a moment to move your head around, finding the place where your head naturally aligns with the spine; your head knows when it finds center. Bring your chin slightly back so that the neck and spine are aligned. Gently gaze past the tip of your nose or a few feet ahead of you on the ground. Open your mouth, and allow your jaw to be soft. Find that place of connection to the ground you stand on. Breathe 5 long breaths through the nose.

Think of finding the tree within you. The spine is the trunk and the roots are your feet, settled into the earth. By pressing firmly into the ground, you are grounding your tree onto the mountain—the earth that you live on. Feel the stability and fluidity that come together because your body is not stagnant; feel it move with the breath.

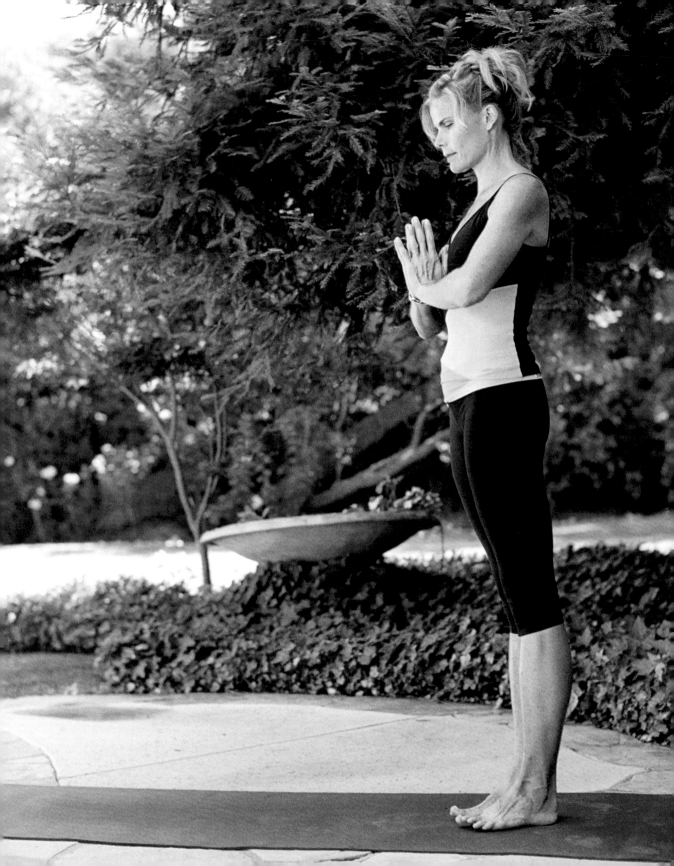

2. Volcano Pose

—Inhale and sweep your arms up from your sides and overhead, gathering up energy from your trunk. Eyes look forward, or, if there is no strain to the neck, look up toward your hands pressed together in gentle prayer pose. Breathe.

—Exhale and slowly hinge at the hips, swan-diving the hands toward the ground. Keep your neck soft. Touch fingertips to the ground or to your knees or shins if that is easier. Inhale and exhale there.

—Inhale and bring your arms up again while raising the body. Engage your thighs so you rise from the strength of your legs and not your back. If it feels better, bend your knees a bit so there is no danger of straining the lower back. Check that your entire foot is connected to the earth in four places: the toes, the ball of the foot, and both sides of your heel are all pressing down.

—Repeat the standing and diving motion 3 times.

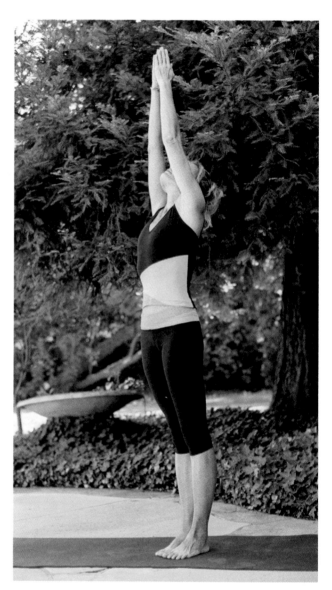

As you sweep arms up, visualize energy as warm light that you are scooping up. As you dive down, imagine it showering all around you.

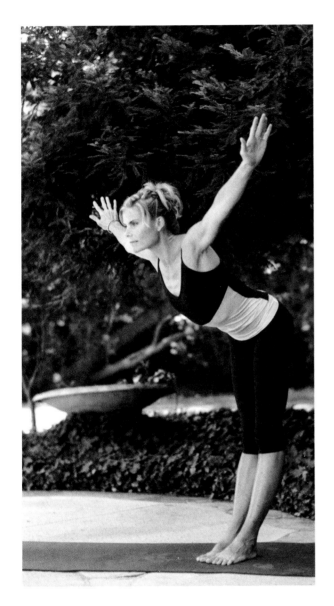

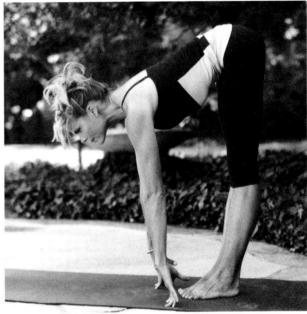

3. Standing Forward Bend

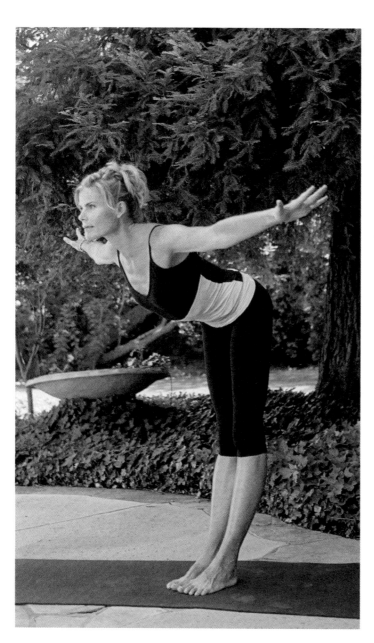

—On the third dive, hold
  your forward bend. Bend
  the knees gently if you
  feel strain in lower back or
  hamstrings.

—Hold your elbows and
  hang. Breathe 3 complete
  breaths.

—Bending the knees,
  roll up slowly to Mountain,
  allowing your head to
  come up last.

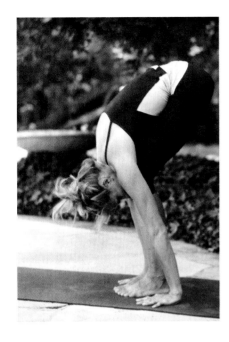

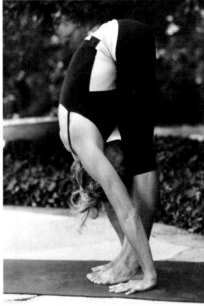

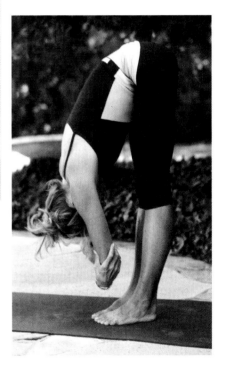

Feel whatever is singing to you in this pose: your hamstrings pulling, your neck softening and lengthening, arms hanging loose from shoulder sockets.

139

4. Lunge and Twist

—From Mountain, inhale to Volcano and
exhale down into Standing Forward Bend.
Place hands or fingertips on the floor (bend
your knees if necessary), and step your right
foot back into a lunge. Get your balance and
look at a spot in front of you.

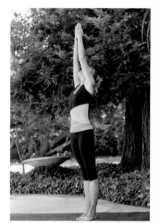

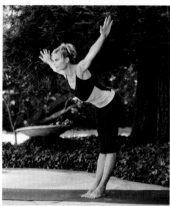

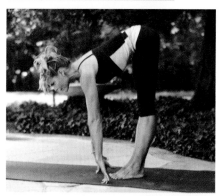

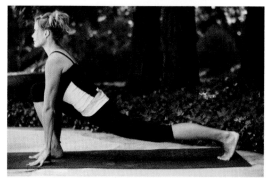

If you feel tension in your neck, notice if you are clenching your jaw.
If that awareness doesn't loosen your neck, then just look at the ground.

—Take your left arm into air, twist your body to follow it, and look up toward the sky.

—Inhale, place the left hand down, and step your right foot to front of the mat to
  Standing Forward Bend. Breathe a full breath.

—Exhale and step your left leg back, and twist your body as the
  right arm goes into the air.

—Place your right hand down so your hands are shoulder-distance apart with palms flat,
  and step your right leg back, shifting your hips up and back into the air.
  Your feet should be parallel and hip-distance apart.

5. Downward-Facing Dog

—Spread your fingers wide, and press your palms and knuckles fully into the ground. Create space between your shoulders and your ears; draw your shoulder blades down your back and lightly in toward your back ribs.

If it's more comfortable for you, widen the feet at first.

—Bend your knees softly with your heels lifted off the floor. Create length in the spine by pressing hands into the floor and lifting your rear end higher, then try to straighten your legs. Firm your outer thighs and rotate the inner thighs inward, which will take the strain away from your lower back.

—Walk in place: bend the left knee and push the right heel to the floor, then switch sides. Repeat several times.

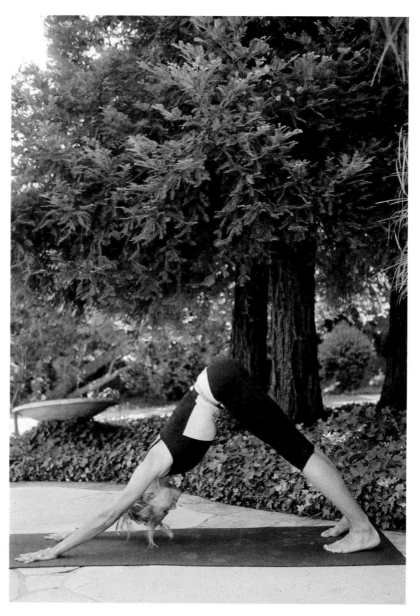

Stretch the calf muscle with each side, then let the shift work into your hips so that your hips and heels shift up and to the right, then up and to the left.

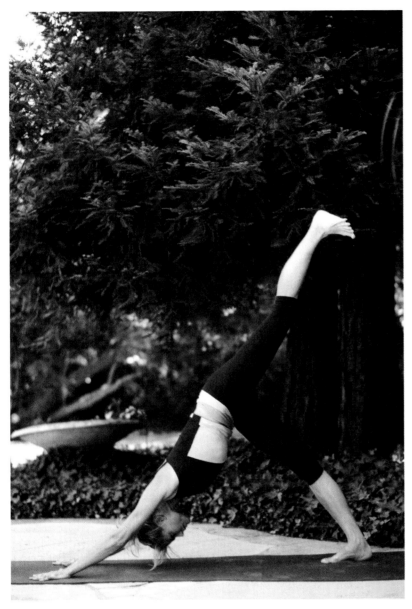

—Inhale and extend your right leg into the air, hipbones parallel to the ground and your knee and foot facing the ground. Breathe 3 breaths. Exhaling, place your right foot down. Inhale and repeat on the left side.

—Extend your right leg into the air again, this time opening your hip out with the leg bent and toe pointing to-ward your buttocks. Breathe 3 breaths, and feel the stretch along the right side of the body from armpit to toe.

Visual aid: a dog, peeing on a bush! Place the right foot down, and repeat on left side.

—Breathe 5 full breaths in Downward-Facing Dog.

—Step your left leg forward, step your right leg forward, and roll up slowly to Mountain.

Exercise

143

6. Sun Salutation

Do the regular version twice or the modified version once, followed by this regular version.

Regular Sun Salutation

—Start in Mountain.

—Inhale, raise your arms up to Volcano.

—Exhale, swan-dive your arms down into a Standing Forward Bend.

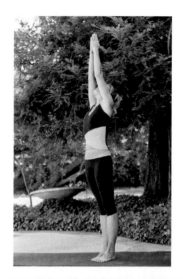

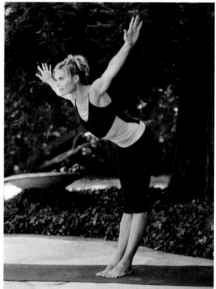

—Inhale, extending your torso forward as long as it can stretch, and place your hands on the floor or legs.

—Exhale, step your right leg back.

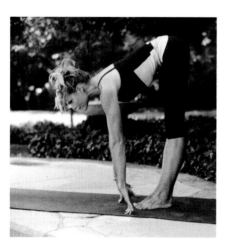

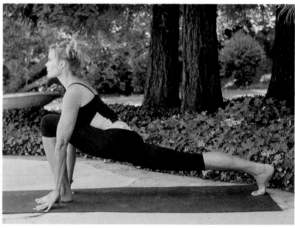

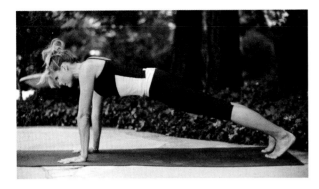

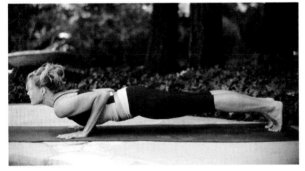

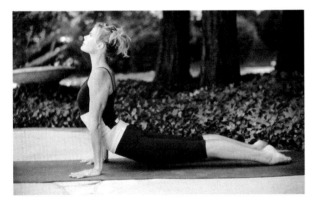

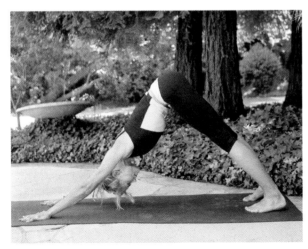

—Then exhale your left leg back straight into Plank, legs off the ground, torso and legs straight, and your shoulders aligned over your wrists

—Take a deep breath, then exhale and slowly bend your elbows until your shoulders are level with your elbows, elbows at your sides, body off the floor, and heels pushing back. This is *Chaturanga Dandasana,* the Push-Up Pose.

—Inhaling, roll over your toes so the front of your foot is on the ground, and pull your hips forward as you press your arms straight, coming into Upward-Facing Dog. Shins are touching the ground, and thighs are raised off the floor. Your arms are straight, and your back is in a slight backbend, and your eyes are gently looking forward or slightly up.

—Exhale, pull your belly into your core, and push back into Downward-Facing Dog.

—Inhale your right foot forward, exhale your left foot forward, and either roll up into Mountain or firmly engage the muscles of your thighs (to avoid pressure on your back) and raise up into Mountain with a flat back.

—Stand in Mountain and observe your breath.

Feel the difference from your first Mountain Pose. How is your breath differ-ent? This time it is probably deeper and more measured. How does your body feel?

Modified Sun Salutation

—Start in Mountain.

—Inhale, raise your arms up to Volcano.

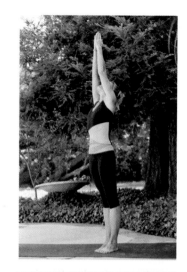

—Exhale, swan-dive your arms down into a
Standing Forward Bend.

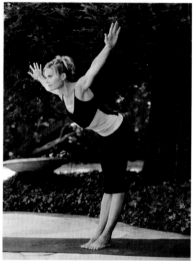

—Inhale, extending your torso forward as long
as it can stretch, and place hands on the
floor if you can. (Bend your knees if necessary, or place your hands on your shins if
necessary.)

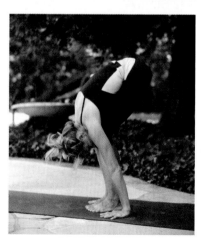

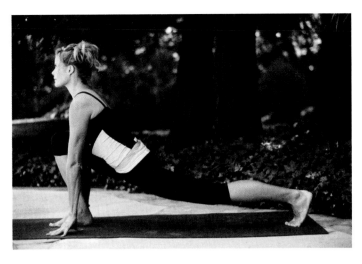

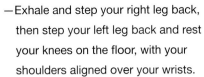—Exhale and step your right leg back, then step your left leg back and rest your knees on the floor, with your shoulders aligned over your wrists.

—Take a deep breath, then exhale and slowly bend your elbows until your shoulders are level with your elbows, elbows at your sides, and release your body to the floor with straight legs.

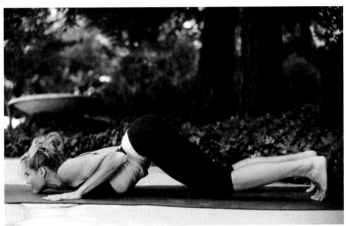

—Press your hips and palms down into the floor, keep your elbows drawing toward your sides, and then inhale and and reach your chest forward and up, drawing your shoulders back and down, to come into Cobra—a modified version of Upward-Facing Dog.

Allow your buttocks to be loose— this is not aerobics class.

—Exhale and press back onto all fours, tucking your toes under, then lifting your hips back and up into Downward-Facing Dog.

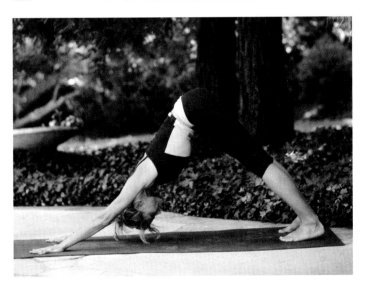

7. Salutation B

—From Mountain, bend your knees and sweep
your arms down to the floor and around
up into the air in front of you, sitting your
buttocks down on an imaginary seat behind
you in Chair Pose. Your hands should be
shoulder-width apart; raise them over your
head if possible. Try to shift your weight
back on your heels. Hold and breathe.

*This is a very powerful pose that challenges
your legs and arms. It is a great place for
observation. Try to detach from any negative
thoughts or sensations and stay in the pose.*

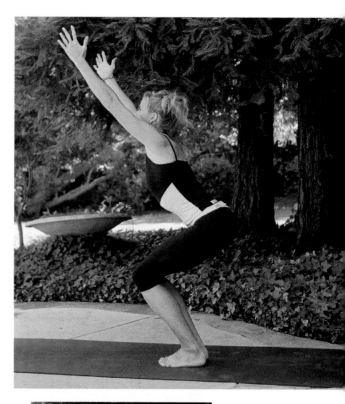

—Exhaling, straighten your legs, and fold
down to Standing Forward Bend. Place
your hands on floor or shins, inhale, and
look up with a flat back.

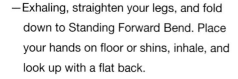

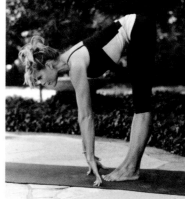

—Bend the knees, place hands on the floor,
and step your right foot back, then your left
foot back into Downward-Facing Dog.

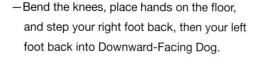

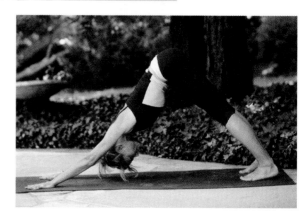

—Inhale and step your right leg forward into a lunge, placing your left foot firmly on the floor, turned in at a forty-five-degree angle. Fully engage the muscles of your left leg, and press the toes into the ground. With your hipbones facing forward, raise your arms above your head into Warrior I. Arms may be shoulder-width apart or palms pressed together. Bend your right knee deeply, trying to get the right thigh parallel with the ground, but do not let the knee move ahead of the toes. Actively engage your whole body, and feel the energy resonating from your feet to your arms through the top of your head. Breathe 3 complete breaths.

Feel the connection that this invigorating pose has to your deep, nasal breath.

—Sweep your arms down to the floor, and step your right foot back into Plank. Exhale and lower slowly into a Push-Up.

—Inhale and press up to Upward-Facing Dog.

—Exhale and roll over your toes, pushing back to Downward-Facing Dog.

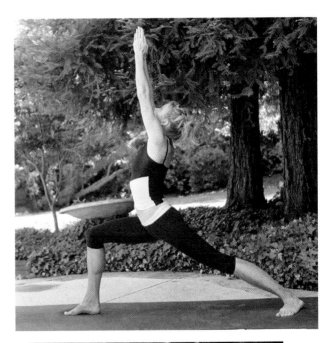

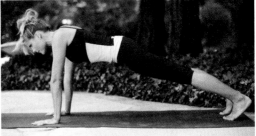

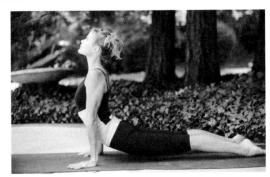

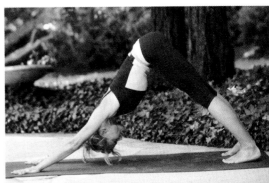

Salutation B

(continued)

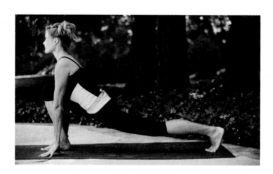

—Repeat the
 sequence on
 the other side,
 stepping your
 left foot forward
 into a lunge
 and lifting into
 Warrior I,
 then down
 through
 Plank to
 Downward-
 Facing Dog.

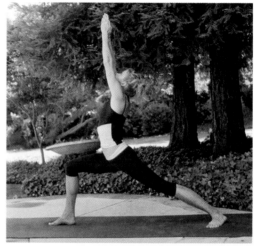

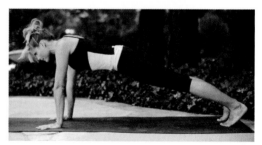

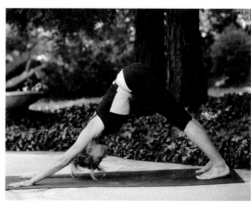

Mariel Hemingway's Healthy Living from the Inside Out

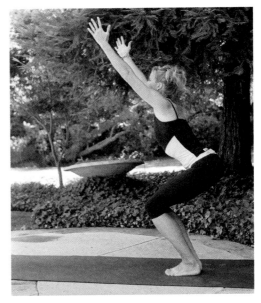

—Step your right foot forward, then your left, and with bent legs sweep your arms up and around on an inhale and come into Chair Pose. Stay for 2 breaths. Stand to Mountain, and bring your hands to prayer position at the chest.

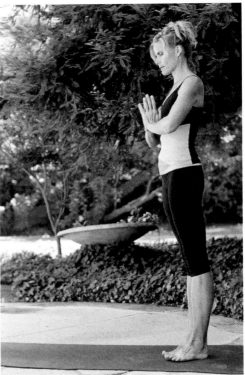

—Repeat Salutation B again. This time, stay in Mountain after completion and examine the feeling of your body. Breathe 5 breaths.

8. Side Angle and Triangle

—From Mountain, step your left leg back into a lunge, placing your left foot firmly on floor at a forty-five-degree angle. With your right knee bent, engage the core muscles and sweep your arms up, barely pausing in Warrior I position, and opening them parallel to the ground, with your hip bones and torso facing the right side of the room. Your arms extend fully from the shoulder blades, your right arm over your right leg, your left arm over your left leg; your head turns right, and your eyes gaze over the right fingertips.
This is Warrior II.
Breathe.

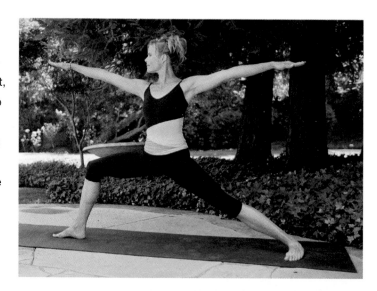

—With the right knee still bent, tip your right side toward the floor, and place your right hand on the ground outside the right foot, or rest your right forearm on your knee. Stretch your left arm up to the sky, and look up at your hand in Side Angle Pose. Breathe, and rotate your left side outward to open the chest. If possible, reach your left hand over your left ear for the full pose. Breathe 3 breaths.

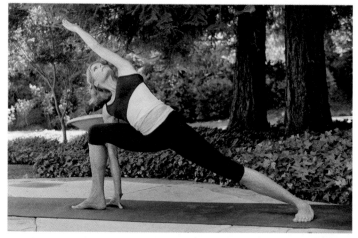

If you feel too much tension in your neck, just look forward.

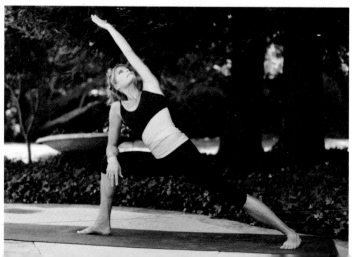

— Bring your left arm straight above you like an arrow to the sky. Inhale and straighten your right leg into Triangle Pose. Your right arm can be touching the floor on the outside of your right leg or holding your shin or knee, depending on your flexibility. Breathe and look up at the left hand.

Keep trying to create space across the chest by rotating it open.

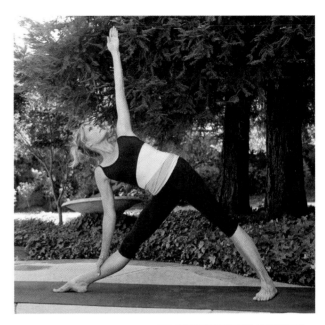

— Place your left hand down on the floor, step your right foot back into Plank, and move through to Downward-Facing Dog.

— Repeat on the other side. Step your left leg forward, raise your torso up into Warrior I, then open to Warrior II with your hip bones and torso facing the left side of the room and your eyes gazing out to the fingertips of your left hand. Move into Side Angle and Triangle on this side. Hold each pose for 3 breaths.

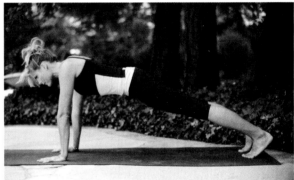

— Place your right hand on the ground, step your left foot back into Plank, and move back into Downward-Facing Dog Pose.

— Step your left leg forward then your right leg forward, and roll up into Mountain. Place your hands together in prayer position at your chest. Breathe.

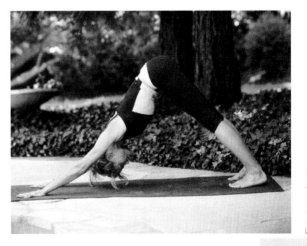

9. Arm Swings

—Stand with your feet hip-width apart. Throw your arms over your head, bending the legs in concert with the up-and-down motion of your arms. Each time you come down, rock backward and forward on your heels with momentum. Make sure you are moving your arms in the sockets, and don't throw your arms out wildly. Do 25 to 50.

—Raise your arms up in Volcano Pose. Stretch up, reach for the sky, and feel your body becoming taller.
Come onto your tiptoes. Balance.
See if from standing on your tiptoes, you can swan-dive your arms down to Standing Forward Bend.

—Make sure your feet are flat on the floor, bend your knees, and sweep your arms up into Chair.

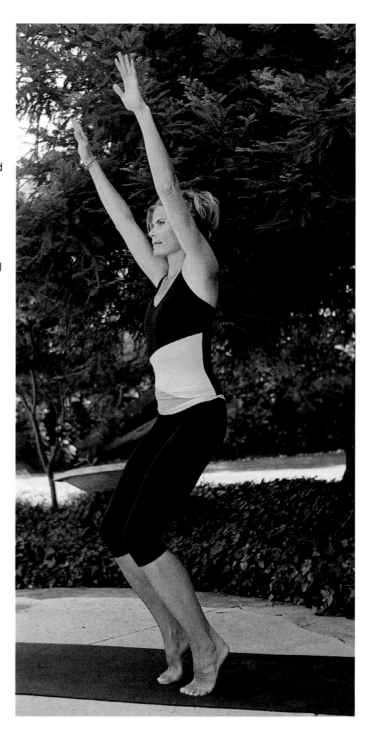

10. Chair

—Feet hip-distance apart, bend your knees as though you are sitting in an invisible chair. Don't bend forward too much. Try to lengthen up your back without straining, slightly tuck your tailbone and take a gentle gaze upwards, raising your arms above your head parallel to your shoulders. Hold Chair for 5 to 8 complete breaths.

Remember how challenging this pose is and how important it is to observe yourself in it.

—Stand up to Mountain with your hands in prayer position in front of your heart. Take a moment to assess the depth and rhythm of your breath.

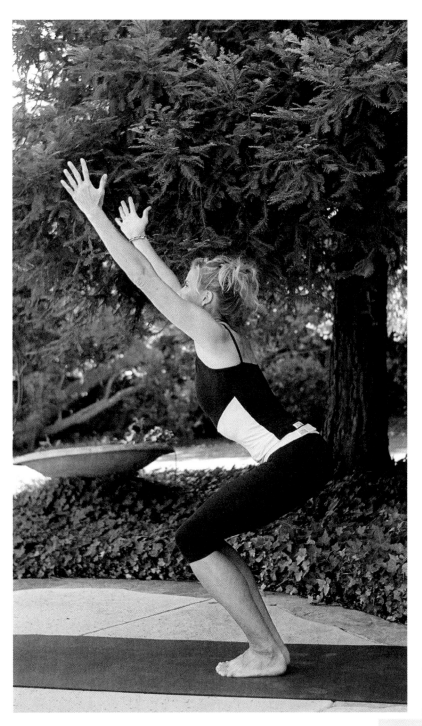

11. Tree Pose

—From Mountain, shift your weight to your right leg, lift your left foot, and place it on the inside of your right ankle or your right calf or, if you are flexible and feeling balanced, the right thigh.

Your body shape resembles the number four.

Place your hands in prayer position, and hold this pose for 8 full nasal breaths.

Play with your balance, and smile like a kid in a play- ground; see the humor in wobbling and falling and know it is no big deal if you don't "stick it."

—Explore the pose further by extending the arms up above your head and then looking up at your hands.

Make light of the idea of fall- ing, and see if you can be comfortable swaying like a tree.

—Put your left foot down, and lift the right foot up. Repeat on this side.

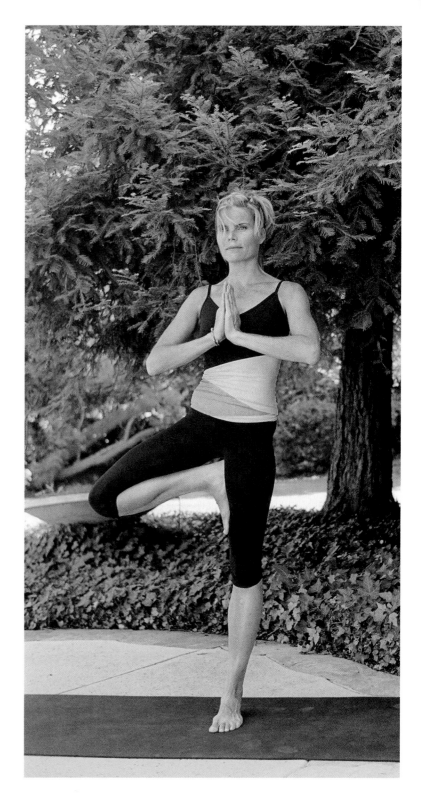

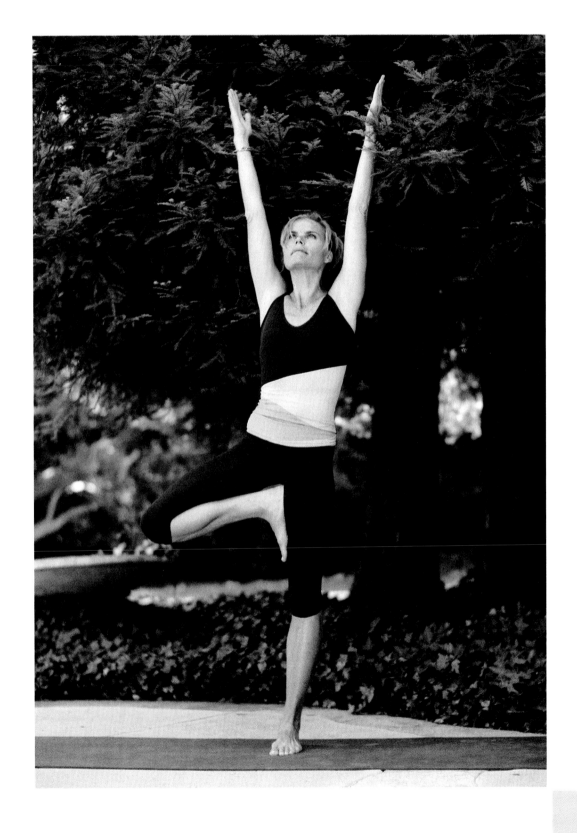

12. Sun Salutation Sequence

—Exhale into Standing Forward Bend, holding your elbows. Bend your knees, and roll up into Mountain.

—Inhale and raise your arms up over head into Volcano, then exhale and swan-dive down to Standing Forward Bend. Step your right foot back, then the left foot back into Downward-Facing Dog, then move forward on an exhale into Plank.

—Roll your body to the right side so that you are holding yourself up with your right arm and the right side of your right foot. Bring your left foot flat to the ground in front of your right knee, making a sideways four, for better balance. Or, stack the left foot on top of the right. Raise your left arm up to the sky, and take a gentle gaze upward. Hold this pose for 3 to 5 breaths.

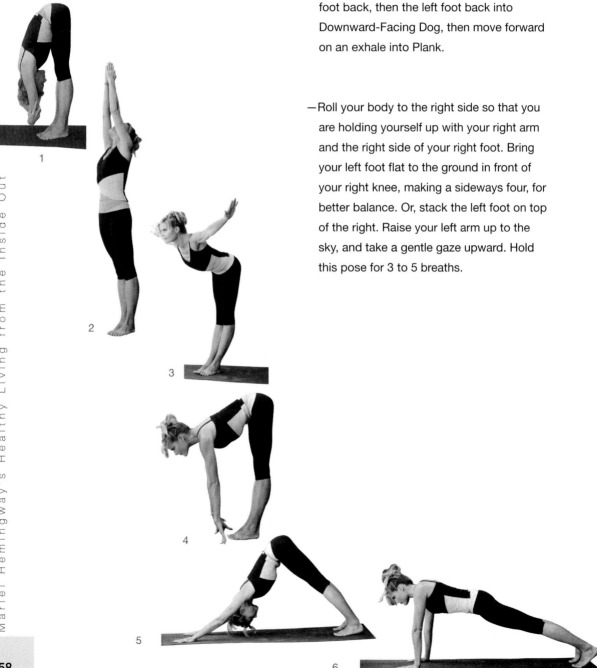

1

2

3

4

5

6

If you feel too much tension in your neck, just look forward.

—Place the left hand down, return to Plank, and roll your body to the left side to repeat the pose on this side.

—Return to Plank, inhale, exhale, and lower to the ground through Push-Up Pose. Inhale up to Upward-Facing Dog, exhale to Downward-Facing Dog. Step the right foot forward, the left foot forward, and roll up to Mountain.

—Repeat the Arm Swings 25 to 50 times. Raise arms up into Volcano. Find your balance on flat feet.

This is a good place to start the five minutes of music in Week 2 of the program. Add freestyle dance moves, or whatever feels good, and turn off the music before the Seated Sequence.

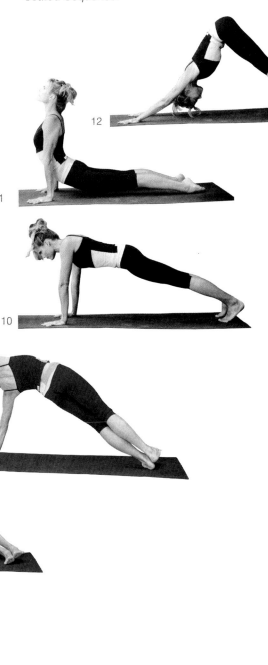

13. Gentle Jumping

—With your feet still hip-width apart, let your arms swing freely by the side of your body, and take some gentle jumps. Roll through your foot as you rise up, and roll down through your foot as you land.

Do not land with a thump; imagine trying to break your fall as though you are trying to quietly sneak up on someone.

This engages and strengthens the muscles of the legs, thighs, and buttocks while opening up the energy channels and stimulating the immune system. Jump for 1 minute, breathing either through your nose or your mouth.

—Spread your feet wide apart, lower your rear end as far as possible into a squat, and press your hands in prayer position at the chest. Press your elbows against the insides of your knees for balance. (See page 119 for an example). Breathe 3 to 5 breaths. Then come to sitting on the ground.

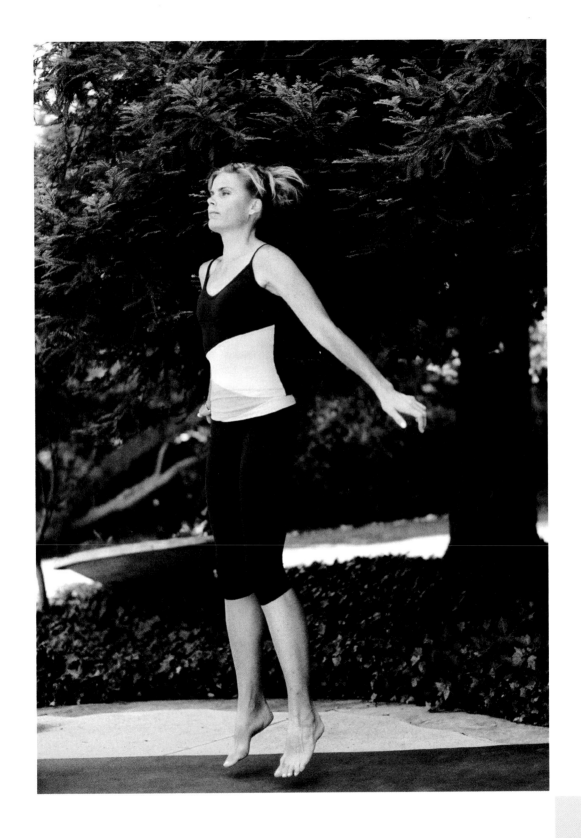

14. Seated Sequence

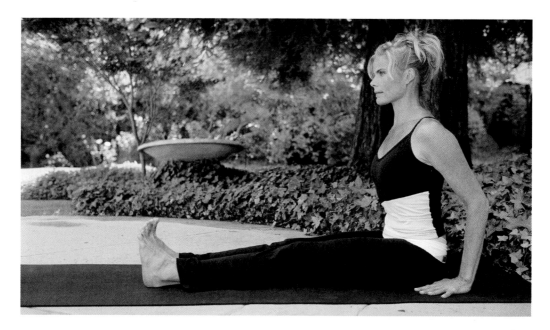

—Extend your legs, and press your hands to the floor, hands behind your hips with your fingers facing toward your body. Sit tall and breathe.

Visual aid: Imagine a string attached to the top of your head pulling up to the ceiling, giving the vertebrae of your spine, which are compressed from sitting all day, a wonderful chance to enjoy some space.

—Draw your knees into Cobbler's Pose by bringing the soles of your feet together as close to the groin as you can, creating a diamond shape. Press the knees toward the ground, and elongate the spine.

Feel the opening of the groin and hips.

Then extend your legs out in front of you. Repeat Cobbler's Pose.

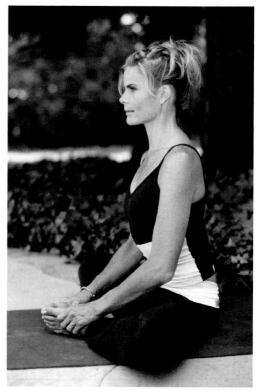

—Sitting up tall, open your legs to Wide-Legged Seated Pose, creating a large V with your legs; then bring your legs back to Cobbler's, then straight to Extended Legs. Repeat this cycle 2 or 3 times.

Notice the abdominal muscles that are working and the flexibility you are gaining in your hips and hamstrings.

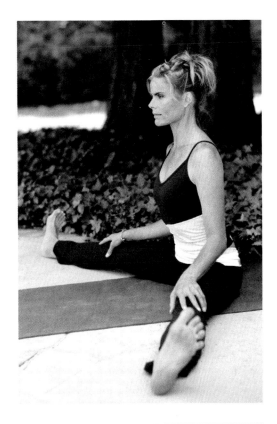

—With your legs extended in front, rock to the right buttock and pull the left buttock away from the heel, then repeat the other side, to create more space. Inhale and reach your arms overhead, exhale and hinge forward from the hips, not the waist. Move your hands toward your toes in Seated Forward Bend, and grasp your shins or your ankles or your toes. Do not curl your back; instead, keep your spine straight.

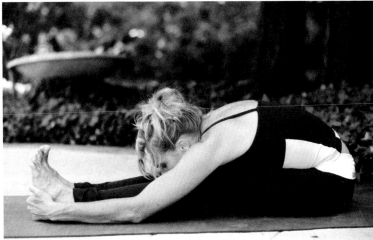

Inhaling, stretch the chest forward, exhaling, lower the body. Set the intention of moving your head toward your legs. Stay for 5 to 8 breaths.

—Come up slowly, and bring your feet back to Cobbler's Pose. Round your belly, creating a hollow in your belly as though you are rounding yourself over a ball in your lap. Now round your spine further forward creating a hollowness to your belly.

—Raise your body, take a breath, and exhale while opening and straightening your legs. Lean to the right, and place your right forearm on the floor if possible and stretch your left arm into the air or, if comfortable, over your left ear. Stretch your entire left side, from your hips up to your left hand, and breathe 3 breaths. Return to the middle and repeat on the other side.

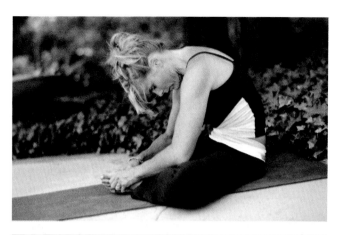

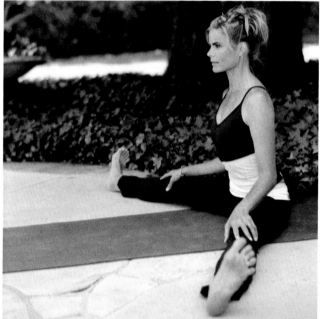

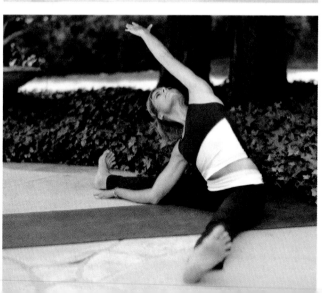

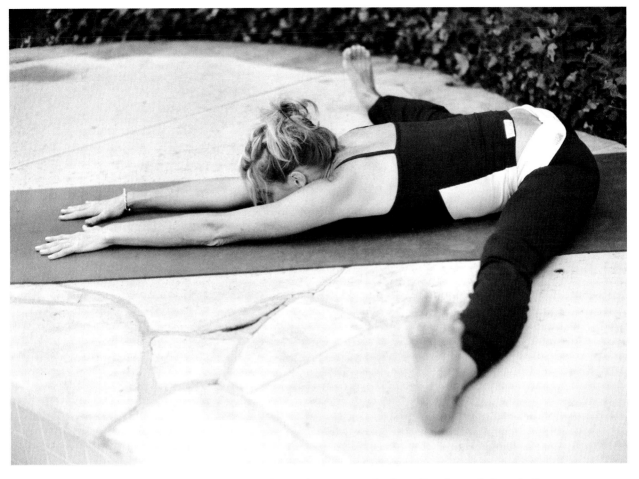

—Sit up, and exhaling, bend forward with your forearms on the floor. Breathe and elongate the spine as you did before, trying not to curl it. Stay for 3 breaths. Come up slowly and, with bent elbows, place your hands on the floor behind you with your fingers facing your body. Inhale, straighten your arms, and arch your back so that your eyes look to the ceiling. Breathe, and feel the stretch in your back. Then lie down on your back.

15. Happy Baby

—Lying on your back, bend your legs and bring thighs toward your chest so the soles of your feet face the ceiling. Grasp the outside of each foot, and gently rock your body to the right and left several times, feeling your spine move against the floor.

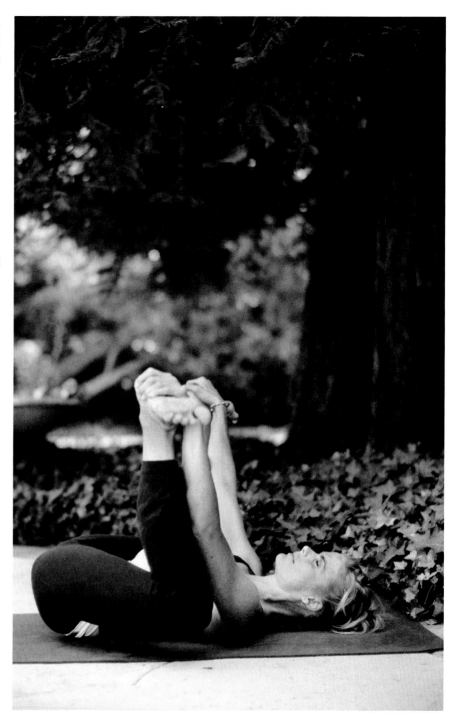

Mariel Hemingway's Healthy Living from the Inside Out

16. Spinal Twist

—Stretch your right leg to the ground, and
draw your left knee in toward the chest
with your right arm. Extend your left arm
out to the side, then pull your left knee to
the ground on the right side of the body,
softly turning your neck to look left. Exhaling, release that knee toward the ground.
Inhale back to center, swap legs, and repeat
the twist on the other side, this time turning
your head to look right.

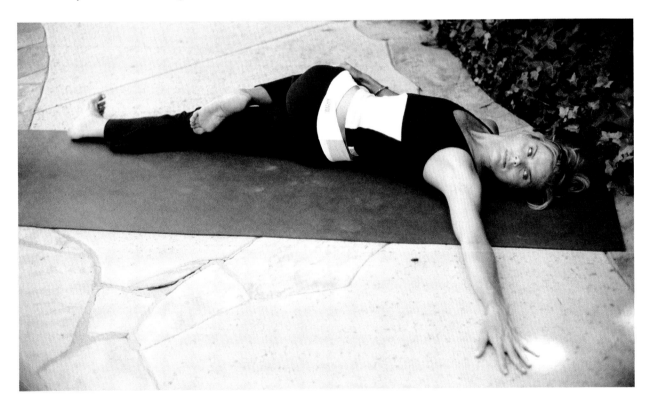

17. Abdominal Curl

—Come back to center with your legs in
Happy Baby Pose again but your hands out-
stretched over your head. Exhale and curl
up, bringing your arms and hands between
your bent knees with your hands flexed
upward, mirroring your feet. Spread your
toes. Hover in that position for 1 long complete breath, engaging your core abdominal
muscles, and then bring your back and neck
to the ground and hold your straight legs an
inch from the ground for a breath. Bring your
legs back to the middle again, and interlace
hands behind head.

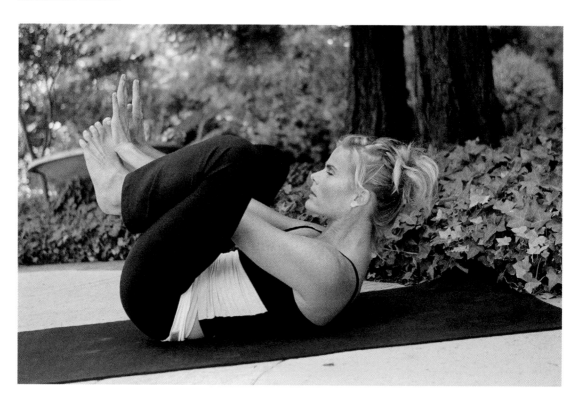

18. Crunches

—With your hands interlaced behind your
head and your knees still bent in the air,
bring your head and shoulders off the floor,
pressing your navel to your spine to create a
hollow belly. On an exhale, twist to the right
side, holding your head with right hand and
extending your left arm out past the right
knee. Inhale to center. Exhale to the left,
reaching your right arm past the left knee.
Repeat 5 complete rounds, then place your
feet on the floor.

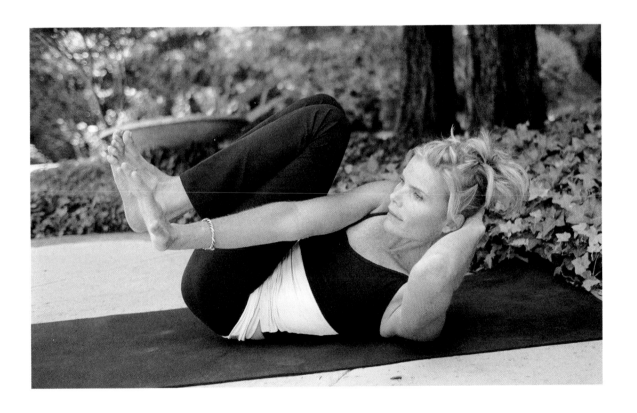

19. Bridge

—Lie on your back, bend your knees, and draw your heels in toward your hips, hip-distance apart. Lay your arms on the floor at your sides. Take a deep breath, and feel how at the bottom of the exhale, the tail-bone tilts up slightly.

—Empty of breath, press your heels down and lift your hips off the floor, following your tailbone up as high as you can comfortably lift your hips.

—Interlace your fingers under your back, and rock gently from side to side so that your shoulders roll under and you feel the outside of your shoulders and arms on the ground, thereby relieving pressure on your neck.

Press your heels firmly down to push your hips up to the ceiling while extending your tailbone toward your knees. Keep your bum soft, and use your feet to keep you up. This will lengthen and protect your lower back.

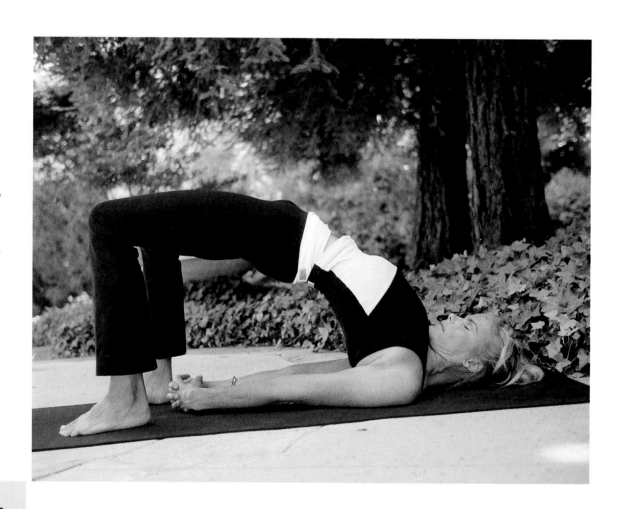

Modification

If that felt good, try this on your second round.

— From Bridge Pose, place your hands on the ground at your ears, fingertips pointing toward the toes, elbows pointing up to the sky. Feet should have outer edges parallel, so you feel slightly pigeon-toed. Stay as relaxed as you can.

— On an exhale, press down into your heels and press down with your hands, pushing your hips up and drawing the crown of your head onto the floor. Inhale, drawing your elbows together and shoulder blades down against the back of your ribs.

— Exhale all your breath out, and on an inhale press your arms and legs as straight as you can. Breathe at least 3 breaths.

— Slowly release, pressing into the inner edges of the feet to control your descent. Gently curl the back to the floor.

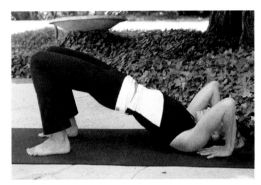

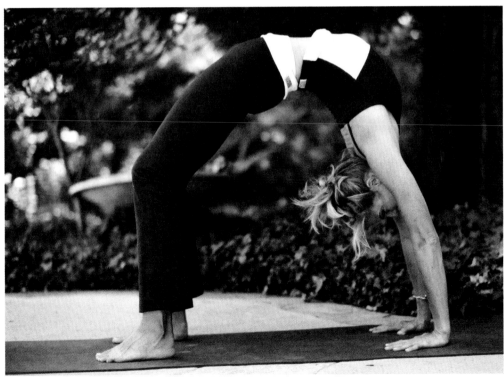

20. Reclined One-Legged Stretch

—Lie on your back with your legs strongly extended. Draw your right knee toward your chest, and hug the right thigh to the belly. If you have a yoga strap, loop it around the right foot. If not, use a towel as a strap. Hold the strap on each side of the foot, and, inhaling, extend foot upward to straighten the leg. Actively push the left thigh down into the floor. Broaden the back of your body flat against the floor. Keep the hands as high on the strap as you can, and keep your head on the floor. Breathe.

—Engage the abdominal muscles, and lift your head and upper shoulders off the floor, reaching your forehead up to your toes. Stay for 3 breaths and release.

—Lower the right leg, and repeat with the left leg lifted.

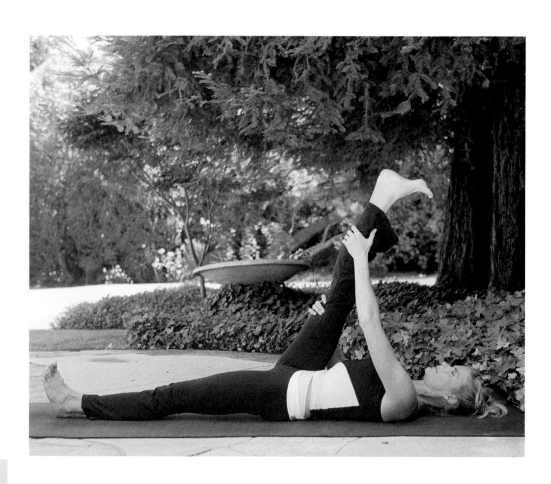

21. Reclined Cobbler's

—Lie on your back, and draw your legs into the Cobbler's diamond shape, your soles together and your feet on the ground. You may need to put some support under your knees, such as thick blankets or folded towels, as not many people can recline with their knees resting on the ground. Use as many as you need to rest in this reclined posture with ease and comfort. Arms lie gently at your sides a few inches away from the body, palms turned up. Feel the opening at your hips and the length of your spine on the floor. Breathe 3 complete breaths.

This pose quiets the nervous system in preparation for the final resting pose.

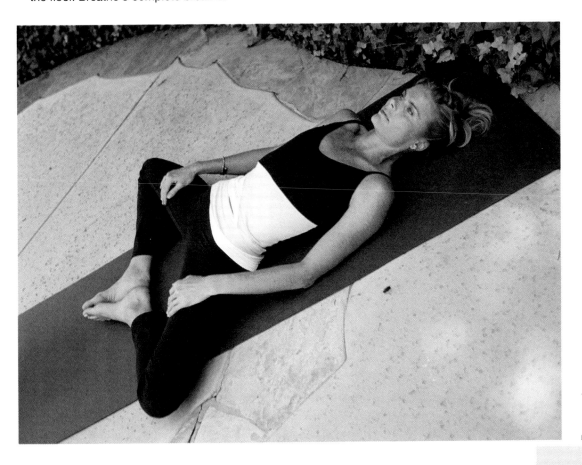

22. Relaxation Pose

—Lie on your back, your body totally released and relaxed. Breathe naturally, with no tension anywhere in your body. Arms lie gently at your side, palms facing up. Legs are spread in a small V, feet rolling easily outward or wherever feels most relaxed. Close your eyes.

—Try to spend 5 minutes in this pose, breathing and simply observing the energy in your body. Let your awareness scan your body from your toes to your head, checking in on how every-thing feels. Let thoughts roll across the mind and out of the mind; do not follow or hang onto them. Remember to let your face soften and melt. Imagine all your senses—sight, smell, taste, touch, and hearing—softening and taking a break from stimulation.

—When you are ready to get up, exhale and roll to one side. Breathe quietly, and on another exhale, push yourself up to sitting with your head coming up last.

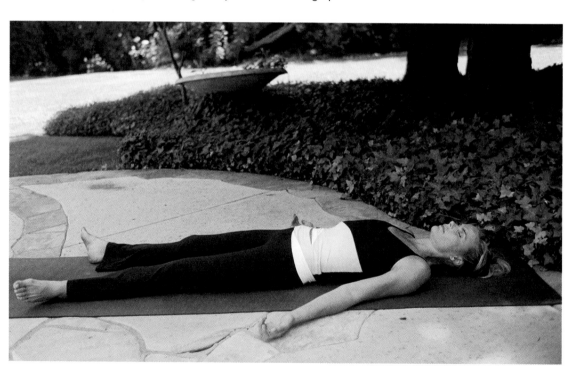

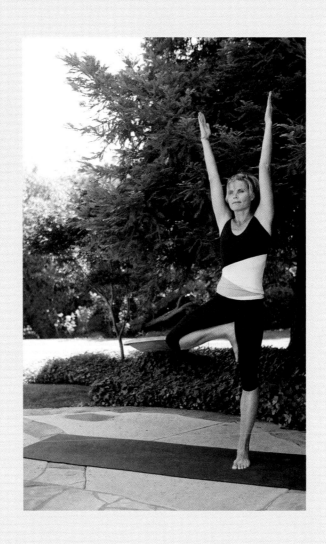

Food

Silence

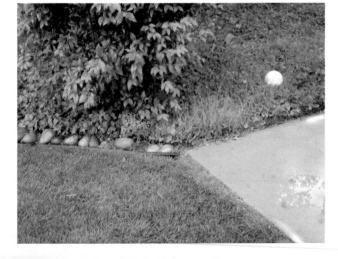

Exercise

Home

Silence

QUESTION: YOU ARE INVITED INTO A SIMPLE, WHITE ROOM CONTAINING NOTHING BUT A COMFORTABLE CHAIR THAT FACES A LARGE WINDOW. IT FRAMES A PATCH OF CLEAR, BLUE SKY. THERE ARE NO OTHER PEOPLE, NO SOUNDS, NOTHING TO READ, TOUCH, OR SMELL. YOU ARE TOLD THAT THERE IS NOTHING YOU NEED DO BUT SIMPLY SIT DOWN AND ENJOY THE ROOM, AND THAT YOU WON'T FALL BEHIND IN YOUR DAY. DO YOU FEEL:

A. Awkward and slightly anxious about the extreme quiet and empty space—it's too quiet in here!

B. Deep relief at the permission to turn off your thoughts and feelings for a spell—your whole body sighs with thanks.

C. Attracted to the idea of doing nothing but hesitant to let go—surely there's something more productive you should be doing?

QUESTION: YOU ARE IN THE MIDDLE OF ANOTHER BUSY DAY WHEN YOU DIS-COVER YOU'VE MISREAD THE TIME OF YOUR NEXT APPOINTMENT. YOU HAVE TEN EXTRA MINUTES BEFORE YOU NEED TO LEAVE YOUR WORKPLACE OR HOME. DO YOU:

A. Flip the computer back on to finish some work or return to your kitchen chores—can't waste a minute!

B. Sit down and make a list of the errands you need to do later, or make a few calls to friends you've been meaning to catch up with—not exactly work, but an efficient use of time.

C. Let the extra time slow you down. You take longer to walk or drive to the appointment, or you spend a few minutes sitting quietly or enjoying the outside before heading off; you're not ac-countable to anyone for these minutes, so why not let them drift by?

LEARNING TO GO TO A QUIET PLACE inside is one of the best gifts you can give yourself. When you turn down the volume, or even press pause on your day for a short while, you slow down the rush, enjoy more of your life, and find more fulfillment.

■ ■ ■

MY DAD TAUGHT ME TO FISH when I was about nine. He was teaching a group of kids, and the truth is I didn't get any special treatment as he never gave out the nitty-gritty dirt on how to fish like a pro, like him. Dad would spend a few minutes teaching a few of us to tie woolly worms and some other odd fish delicacies on a line, but if the fishing was particularly good, he left me alone on the bank with a rod and some flies and I was meant to figure it out on my own. One of the reasons he was such a poor fishing teacher was because his father, Ernest, wouldn't teach him to fish as a kid and so he taught himself, which I suspect is what he thought all of us should do as well. (It didn't occur to him that his three daughters might not be quite the self-starters he'd been at their age.) But the true reason he couldn't teach others was that he fished as easily as he breathed. There was nothing learned about it. It was who he was: the river was his haven, nature was his church, and fishing was his service. He became still and quiet on the stream, and he stayed there for hours, losing track of time, meditating on the nature of the wind and the feel of the water against his legs in his waders. He loved the sun and the cold equally, and with a rod and fly he celebrated the newness of the day. I watched and learned as I sat on the bank, absorbing all that he did.

Without realizing it, my dad was teaching me how to be still. He was showing me by example how to listen to "nothing" in a world that was filled with noise. All my chattering, nine-year-old thoughts would drop away, and I'd simply notice the world I was in. I'd hear grasshoppers chirping and the bite of a trout on a fishing line or the fish's flips on the surface of the silver creek. I'd hear the magpies' belligerent shrieks and the rustle of groundhogs in the sagebrush. Then a mouse rustling, a rabbit hopping, and a cacophony of dry leaves being stressed by gusts of wind. All these sounds became important to me as I sat motionless on the stream bank, patiently waiting for my father to finish his sermon to the fish. While fishing never became my thing, the sensation of stillness by that river became imprinted on every cell of me because in those moments I experienced peace and presence. Even today when I am not able to be in the outdoors, I go deep inside myself when meditating and remember the creek sounds. I follow them through my veins, and they are soothing. They fill my internal environment with peace. I take some time every day to sit in silence because the ultimate benefits of life come from being quiet and taking the time to feel how you feel inside.

■　■　■

THE ABILITY TO ACCESS THE PEACE within is one of the most valuable skills you can develop. It helps you move calmly forward in your life without getting derailed by stress. It helps you to feel more rested and restored by day and to sleep better at night. It gives you a deep well of patience so that you can respond to situations moderately instead of reacting emotionally. And it helps you get rid of some of the dead weight from your past that may be holding you back from happiness.

As we've seen so far, inner peace is not out of reach. You start to create inner peace when you eat in such a way that you create a clean internal environment. Then you increase the peace when you use exercise to shed stress, toxins, and superfluous thoughts. Yet the true benefits come when you take this project one step further inward and you practice having a quiet mind. When you deliberately choose silence in different ways throughout your day, you begin to build a core of calm deep at your center that will support you no matter what circumstances arise.

Wonderful things come from silence. It allows more to be revealed: during conversation, if one person keeps quiet rather than talking, the other person will inevitably say more. Silence allows things to have their full significance—think how when a great orator speaks, the quiet between her phrases carries as much weight as her words. And silence always rewards you with new discoveries. When you allow yourself to be silent outdoors, you invariably begin to hear sounds you'd never have heard if you were talking, just as I heard them on my childhood fishing expeditions.

It's the same when you cultivate silence in your mind. Aspects of yourself are revealed that you may not have noticed otherwise. Needs are prioritized, and excess demands can be dropped; you begin to see what is most significant and what is less. And you begin to notice more about the individual moments of your life. You become more present in your day as it happens rather than feeling swept along by its relentless pace and dumped out at bedtime, totally exhausted. As I first learned on the stream banks in Idaho, becoming comfortable with quiet helps you observe your life while you live it. Silence allows you to step back from the action and reflect on it rather than being

consumed by it. Though it can't be seen or touched, it's a cornerstone of the balanced life: the habit of silence will lead you to your peace.

Of course, it took me a long time to remember what I'd understood intuitively at age nine. Like many of life's truths, it was too simple—or perhaps just too subtle—for me to take seriously in my youth. Sitting still and doing nothing in order to remedy fear and anxiety was way too easy for a Hemingway. For years I tried to earn my peace the hardest way possible. Feeding myself inadequately created a kind of faux peace—the spaciness and fatigue that come from being undernourished most of the day. Working out to the point of exhaustion mellowed my mind—but mainly because I was too tired to think straight. It was only after I started regularly attending yoga classes in my twenties that the lightbulb went off. There might be a slower, quieter, and more sustainable road to peace. Lying in the Relaxation Pose at the end of each session was heaven: I would dive into the silence within me like a thirsty hiker at a lake.

What I discovered was that a quiet mind is a spacious mind. When I gave myself permission to lie there on my back without thinking, my normal mental clutter dropped away, my self-criticism dissolved, and in their place was relief. It was deeply restful yet different from sleep; I was not conked out but instead aware of this great tranquillity I'd found. In those ten minutes at the end of a class, things simply quieted. Like tap water that's cloudy when poured but crystal clear after it sits, the inner contents settled into clarity.

Discovering how much silence and space I had inside was like finding a whole other room in my house—a place to go that was just for me, where I could close the door on all the effort that my career and my marriage entailed and get some separation from pressing concerns of the day. Yet those ten minutes were way too short. A couple of hours after the class finished, I'd be back to where I started. Even though the teacher would always end the relaxation period by telling us students to "take this feeling off the mat and into the rest of your day," I secretly thought, "Yeah, right." It was one thing to be peaceful in the sanctuary of a yoga studio, and quite another to stay that way on the streets of New York City or in a heated debate with my husband.

Yet my curiosity was piqued: Why did I feel so good after yoga, and how could I make it last longer? As an experiment, I began to apply some of the techniques I'd learned in yoga class to the rest of my life. One, I made a conscious effort to notice my breath throughout the day; two, I tried observing what was happening without reacting to it; and three, I started taking more time to check in with how I was feeling and why. These were things I could do easily, no matter where I was or what was going on around me. I could do these things in hectic city streets, I could do them when my husband and I were at odds, and I could do them in the middle of a film shoot. Their effect surprised me: they worked for regular life as effectively as they did for exercise. By training my brain just as I had been training my body, I was able to find some space inside and step back from stressful circumstances.

These simple techniques, which are often referred to collectively as the practice of mindfulness, were subtle yet powerful teachers for me. Bringing my attention back to the task at hand, be it chopping vegetables, walking the dog, or even showering, was a way of becoming more present in my life as it was unfolding. I was noticing more of the moments rather than speeding through them in order to get to more important things. They slowed down the pace of my day ever so slightly, as if they were

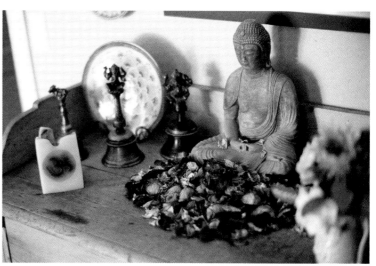

a remedy for the maxed-out modern condition (not to mention the dilemma of being a working wife or mom). I realized that with so much activity going on from dawn to dusk, if we don't give ourselves time to observe and reflect, we can miss out on half our lives because we're too busy to process them. (Who hasn't had that horrible realization at the end of the week—*what, it's Friday already?*—and then been stricken by fears that time is going by too quickly?) By living mindfully, I found more time.

Find quiet, find time. When your life is passing you by in a rush, you experience very little of it. When you slow down and feel the presence of yourself inside and take time with your activities, you create more time. You don't have the need to fill every moment. What seems important when you're in a frenzy of activity loses its power after a few minutes of silence. Is it really necessary to run to the mall and get a T-shirt that you saw in a magazine—will it solve any problems? Or can you wait to do that pile of ironing—you waited this long, so what is another few hours? Silence helps prioritize your actions. It also keeps you from making habitual choices that are not in your best interest, like having a bowl of ice cream when you are not hungry or it is not a day for a treat and you may be doing it for the wrong reasons. Giving yourself time separates you from your emotions, your patterns, and your knee-jerk reactions to desires.

QUESTION: AS YOU READ THIS CHAPTER, HOW FREQUENTLY DOES YOUR MIND SKIP TO ANOTHER TOPIC?

Do you keep thinking of other things you need to do right now? Do you frequently find that you've stopped reading and are daydreaming about someone or something else? Do you keep getting up to make a cup of tea or water the plants or make a phone call?

EACH TIME A THOUGHT, desire, or task pops into your mind as you read, notice it arriving. Pause, breathe, and ask yourself, "Could I just let it wait?" If your mind instinctively says no, just ask the question again. Let a long breath chop the thought off at the root. Notice if it's hard for you to say, "Yes, it could wait." Likewise, notice if it seems charming and fun to ignore the other tasks and stay with the words on the page.

If it's hard to let go of the thoughts that pop up, keep a piece of scrap paper and a pen by your side as you read. When the thought, desire, or task pops into your head, write down the single word that distracts—*tea, plant, Stephen*—and bring your attention back to the book. Letting go of the thought in a physical way by putting it on paper will lessen its power. When you feel satisfied with the amount of reading you have done, close the book and glance at the list to see which of those "urgent" tasks you still want to do. Follow through on those that still appeal.

Practice using the "Could I let it wait?" question during any activity in which you get distracted, such as working, writing, cleaning the house, paying bills—or even during an exercise session if you get tempted to cut out early and return phone calls. If you feel like you never have quite enough time, this will help you be more conscious of the small instances when you are losing time.

The more that I practiced mindful actions in my day-to-day life, the more I became convinced that in this space of inner quiet, my emotional pain and anxiety lost their power. The yoga relaxation reminded me of that nature feeling I'd had on the riverbanks: expansive, accepting, and okay with the world. The ability to get there again must still be inside me, I figured, but I just needed a bit of direction to find my way back. So I explored how to "take the peace off the mat" in more structured ways. When I was pregnant with my first daughter, Dree, I bought a guided meditation tape called *Opening to Receive.* I was uneducated about what meditation was and how exactly to go about it, so I plopped down on the couch and listened to this dreamy tape every afternoon. Not surprisingly, I did a lot of guided sleeping at first. But the guidance helped me to surrender to a softer state, at least to the extent that I was able to at that time.

As a mother-to-be, I instinctively knew that I wanted to find a calm and peaceful way to bring a child into the world. I knew that my upbringing was challenging and that if I wasn't careful, I would habitually fall into the practices I'd learned from my mother—her I'm-always-suffering attitude, her impatience with her husband and kids, and her unexpressed frustrations with life. I wanted to shed the patterns of my genetics. There were just too many members of my clan who had checked out of life through destructive behavior. With my own escapist tendencies popping up more and more—albeit through exercise and lettuce diets, not alcohol and drugs—it felt imperative to learn some way of checking in and staying present, especially as I created a brand-new family of my own. Even though I was meditat-

ing to a tape, it was a beginning; I felt able to look at myself for the first time. I was struck by how silent contemplation provided moments in which to feel unjudged and calm.

I continued with this simple relaxation practice for a few years. After the birth of my second daughter, Langley, I became more committed to my physical yoga practice, and it led me toward another branch of yoga called Kriya, a seated meditation technique that develops concentration and quiet mind. For the last fifteen years this technique has been my method of choice for beginning and ending my day with silence and reflection. It is just one of many ways that a person can choose to sit in silence and pause from activity; there are as many ways to sit still as there are leaves on a tree. It happens to be what works for me.

My daily meditation practice has become a spiritual practice. Just as my father used fishing to commune with nature, meditation is a sacred time for me to feel connected to something bigger than myself. This may or may not be another person's experience— I think that whatever arises when you regularly retreat inside yourself is your own business and nobody else's. But when I ask others about the pragmatic effects of a regular silent practice, their answers are often similar. They feel themselves changing: their mundane chores become less mundane; the rhythm of life seems to be calmer and their sleep is more satisfying; their gratitude increases, their acceptance of *things as they are right now* increases, and their relationships move toward greater harmony. During challenging moments when they feel overwhelmed or depressed, quietly checking in helps them regain stability. Through silent contemplation, their powers of concentration and focus have grown—and in this day of information overload and wall-to-wall technology, who doesn't want that?

For me, the small act of sitting quietly helps to temper any panic about the big-picture things that are out of my control. It dissolves much of the pain held over from my past and leads me to be aware of the present instead of worrying about the future. It brings me back again and again to a simple question: What is going on right here, right now, and what realistically can I change to make things better? Meditation is not miraculous; it is humbling. It always reminds me that even if I am on a journey toward the big goals, there's no point worrying about them. What I am most in control of are the small, good decisions I make each day.

I've tried many things in my search to feel saner, stronger, healthier, and happier. In my youth I spent a lot of money and time on healers and doctors and experts. Yet the best lessons of life have come from something that is completely free: simply being silent. Turning inward rather than constantly seeking outsiders' guidance is what helped me become the expert on myself. Little by little, I learned to hear my own inner wisdom and trust what it was telling me, which helped on all fronts, from family life to filmmaking. And becoming more aware of what I could reasonably do with my time, instead of thinking I should always be trying more and working harder, made me infinitely kinder to myself. That's why I think that if you never get quiet, you miss a lot of life's lessons.

This section of the program is dedicated to accessing that quiet zone through small actions that fit into your everyday life, no matter how crowded with activity and responsibility it may be. It's not about devoting masses of time to the project but rather using a few moments differently. First, learn to "Trust the Silence" by resisting the temptation to switch on sound and deliberately choosing quiet when you might otherwise have noise. Second, learn ways to "Shed the Stress" by adjusting your reactions to stressful situations and doing exercises that restore calm. Third, "Sit Down and Shut Up": Bring curiosity to a cushion, and explore how it feels to devote a few minutes of the day to doing nothing at all. And fourth, with "The Quiet Power Tool," discover how silent practices like meditation and mindful behavior give you insight into your life and help you create a happier existence. The practices in this section may be subtle, but they are immensely important and empowering, especially in a world that seems to turn quicker every year. They are moderate actions that any of us can take to recover, rest, and restore ourselves on an ongoing basis.

In the Food and Exercise sections of the program, you are building up awareness of what makes you feel good and what does not. Now you begin to peel the layers of the onion and see a little deeper. It's unavoidable: when you bring more silence into your life, you get to know yourself better. You have moments of clarity that take you below the constant stream of thoughts and concerns on the surface of your mind. You get some answers to the questions *Who am I?* and *Why do I do what I do?* Building a balanced and peaceful life is, as we've seen, not just about following some tips in this or any other book. It comes from acquiring a certain amount of self-knowledge. On this journey to knowing yourself better, I believe that silence is where the most potent transformation can occur.

It's also a place you can return to when you need to make sense of your life. Moments of stress will hit you when your life feels stupid to you or you don't know what your purpose is. They strike me just as frequently as anyone else. Nobody lives in a state of constant nirvana; we all face moments of drudgery or confusion. The key to calm is finding satisfaction or even beauty in the modest daily moments rather than finding them only in the dramatic highlights. Don't fall into the trap of waiting for some extreme makeover to give you a better life; make your current life better by finding peace in small ways every day.

Our true home is in the present moment. To live in the present moment is a miracle. The miracle is not to walk on water. The miracle is to walk on the green Earth in the present moment, to appreciate the peace and beauty that are available now. Peace is all around us—in the world and in nature—and within us—in our bodies and our spirits. Once we learn to touch this peace, we will be healed and transformed. It is not a matter of faith, it is a matter of practice. We need only to find ways to bring our body and mind back to the present moment so we can touch what is refreshing, healing, and wondrous.

—THICH NHAT HANH

Give Peace a Chance

It can seem so intimidating to speak of quiet-mind practices. Words like *mindfulness* and *meditation* can sound like things that *other* people do, not you. If you're thinking, "I can't do that. My mind won't be still," know that this is the very reason you are learning these practices in conjunction with changing your eating habits and bringing a new focus to exercise and creating a physical space in your home to be still.

The new eating habits help turn the volume down in your internal environment. Getting off the caffeine, sugar, and junk-food swings and fueling yourself with the slow and sustained energy of wholesome foods creates a clean and quiet chemistry. Plus, when you cook and consume your meals in a slower and more deliberate way, you are eating with mindfulness. The new exercise habits train the brain to focus on what is happening in the present moment—the breath and bodily sensations occurring in this instant—instead of roaming from thought to thought about what might happen tomorrow or already happened yesterday.

When you put effort into these two areas, therefore, you have already laid the way for this third area of quiet-mind practices. The biggest obstacle is likely your own resistance. The little devil on your shoulder might say, "What is the point of allotting time to something that I can't see or touch or prove makes me thinner or prettier or better?" Don't listen to it. The trick with these practices is to deprogram that part of you that believes that something simple is not valuable. We believe that if something doesn't take lots of effort or produce a spectacular success that it doesn't count for much. But following that line of thinking has made us more stressed, so let's just trust that for the duration of this program, there's a reason you are investigating being quiet. Think of it as prescribed downtime: moments in which the goodness of what you're doing over the course of this 30-Day Program can take shape. (And by the way, people will notice you look calmer, lighter in spirit, and probably younger because you are not tight with tension.)

Trust the Silence

THERE'S A LITTLE EXERCISE I used to do during public speaking appearances about health and wellness. In the middle of the talk I'd fall silent and simply stand on the podium, looking at the audience. Five seconds of silence would pass; people looked at me expectantly. Then ten seconds—a few quizzical expressions. *Is the mike broken?* Twenty seconds. Raised eyebrows and nudging elbows—*she's totally forgotten her speech!* Thirty seconds. Now people were uncomfortable and squirming in their seats. They had that hot-under-the-collar look. *Something's really wrong here!* And then I'd finally say, "This is one of the most important components of a balanced life. Silence. So why are you all uneasy with it?"

The answer is that we've been trained to fill silence up, and we do it well. Put your hand up if you frequently walk into your home and switch on music or the TV. Or if you get in your car and automatically flip on the radio. If you walk or take public transportation rather than drive, maybe you stick in your iPod ear buds and turn on the tunes before you hit the street (that little white box is today's don't-leave-home-without-it accessory). We have become so accustomed to noise and activity that when that noise is taken away, the silence can be jarring. Suddenly we go from filled up, switched on, entertained, or distracted to nothing. No sound. No distraction. The silence, to our unaccustomed ears, seems deafening.

Nothingness is not a state we are comfortable with. We have learned to be oriented toward action, success, and achievement. Productivity is prized—in fact, busyness is equated with importance: she who has more meetings and more demands on her plate is often assumed to be more of a power player. (Have you ever known people who boast about how little sleep they get because their life is so hectic?) Doing nothing and surrendering to silence, on the other hand, carries little value. That is what I saw when I zipped my lip during the talk. The quiet in the room sparked in people that awkward fear of wasting time. Doing nothing pushes all our buttons: it suggests that somehow we've failed.

Yet I think the opposite is true. There is something fabulous about being in a big group of people and not hearing the noise and madness. If it makes us uncomfortable, then let's be uncomfortable. See what that discomfort brings up, and use it to learn something about yourself. When you choose silence over noise in any situation—whether it's in a group or alone at home—you are not being unproductive. On the contrary, you give yourself permission to rest for a moment and stop trying to control every part of life. You get a breather.

Not long ago I was in northern India, where I was fortunate enough to spend time visiting a community of Buddhist monks. It struck me how they prize silence. They speak only when it's necessary, and they speak only kindly. The value they put on silence is a fundamental to their beatific states. Before we do anything else to bring calm and serenity to our minds, we must learn to prize silence in our external environments. Quiet is something that is rightfully ours, not something to avoid. It was quiet in the womb, it will be quiet at the end of our lives, but in trying to squeeze more experiences out of all the years in between, we have become compulsive about filling up the quiet at all costs. We keep the information pouring in and the stimulation switched on, perhaps because we have a desperate fear of boredom or maybe even a fear of running out of time. The activity and noise reassure us that we're living to the fullest during our brief tenure here.

Yet if we can drop the idea that silence is an emptiness that should be filled, and learn to enjoy it for the respite it offers, we'll start to move toward greater calm inside. Instead of being suspicious of silence, we need to learn to prize it and use it wisely.

QUESTIONS: JUST AS YOU LOOKED AT WHY YOU AUTOMATICALLY MIGHT SWITCH ON MUSIC TO EXERCISE,

LOOK AT HOW YOU ACT IN THE REST OF YOUR LIFE.

IF YOU NOTICE THAT YOU TEND TO SWITCH ON STIMULATION EVERY CHANCE YOU GET, ASK YOURSELF IF YOU'RE RESISTING SILENCE WITHOUT REALIZING IT.

IS BEING WITH YOURSELF NOT EXCITING ENOUGH, OR DO YOU HATE BEING BORED?

Do you multitask in any the following ways: Cooking while watching TV?

Enjoying a cup of tea while listening to talk radio?

Filing paperwork with a rock CD playing or working on the computer with Internet radio streaming through?

IT IS TRUE that music and media can take the drudgery out of menial tasks, but our goal here is to adjust our ears to a new norm, quiet, and start training ourselves to do one thing at a time. Try stripping out the sound and focusing on the primary action alone. Instead of filling up the silence, why not let the silence fill us for a change?

We operate under the premise that noise brings with it new clarity and new stimulation and fun. But noise so often brings confusion, another layer of activity that muddles what we are trying to do. Begin to notice whether noise in your day is adding to your quality of life or adding confusion.

Silence

Exercise: Sacred Morning, Sacred Evening

My grandfather Ernest claimed that he saw every sunrise of his adult life; he always awoke early to write in those silent magic hours of the day, before the world got busy. You don't have to be a writer to find something special in starting your day with quiet. For one week, commit to starting *and ending* the day in a quiet environment: no TV, radio, or music for the first thirty minutes you're awake, and none for the last. Use this quiet time to mindfully go about your morning and evening. Notice if you feel different during your day after a calm start, or if it's easier to wind down into restful sleep.

TIP If you find that silence in the home gnaws at you and makes you uneasy, and you are tempted to just give up and turn on the morning show instead, try to "release the resistance" to it, just as we have practiced in earlier segments. First, try to locate the sensation of unease in your body. Sit with it for a moment, and breathe into it. Ask yourself, "Can I accept this feeling of unease/irritation/frustration?" Repeat the question several times until you find that you answer yes. Then simply ask yourself, "Can I let it go?" By releasing some of the resistance in your mind and heart, you may find that the reality of the situation is easier to live with than you think.

Exercise: A Day Without a Cell Phone

Pick one day this week to be free of your phone and e-mail or pager and, ideally, to interact minimally with other people. Plan ahead, and if you have children, see if you can get someone to watch them for a bit. (If that's not possible, you can certainly do a technology-free day while in the company of your kids.) Sunday is often the best day to do this, especially if you can go somewhere quiet for part of it, like to a museum, to a bookstore, or for an extra long walk. No matter what you do with your day, put the phone away. Tell friends and family you will be back in service later. (If you do have small kids, switch off your ringer and let your voicemail pick up any calls, which you can check if they come from important numbers.) Try using some of this time to do various segments of the 30-Day Program: buying and cooking healthy food for the week ahead; doing your yoga practice; making changes to your living space; and so on. Notice whether the day feels longer or shorter. Notice if being with yourself is enjoyable, neutral, or perhaps difficult. What kind of thoughts and feelings come up when it's no one but you?

BONUS: Make this day a Time Fast as well. Do not wear a watch or any other gadget that tells you the time. Turn alarm clocks to face away. Allow the day to unfold at the pace it unfolds. Let every task take as long as it needs to take. Eat when you are hungry, not when the clock says lunch. Notice how often you feel an impulse to know what time it is. Constantly checking the time can serve to remind you that you don't have enough of it. See how it feels to operate at a natural pace.

Society is organized in such a way that even when we have some leisure time, we don't know how to use it to get back in touch with ourselves. We have millions of ways to lose this precious time—we turn on the TV or pick up the telephone, or start the car and go somewhere. We are not used to being with ourselves, and we act as if we don't like ourselves and are trying to escape from ourselves.

—THICH NHAT HANH, *Being Peace*

Now that you've turned down the volume in your external environment, it's time to start turning down the volume on yourself. In order to build a core of calm inside, you must learn how to still the rush of thoughts and emotions that constantly flood your mind. Just as with the noisy food we talked about, if you can clear out some of the superfluous mental activity, you can better maintain a state of steady, sustained calm.

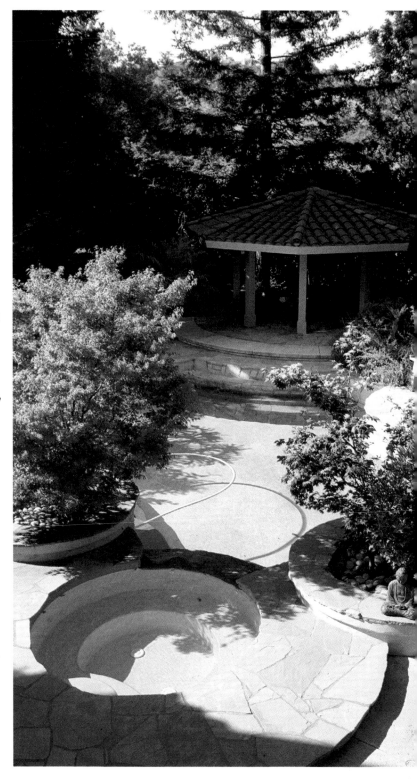

Shed the Stress

QUESTION: HOW DOES AN EPISODE OF UNEXPECTED PRESSURE MAKE YOU FEEL?

A. My brain goes into a whir of high speed to control the situation, and I don't even feel anything in my body until later.

B. I feel surges of anger and frustration in my physical body: my heart rate increases, and I get tight inside.

C. I want to hide and not have to deal. I feel physically shut down, like I'm stuck and can't move.

D. I wish I had a better way of dealing.

QUESTION: AFTER A CONFRONTATION THAT PUSHES ALL YOUR BUTTONS, WHAT DO YOU DO?

A. Reach for a glass of wine, cocktail, or cupcake.

B. Want to yell at someone or something to get the frustration out.

C. Tune out with some kind of entertainment.

D. Go shopping and get some retail therapy.

E. Wish I had a better way of dealing.

PRACTICING CALM during low-key parts of your day is one thing; keeping your cool when the pressure builds is another. In order to truly take care of yourself, it's important to look at the way you respond to stress. If you can acquire a few tools that enable you to deal with unexpected situations in a moderate and quiet manner, you can dispel stress kindly rather than reacting to it, feeding it, and making it worse. You can't always change the circumstances you find yourself in, but you can change your reaction to them.

Consider the ways you react to pressurized situations. Do your reactions turn up the pressure in your body and mind? You might lash out and yell or argue, as if putting your feelings out there will free you from pain. But all that does is stress your physiological state more; your heart rate increases, muscles tighten, your breath gets tight. Perhaps you turn to a stimulant—a coffee or cigarette to help you think straight, a cocktail to take the edge off anger, or some junk food to soothe hurt spirits. Yet these things do the opposite of dispelling stress: caffeine and sugar agitate your chemistry and help to release stress hormones. The crash after consuming noisy foods can make you feel headachy, dulled, and exhausted. If you respond to stress by curling up in a ball and trying not to feel it, this too is rarely helpful. What is needed is a change or a shift, and being immobilized simply sinks you farther into a funk.

When I face a situation that is about to spark a stressful response in my body and mind, I actively turn toward silence to find a solution. Quiet is the cure. Doing a conscious exercise when things get nasty rather than staying with the stress and letting it build—or feeding it by thinking and stewing about what happened—is like twisting the cap off a bottle of soda instead of shaking it. The energy gets released instead of building up until it explodes. I've had to train myself to do this because my natural tendency is to overthink and overanalyze. But then I remind myself that all things shift, including negative feelings, and that I can hasten that shift by breathing and consciously relaxing.

This puts me in a good position to take whatever action is necessary. I lose some of the tension and anxiety and go straight toward the cause of the problem, making whatever change is needed to solve it. And I've found that peace is infectious: if I approach the issue in a peaceful frame of mind and with at least a little bit of joy in my heart, the other parties involved almost always mirror that, and the interaction becomes less trying.

Getting quiet might seem too subtle of a response in times of urgency, and the overwhelming instinct may be to shout and scream or have a double vodka and tonic. But in fact, going deep inside yourself brings about the most change in your feelings. You might doubt that it will work, but you have to make yourself do it. Even if you only remember to do it after you've already blown your stack, know that some conscious silent exercises will bring you back into balance.

WHAT IS STRESS?

We've all been stuck in traffic and watched people react differently to it. One person may take it in stride while someone else is totally freaking out. Why is that? Because one person is fighting the situation, and the other is accepting it as it is. Technically, stress doesn't exist. There is no such thing as an inherently stressful situation. A situation exists, and your response to it can either be stressed—the fight-or-flight reaction—or not stressed. Your reaction to an event is your choice; what upsets you does not necessarily upset the person next to you. When it comes to feeling stress, you have a choice: you can go there or not.

I believe that stressful responses come from one thing: a resistance to unexpected change. I realize as I get older that I have no control over things that I thought surely I could control. Even if an event is firmly inked in the schedule, there's no guarantee it will happen. Even if I'm sure I've figured out how to make something work, there's no assurance it will pan out as planned. The natural way of the world is always going to be a bit curvy, so why do we keep trying to go forward in a straight line and fight like banshees when we get knocked off course? Stress comes when the idea of having to adapt to a new circumstance makes you angry, fearful, or irked. If you are loose and flexible and can bend in the wind, your stress level is much lower. If you can lose the resistance, you can lose the stress.

To be flexible, it helps to have some tools that give you power to change your state: you know that whatever comes up, you will be able

The Health Risks of Stress

Stress makes you sick—and there is a proven physiological reason for it. Our bodies are built to respond to dangerous situations with lightning-quick physical reactions. Our Stone-Age ancestors evolved the fight-or-flight response in order to escape from saber-toothed tigers and other predators, and that response is still part of our complex physiology today. When our senses register an imminent threat, our body goes into red alert. Adrenal glands shoot out stress hormones so that we can either turn and fight or take flight as fast as possible. Our heart pumps two or three times its normal speed, coagulants are released into the blood to thicken it so it can clot if we are injured, and our surface blood vessels close for extra protection against wounds (which causes our blood pressure to soar). Lactic acid floods our muscles so they tighten in preparation for sudden movement. All nonurgent functions like digestion, sexual response, and most important of all, immune system functioning, shut down temporarily so that energy is available for our urgent needs. (We may have the impulse to shed any waste in our systems too, to make us lighter for a quick getaway.)

Of course, marauding predators rarely besiege us today; the vast majority of stress-inducing situations we encounter are far from life threatening. Yet if something triggers a sudden surge of fear or anger in us, the body will jump to emergency mode regardless of the cause; it doesn't know the difference between the threat of tigers and the threat of being late for a job interview. That's why seemingly mundane things like a traffic jam or an adversarial meeting with a coworker can cause such physical distress. Over time, if we experience this stress response frequently, even at low levels, its impact accumulates. For starters, it is physically exhausting to go into fight-or-flight mode; afterward, you need to fall into fatigue in order to repair. The toll that it takes on our bodies may bring about physical and mental symptoms such as acute anxiety, panic attacks, restlessness, insomnia, as well as heart disease, immune and sexual dysfunction, and migraine headaches. Even if these conditions don't occur, exposure to steady streams of stress will affect your emotional state and your relationships. If adrenaline surges in your system all day long, by the time you get home you might be impatient and irritable with those around you.

It is common in this era for people to turn to pharmaceutical drugs in order to remedy these physical and mental symptoms. Yet in many cases it is possible to shift our physiological, mental, and emotional states ourselves. We can learn to trigger the "relaxation response," a physiological response that slows our heart rate, calms the nerves, and lowers blood pressure. Deliberately practicing stress-busting techniques will trigger this response and help you avoid the constant high level of stress that, when ignored, can drastically compromise your health and well-being.

to shift back to center and feel okay. Here are four stress-busting techniques to change your physical, mental, and emotional responses when in states of stress. They are arranged in order of magnitude from simple anxiety on up to panic.

State: Anxious, Irritable, Flighty

Stress-Buster: Relaxation Breath

Yoga teaches us that we breathe too fast in our culture, which leads to elevated physical and mental states—not only faster heart-beats and higher blood pressure but also too many thoughts, including too many negative thoughts. By slowing down the breath, you therefore calm the body state and slow the mind. You initiate the relaxation response.

Yogis believe that breath is the bridge between mind and body. Developing aware-ness of the breath takes us out of our thinking heads and into our feeling bodies. In other words, by focusing on our breath we become more present in our body and less dominated by our ego and mind. Furthermore, yogis say that breath is how you bring *prana*—the vital life energy of the universe, what Chinese tradi-tions call *chi*—into your body. That's why if you skimp on your breath, taking only tiny sips of it like a guppy in a bowl, you are constrict-ing your relationship to the world. (Yogis also say prana can be absorbed only through the nose—another good reason to inhale through the nose, not the mouth.) In stressful situations our tendency is to tighten up and constrict, like hedgehogs rolling into a ball to protect them-selves. Using relaxation breath expands you

so that you can find a new, better state. Each inhale invites a better state of body and mind.

HOW TO: Diaphragmatic breaths will help you enter a calm and introspective state. They will slow down the breath and heart rate and cut off emotions before they can rise up and flood your mind. Diaphragmatic breathing is slightly different from what you learned in the exercise section. Sit comfortably and soften your gaze or close your eyes. As you slowly inhale through the nose, let the rib cage expand and pull in the belly; this pulls the diaphragm (the muscle between the chest and abdomen) downward so there is more space in the upper body. Pause for a moment at the top of the breath. As you exhale, let the belly expand outward gently. Do this in a slow, rhythmic way for one minute whenever you find your mind getting anxious. Diaphragmatic breathing creates the inward-looking state suitable for con-templation and reflection. On your inhale, feel your heart expanding, which is a way to get out of your head and into your body, thus calming the mind.

TIP Use this breath proactively to avoid stress. Do it for three minutes before entering a situation that you know causes you to get emotional, anxious, or constricted, for example, waiting for take-off on an airplane, before a big meeting or presentation, before a discussion with a spouse, partner, or family members, or on your way to pick up a carload of hyper-excited kids.

Stress-Buster: The Balanced Breath

When you feel unsettled and flighty, try doing alternate-nostril breathing for two minutes. It is a yogic breath that helps to balance the right and left hemispheres of the brain and is often done in preparation for deep relaxation or meditation. Raise your right hand to your face, and place your thumb on your right nostril and your pinky and ring finger lightly on your left nostril. Hold your right nostril closed, and inhale slowly up your left nostril. Pause, and while your lungs are full of air, press the left nostril closed while lightening the pressure on the right one. Exhale slowly out your right nostril, then inhale up your right nostril, pause, and while your lungs are full of air, switch your fingers so that your right nostril is closed again. Exhale. Do ten cycles of this breath at first, adding length as you get comfortable. Try this in the early morning before meditating, before bed to wind down a busy mind, or any time that you need to reset your thoughts.

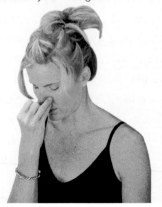

State: Stuck in a Rut, Foggy-Headed, Down in the Dumps

Stress-Buster: Get Walking

The Indian philosopher Krishnamurti said that whenever he felt stress, it was time to get up and walk. (When asked what he thought about when he walked, he said, "Walking.") Get moving, get breathing, and walk around the block. The simple act of changing your environment can start to change the mood. Often the very time you don't want to move—wanting to curl into yourself, retreat onto the couch, and lose yourself in TV—is the time when you need to make the effort to move. That's the time to say, "No. I'm getting up. I'm walking out the door, and I'm going to at least walk around the block. I'm going to take myself out of this situation because I have to." It may be that the energy of the room or of other people is dragging you down and getting you stuck. The only way to get unstuck is to shift yourself into a different state. In addition, walking by its very nature curbs your tendency to panic and seek instant change (which only leads to more frustration). There's only so far you can get on foot; walking gives you a healthy reality check: *"What can I realistically achieve today?"*

State: Maxed Out, Exhausted, at Low Ebb

Stress-Buster: Restorative Pose

Lying on your back on the floor with your legs up the wall may look goofy to your coworkers or kids, but it is one of the best things you can do for your body. Yoga features many kinds of inverted (upside-down) poses because they trigger a physiological calming response in the nervous system. Putting your legs up the wall stimulates receptors in your heart and neck, causing them to send messages to your brain via the nerves to slow down your heart rate and lower your blood pressure. This healing and restorative pose creates tranquillity in your mind and body and subtly energizes you so that when you stand up you can get on with what you need to do. (Plus, it gets that pesky bloating out of your legs.)

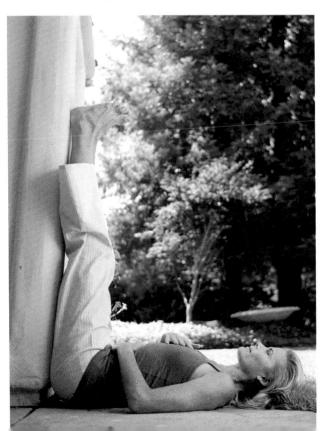

USE FOR: After things have gotten trying and you feel you've been through the wringer. If the day has done a number on you and you want to leave thoughts of it behind before nightfall.

HOW TO: Turn off noise, and reduce distraction in the room if possible. Dim the lights if you can. Place a firm pillow six inches from wall, under your lower back, then place a folded blanket under your spine and head. To enter the pose, sit on the center of the pillow with your side facing the wall. Press your hands down onto the pillow to hold it in place, then swing your legs up and onto the wall as you lie down with your back on the folded blanket. Scoot your pelvis on the pillow so that the very bottom of your tailbone is hanging off the pillow (this will give your pelvis a slight backbend). Make sure your spine and head are completely supported, and keep your legs lightly activated by pressing gently into the wall. Do this for between 1 and 3 minutes. A scarf draped over your eyes enhances the experience.

CHAIR MODIFICATION: If putting your legs up the wall is uncomfortable, start by putting them over a chair. Place a firm pillow or folded blankets on the floor, about one foot from a chair. Place another thin blanket or pillow on the floor for your head. Begin by sitting as above. Swing your legs up over the chair seat, and lay your shoulders on the floor with your head on the thin pillow and the bottom of your tailbone hanging off the firm pillow. If you don't feel comfortable, move the chair farther away from your tailbone.

Silence

TIP The yoga posture known as Child's Pose is another instant calmer for out-of-control emotions. The forward bend will soothe the nervous system and allow your mind to turn gently inward. Sit on your shins with your feet slightly apart. Let your bottom sit on the floor between your feet. Then simply curl forward to rest your forehead on the floor, with your arms at your sides. Breathe quietly for a few minutes, and let your thoughts go. The position offers comfort and a feeling of security. Stretch your arms on the floor in front of your head if that feels good. Even if the only pose you do is this one for a few minutes a day, you have initiated a yoga and meditation practice.

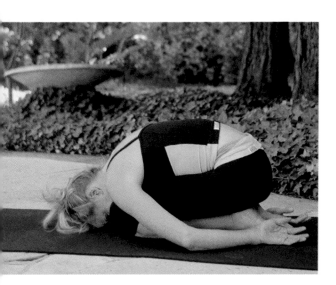

TIP If you feel conflicted about wasting time, softly repeat the affirmation, "The world can wait." Grant yourself permission to take this time-out, knowing that you and everyone else will benefit if you attend to yourself for a few minutes.

Picture Your Oasis

Everyone has his or her own idea of a personal oasis—the ultimate refuge that would feel most restful, restorative, and soothing. When life gets rough, lie down if you can, close your eyes, breathe with calm and quiet, and ask yourself where that place is for you. Is it a place from childhood, is it an imaginary place, is it somewhere in your current life that you wish you could be, like at home on your bed? In my case, I go to a high mountaintop, since I grew up in mountains and for me it's very powerful to feel like I've arrived at the top. For other people it may be the ocean, watching the tides flow in and out, or on a lakeside at twilight. You want a place that makes you feel empowered and free and that reminds you that in the greater world, things come and go constantly. Spend a few minutes sitting or lying down, and focus on this place, bringing all the details to life and noticing all the sensations in it. On a mountaintop you may see clouds skittering across the sky, and you watch them roll out and move out. At the ocean you will see waves constantly refreshing themselves. Near a lake at twilight, the evening comes on with the sound of crickets. Let the scene inspire trust in you that all situations change, no matter how stuck you think you are in a stressful situation. Your body and mind will calm immensely. Do it for as long as you need. It is a good one to do before falling asleep.

State: Fearful, Panicked, Disempowered

Stress-Buster: Visualize Your Oasis

Sometimes you need to stop the world for a few moments and go off to a better place. Doing a creative visualization exercise in which you imagine yourself in a setting that restores and soothes is very healing. It's a great way to learn how to relax and instantly focus your attention inward, which makes it a good preliminary exercise for meditation.

■ ■ ■

OUTSIDE KETCHUM, IDAHO, where I grew up, was a gnarly run on the local Baldy Mountain. I never really ran it because it was all uphill. It was vicious. In the summertime I'd half-run, half-speed-walk it as part of the high school ski team, and frequently I went back there alone to escape from the drama in my home. Hills were always a draw to me because even though they were hard to get up, you always reached an end and could feel a sense of completion. I loved getting to the top of Baldy, arriving at an enormous vista, a place where I could see. It made everything clear. So when I go to my special place of peace in my mind today, it's always at the top of that mountain, looking over a familiar sight: the Sawtooth Mountains towering high, and the flat valley down below dotted with little houses and roads. I imagine the cool breeze on my skin, the way temperature can change from one gust to the next. I hear the sound of new weather blowing in. This visualization always makes me feel empowered and safe, and I know that new inspiration and faith will come to me there, just as it did when I was a teen.

You Deserve Peace

It can be hard for women to devote time to themselves. We often have so many responsibilities and demands on our time that we feel pulled apart at the seams. Finding more minutes to devote to our well-being can seem like an indulgence. Yet it's important to recast these practices in a new light: they are neither indulgent nor terribly time consuming. Silence in all its manifestations can be an extremely serviceable tool for some of the hardest jobs: being a mom, being a wife, working plus keeping a home together, or simply being on your own and staying healthy and happy. Taking a few minutes to find that peaceful place inside keeps us from flying off the handle, or if we do fly off the handle, it helps us recover our cool. It helps us start the day with enthusiasm and end it with acceptance. And it helps enormously in crises.

Too often women push themselves to keep going so that the only time they sit down and rest is when they're exhausted, burned out, or sidelined with sickness. In fact, many spiritual teachers say it's pain that gets you to stop, meditate, and beg for help because pain is the only thing that slows you down. But we can create a better way of doing things, a more proactive and preventive way, taking time to cultivate a little more peace every day so we don't have to experience pain before taking stock of our lives. For any woman, making quiet a part of her lifestyle should be considered part of her preventive health-care plan: something that takes minimal expenditure upfront but gives major payback later.

Step back from the drama of your life, and you often see that your problems repeat themselves: the same things come up time after time, and you respond to them in the same stressful ways. Learning better responses to your problems doesn't mean that life becomes instantly pain free. You still have to put in the effort. But it does mean that you have a set of tools that work to combat stress, and you can try different techniques to keep plugging away at the problems. Even if a deeply seated issue is holding you back from happiness, you just keep using your tools, chipping away at it. And suddenly one moment you'll discover, "Oh, wow! These clouds are moving on!" It is wonderfully empowering to take responsibility for your emotional well-being.

Sometimes all you need is a hug or a few words of comfort. But do you always get those hugs and comforting words from your partner, your friends, your kids? Of course not. So when you don't get the support you need in the "right" way, you need to make the right way for you. Find your space, take a walk, or in my case sit in the car for as long as it takes for the energy to shift.

Last Christmas, a truckload of stress hit me at once. My body was injured, my teenagers were having meltdowns, my husband and I were clashing, there were too many people in the house, and old memories were for some un-known reason rising

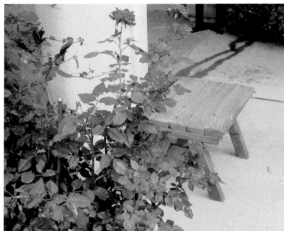

up to haunt me. It all got to be too much, and the panic rose in me as it sometimes does for any woman with a family—I want out of this, Calgon, take me away! But it was Christmas Eve, and the only thing I could do was escape to find a place to be alone. I walked outside in a snowstorm and sat in my parked, cold car meditating and releasing my anxiety until I felt I could go inside again with a clear and level head. My resentment had lessened, and the world was okay again.

Sometimes we have to nurture ourselves by ourselves. You may think you want the week off, but sometimes all you need is a little time to let the mind rest and the pity party die off and for everyone, especially you, to get back to normal, and then you feel like you have had a minivacation. Just sit with your problem long enough with the knowledge that everything changes and the intention that all will be well soon. You have the right to take an hour or two alone to do what you can so that you don't explode, and likely when you return things will have settled down. But take your time, and do it without guilt, for guilt will keep you feeling awful and you won't get the relief you need.

We have to know we are loved and valued beyond belief and that our family would not be happy without us, as we sometimes think they would. When we find some peace in our silent prac-tice, we find some perspective on our personal life. We are reassured that the laughs usually outweigh the tears and that having a balanced family means you get it all: pain, laughter, injuries, and bliss. That is the very nature of balance. If you know you can take care of your mental and emotional state, you are reassured that you need to don't throw it all away when life seems too much. If you can just sit quietly, trusting that all things come to balance, and surrender some control, then you are finding your way.

Sit Down and Shut Up

ONCE YOU HAVE BEGUN to bring awareness to breath and quiet, it's not as hard as you might think to create a seated meditation practice. The benefits of taking a few minutes to deliberately sit in silence at the same time every day are manifold. If noise creates confusion, then silence creates clarity. Your body and mind get a chance to unwind every day and unload whatever small stresses accumulate. Your cells begin to memorize what it feels like to be in this calmer physiological state, with its slower breathing, slower heart rate, softer muscles, and other effects of the relaxation response's "rest and digest" mode. After a while, a calmer, less reactive state becomes your new bottom line: it's where you start from most of the time, not a special state that you get to only through deep concentration. This will affect every part of your life. Your intuition grows and your creativity expands because good ideas float up to the surface when you get still inside. You are able to be more spontaneous, and even self-esteem gets a boost. Meditation develops awareness—a quality bigger than the thinking mind.

One of the teachers with whom I regularly sit has told me that women find meditation easier than men because we are more comfortable with letting go of our egos and just being with whatever comes up. At the same time, feelings of hurt or pain or joy can take center stage in our experience and cloud our perception of the truth. While men feel anger, they are prone to holding onto their egos and often stuff their emotions. Meditation helps women step back a bit from surges of feeling and calmly respond to situations without judging or reacting to them. When we have a spacious and quieter mind, we can develop the habit of looking before reacting—we literally get some space between ourselves and the issues in our lives. It doesn't make difficult issues less difficult, but it makes dealing with difficulties easier because a meditation practice helps you to observe your life's problems instead of becoming them.

Having a regular, daily meditation practice is like digging a well. Each time you do it, you get closer to a source of compassion and patience until at some point you will be able to drink from it any time at all. But notice I said a water well, not a gold mine. You don't automatically hit an immediate, blissful, wonderful state when you meditate. It is a constant journey, an exploration into yourself.

Sitting can be a very nurturing experience as well. On those days when you feel lonely or have the blues, take to a comfortable spot to sit in silence. Consider that you are breathing in atoms of air that have traveled in and out of untold numbers of other people—you are literally sharing the basic element of life with your fellow women and men. By doing nothing more than breathing, we experience a sweet moment of intimacy in a world that can sometimes seem huge and lonely.

Until fairly recently in our culture, meditation practices were always attached to some religious beliefs or Eastern philosophy. But today people are starting to realize that meditation is simply a technique. It is a practice that helps you rest and restore, to gather insight into your existence, and to stay present. No special belief system, lifestyle, or larger idea is necessary in order to benefit from it. Increasingly I find that interest in meditation transcends cultural barriers because we all have the same problems.

To state it simply, to meditate means to concentrate the mind on an object—be it the breath, a word, or even an object—then to move into a relaxed awareness of that object, and finally, to let go of it completely so that you can restfully and peacefully exist in a state without active thought and stimulation. Many people ask, "How can you have 'no thoughts' in meditation?" You still have thoughts, but if you don't hold on to them and instead keep returning to the empty space, you are meditating. In essence, meditation is a practice of harnessing the mind so that your thoughts don't run wild and lead you where they will. When the mind is gently harnessed, you can let it be for a while—you simply stop using it—and let that quieter, more ineffable quality of awareness take over. That's when your whole self gets a chance to rest and restore.

Physiologically, there is good reason for doing the practice. In my tradition, Kriya yoga, we say that slowing down the breath is a way to lower the toxic load on the body. Since mental activity creates a faster pulse and breath rate, when you are thinking lots of thoughts the whole system has to work harder to shed carbon dioxide and take in more oxygen. Levels of activity in the body stay elevated. Meditation lets the body come down from those elevated levels for a set amount of time every day. It offers relief from being so mentally and physically active.

In sleep, you might spend much of your night dreaming with an active mind; it's why you can wake up in the morning feeling so fatigued. Meditation helps your mind and body sink to a deeper level of rest so that afterward you feel renewed and refreshed. A regular practice will help you have more energy in your day and sleep better at night, which is a key to achieving ongoing well-being. (It's also a key to staying slim: too little sleep results in disturbed levels of the hormones that control appetite, making you hungrier.)

Some people say that the feeling of meditation is similar to that moment between waking and sleeping; you feel effortlessly comfortable and peaceful yet aware of all that you're feeling. When the practice becomes a constant in your life, you will find that the benefits fill your spirit, not just your body. You might feel a great joy emanating from within. Any extreme desires for external stimulation, entertainment, and distraction begin to fade; addictions lose their power, and you feel more complete within yourself. That sense of harmony within yourself—body, mind, and spirit coexisting rather than struggling for dominance—is one of the greatest gifts that the practice delivers.

But to start with, meditation is about getting into the habit of simply sitting still and resting the body and mind. My friend and collaborator on the *Yoga Now* DVD series, Rodney Yee, said he considers meditating a treat because he goes to a place in his psyche and in his body that he's not allowed to go any other time during the day.

CREATING YOUR PRACTICE

HOW MUCH: In meditation, it's good to start small. If you're a type-A personality who thinks the longer you do something, the more payoff you'll get, check those tendencies now. Most people start by trying to sit for too long, and then when they don't get immediate results or they get distracted and uncomfortable, they quit. In this program you will sit for three minutes a day for the first week, five minutes the second week, seven minutes the third week, and ten minutes or beyond—up to twenty minutes if it feels good—the fourth week.

WHEN: As for when to do this, it is up to you. Many people are stronger in the morning after waking up, before the thoughts of the day have begun to flood their minds. Doing a few minutes first thing—before you've eaten breakfast or drunk any caffeine—will set your day up nicely. (It's especially good if you have a big day ahead.) But if that doesn't feel right, evening might work well for you. Some people say that meditating before bedtime makes them too energized to sleep; you will have to experiment with different times of day to see what works best for you. (Don't forget the option of doing it in the middle of the day or between day and evening.) Ultimately, you should aim to meditate at the same time and the same place every day. As with any ritual, the power comes from consistency and repetition.

TIP Meditating after a workout can be particularly powerful because your physical body has had a chance to unwind and burn off excess energy. By the time you have finished a walk or yoga practice, your body is eager to rest and restore, making the transition into a meditative state even easier. Even if you have a regular morning or evening meditation, try doing a short, seated session after a workout at least once a week and see how it feels.

WHERE: Find a space in your home that is quiet and free of clutter. Even with your eyes closed, you will sense if you are in a disturbed, messy space, and it will make you anxious. Try out various rooms in your home to see what feels good. If your bedroom is your haven, it can be a great place to meditate, but don't get too cozy in bed as you may fall asleep. Try sitting on the edge of the bed, or bring a chair into the room. Light should be low, not bright. Close the door so you feel you won't be disturbed, and unplug or turn off phones and media.

SET YOUR BOUNDARIES: If you live in a busy household, it may be challenging to get the space and quiet you need. It's important to ask for the time. Assuming that you respect the needs of your family members (or roommates), then they should respect that you need a few minutes in a room to yourself and should try to keep their noise levels down in the rest of the house. I am tough about that in my own home. I make a big announcement, "I'm meditating now," and retreat to my bedroom. It's understood that my kids keep their music to a reasonable level downstairs and don't come looking for me until I'm done.

TIP Using earplugs can be helpful if excessive noise is coming from the indoors or outdoors. Earplugs don't muffle every sound, but they do take the edge off noise so that you can draw your attention inward; for me, the experience is almost womblike, listening to the inside of my body and then going deep into meditation. However, don't get addicted to using earplugs because one of the greatest aspects of a practice is to be able to access your inner quiet when there is activity around you. Rest assured that even if at first the sounds of birds chirping or cars passing drive you crazy, you will learn not to notice them.

SMALL CHILDREN: If you are the sole caretaker of your kids and they are too young to occupy themselves, try inviting them to be quiet with you. Try using the old "Mommy's doing what she wants to do right now, and then we'll do what you want to do" technique. When my girls were small, I would get them to sit on the carpet with me for a few minutes and practice being still. A lot of times they'd just fall asleep, which was great. Other times they'd run rampant—they told me later they used to amuse themselves by making ridiculous expressions right in front of my face. If your kids are very young, it will be harder. Try doing your session during their naptime, or if that's not possible, squeeze in a few moments sitting next to their crib or playpen and accept their noises without getting frustrated.

Method:

Posture

Sit on the edge of a chair without leaning your back against the chair back. (Leaning your whole back body against support can make you too relaxed to focus.) Keep both feet solid on the ground; feel the earth beneath your toes and heels, feel your spine straight. Wiggle your neck and shoulders until you feel your torso is positioned directly above your hips, with your seat lying heavy on the chair. Hands may rest on the thighs near the hip creases, with your palms softly opened upward. Try to place your hands comfortably without strain. At first you may want to place a watch in the palm of hand so you can glance at it as you go. Do not use a loud alarm clock to set your meditation time; it is unnecessarily jarring. You don't have to be absolutely strict about keeping the time.

To begin, hold your hand out in front of your face about two feet away from your nose and fix your gaze on the index finger. Follow your finger as it moves toward the nose so you go cross-eyed as it comes very close, and then shut your eyes. This will focus your attention on the spot between your eyebrows, and the effect is to very gently blank your mind. This spot between your eyes is the empty space, and it is always there for your focus to return to. Every time you start thinking and getting too active in your mind during the session, pull your awareness back to this empty space between the eyes.

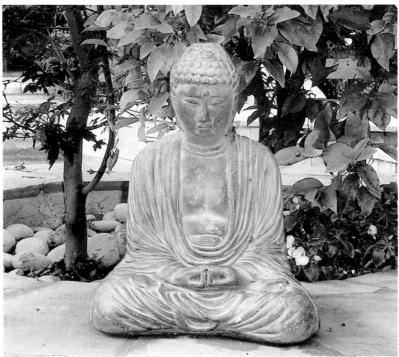

Start the session by inhaling through your nose to a count of eight, holding your breath for eight counts, then releasing the breath for eight counts, until you feel your breath calming down and finding a gentle pace. Then simply begin breathing softly without force, a natural breath. Invite the mind to get quiet. Breathe and settle slower; you may even talk to yourself slowly as though you are bringing the body to a halt.

As you breathe, notice if you feel physical resistance. Is your body twitching, tight, fighting the still posture? Don't adjust your posture; stay still. Then, notice how your mind wants

to literally take you to task. Thoughts such as, "Get up and take care of that carpet stain, right now!" or "Hmm, do I have enough butter for dinner tonight?" may force their way in. The mind wants you to begin doing something, but just notice the thought, tell it to go away, and watch it dissipate. You will see the thought lose its urgency. If the thought is important enough, you will remember it later with plenty of time to have it taken care of. The thoughts will keep coming, and you will keep having to ask if it is truly important and tell the thoughts that you will address them later.

While inhaling and exhaling naturally, allow yourself to sense how you feel inside. Don't think about it, just observe what's going on in your body and allow yourself to feel everything. Imagine following your breath on a journey into your nostrils, down the windpipe, and into your lungs. Visualize the air as light that is traveling into the bloodstream and up and down your spine, which is your source of energy and power. See if you can be the director of your breath, guiding its path inside your body and mind. Any place that you feel discomfort, imagine the breath softening that stuck energy until it melts into a soft stream of water that flows into nothingness. Take your breath through the whole body, and keep breaking the blockages by imagining them turning to water or maybe to dust, which blows away. Now bring your awareness back to that empty space between the eyes, and simply breathe quietly. See if you can enjoy a period with no thoughts and no physical sensations. After several minutes, bring your awareness back into your body and the physical world around you. Sit for several moments noticing sounds and feelings, then slowly open your eyes. You may also be filled with a wonderful feeling of peace.

If there is a persistent thought that keeps distracting you or a problem that your mind wants to solve and that is keeping you from getting quiet, imagine placing that thought on a platter in front of you. Give it a box, a colored wrapping, and a ribbon and ask that your inner self—the one that truly has your best interests at heart—to take the box away and return to you at some later point with a solution. Don't ask how you wish it to be revealed, but tell yourself that you trust that you will be given guidance at the appropriate time and when it will have the most impact. More than likely the thought or obsession has taken so much of your thinking time already that it has exhausted your conscious possibilities. So giving it

away is not being irresponsible; you are giving the thought or problem to your intuition and inner guide—that part of you that knows what to do. Surrender to the idea that the resolution will come naturally at some point in the future, if you will only stop controlling the need to know the answer now.

If there are pronounced sensations in your physical body that are calling for your attention and making it hard to focus on that empty space between your eyes, then try to imagine an imaginary boundary around the part of your body that is feeling sensations. Visually seal it off, picture it getting enclosed by a colored band or light field, know that you can leave it safely, and bring your attention back to the empty space between your eyes. Sensations in your body are not bad; don't get angry that you have them. It is fine to observe them. What you want to avoid is having an emotional reaction to the sensation, which can then trigger that pesky stream of thoughts. ("My hip hurts again. . . . Gosh, I am getting old. . . . What have I done with my life?") If true pain hits you due to the way you're sitting, then of course you should move. But if it's simply discomfort, try to "seal it off" and know that your body will be fine for a few minutes without your actively thinking about it.

In meditation, surrendering control of the experience is key. I was a clock watcher for a long time. I always wanted to know how long I'd been sitting there. Had I done enough yet? Was I correct in guessing how many minutes had passed? But eventually I began to instinctively know how many minutes I'd been sitting and I could let go of looking at the clock. The whole process started to take less and less effort.

That said, there is a certain amount of persistence involved in the practice of meditation. Sometimes I get a wonderful sensation of tranquillity and serenity afterward, and sometimes nothing. Zilch. Zippo. My journey with meditation has taught me acceptance because I've had to accept the unremarkable sessions along with the sensational ones. My tendency is to always strive for the best session ever, with the most powerful results, and to be dissatisfied by the ordinary. Yet I have learned to keep showing up and trusting the practice because for the most part the outcome is experienced after the session, when I am calmer and more stress free in my daily life. That's where the extraordinary lies. Furthermore, I trust in it because I have seen how much it has transformed me. And from time to time there is a breakthrough during the session itself, just like with physical workouts when suddenly running becomes easy and free. I feel an energy move through my body, and I reach a new level of perception about myself, and I go, "Okay, so this is what it's all about!" I have to admit, I find those moments very exciting.

TIP Taking it further: It won't harm you to sit for longer. For beginners, anywhere between five minutes and thirty minutes is beneficial. If you feel focused and aware and you're doing the practice with enthusiasm and not because you think you must, then keep going for longer. It won't hurt you to explore the effects.

■   ■   ■

Commitment Issues

The true benefit of meditation comes when you do it every day. But remember at the root of all the quiet-mind practices is kindness. If you don't have time to sit or you forget to sit, don't berate yourself for screwing up. Acknowledge that sometimes it's just not going to happen. First, let go of the resistance and frustration, and then consider how else you can get your quiet-mind time. Just as with exercise, finding balance in a busy life may mean improvising. Be creative and kind to yourself, and find the outlet in the things you have to do. See your laundry folding as a meditation; see your housecleaning as your walk. Tell yourself, "This is my walk today. This is my meditation today." Bring the same intention and quiet mind to these practices, and know that you are not getting off track.

I AM NOT A GREAT MEDITATOR. It's not always easy for me, but I am disciplined, so regardless of how I feel I meditate daily. And more often than not I struggle with my thoughts and often with my body. I am uncomfortable sometimes, and yet if I hang in there I usually get past the discomfort and into a state of deep calm. I realize that I have resistance to believing that I can feel that good, that taken care of, or that much love and joy. The ability to receive is the most difficult for us. We think we have to earn the right to have joy in our meditation. We turn our belief into "It's hard!" because deep down, at least for me, I'm thinking that if it feels so good I don't deserve it. But the healing and the joy are right at our fingertips. They are all around us; we are never away from our peace and joy or love and bliss.

Customize Your Practice

There is no right or wrong way to meditate, but there are other elements you can bring in to your technique to aid you. Most people eventually hit on the type of practice that works well for them. Since this program is all about experimentation, consider trying some of the following:

MUSIC. Relaxing music, particularly if it's composed specifically to aid meditation, can be very helpful at the beginning stage. Don't let it become a crutch because you want to move away from music eventually and get used to sitting in silence, but it can be a very pleasurable way to start. Look for CDs and Internet radio stations dedicated to new age, ambient, and classical genres.

CHANTING is also used in many meditation practices. One great teacher is Dr. Dharma Singh, who sells chanting CDs on his Web site. I find chanting different than listening to music; it is a strong way to focus the mind and bring physical and mental healing to yourself. It is powerful in its ability to transform us.

MANTRA. Using a mantra may help you get focused and settled. A mantra is a word or phrase that you repeat softly in your mind to help focus your attention. It can be any word or words that inspire you, though two syllables are helpful, as they lend a kind of rhythm to your practice. Personally I think Eastern words have a better lilt as a mantra: the Sanskrit phrase *Om shanti* essentially means, "Peace, peace." (*Om* is considered the primal sound of the universe; *shanti* means peace.) If the word *amen* or another word with spiritual significance moves you, try that.

COUNTING NUMBERS. If you find it very hard to keep your mind quiet during meditation, try this technique. As you breathe, begin to count slowly from one to ten in your mind. Each time a thought pops up, begin the count at "one" again. At first you may not get further than "two" or "three" before returning to "one." Do it with lightness and no expectations, and simply focus on the sound of the words in your mind. Let your body sink into relaxed awareness.

OPEN-EYE MEDITATION. An alternative method for focusing the awareness is to look at an object before you with a softly focused gaze. It could be a flower, a picture, a candle, or some other beautiful object that pleases you. Do not stare aggressively at it, but let your eyes settle on the object and simply keep noticing it. Do not have active thoughts about how it looks or what it means. Bring your awareness back to its color and shape again and again.

TREAT YOURSELF: *A meditation cushion, seat, or bench can make your practice more comfortable and special (see Index of Products).*

I believe that ultimately you find the thing that makes your experience of meditation work for you. It is a process of discovery. The practice is experimental by nature: each time you sit, you observe how you respond today. If this basic technique makes you curious to learn more, it is simple to engage in some spiritual window-shopping. Attend classes or workshops, or rent DVDs and CDs that teach different kinds of meditation, just as you might shop to find a type of yoga practice that suits. Different types of meditation have different effects; some are more energizing, and some are more tranquilizing. Not everyone finds seated meditation as appealing as I do. Some find it easier to relax and focus the mind in movement. If that's you, then the Chinese healing arts of qigung and tai chi, which combine physical movement, quiet mind, and an awareness of energy, may appeal. Your exploration can start here, however, with a few minutes a day of sitting down and shutting up. Commit to it for thirty days, and see where that takes you.

There is a facet of meditation that is outside the realm of rationality and logic and science. When you feel the peace, see if you can feel more than that. Maybe you find deep joy there too, or something more. Joy is there; just give yourself permission to feel it. I believe that when you touch joy in your quietest moments, you are feeling unconditional love. You might consider it coming from your belief in God or from your own self, or from your devotion to Jesus or Muhammad or maybe simply Mother Nature. Wherever the feeling comes from, it is yours and it is there to heal you and love you. Allow it to rise up and flood through every part of you. This is the ultimate benefit of meditation: you drop so much of the noise and clutter that keeps you from being kind to yourself and feeling the best feelings inside. I love the idea that we are all the same under one god and that whatever our beliefs may be, what all of us want is to get back to that joy both now and at the end of our lives. Finding peace or bliss or love inside ourselves has no color and no religion. There is no need to define it. It is like the taste you have in decorating your home: just follow what makes you feel comfortable, what makes you feel calm and loved.

My sense of god manifests most powerfully in nature. I must get outdoors and smell and feel the wild; otherwise I don't feel stable. But we can all find something that gives us that sense of inner home—the place that is always present and nurturing in every way. It doesn't have to be a belief in any god or any religious figure; the inner guide is always there, waiting for you to meet it in silence.

The Quiet Power Tool

QUESTION: WHICH WOULD IMPROVE YOUR QUALITY OF LIFE MORE:
BEING BUSIER AND MORE PRODUCTIVE, OR UNDERSTANDING YOURSELF,
RELATING BETTER TO LOVED ONES, AND FINDING JOY IN WHAT IS
ALREADY AROUND YOU?

CREATING SILENCE within will play out in your daily life and your relationships in profound ways. Silence has subtle power. The more you bring moments of it into your life, the more it reveals its importance. Learning to pause and quietly reflect before I take action has allowed me to access reservoirs of patience and compassion that I didn't know I had. I am more patient and compassionate with my family, and I am infinitely more patient and compassionate with myself.

That's why this nothingness—the thing you can't see or hold—ultimately has the power to transform your life. If, on occasion, in place of thinking or talking, you are simply observing and noticing, you create something of an open field in which new realizations can find you. There is no formula or equation for this; let's just call it growth. But just as sitting on that riverbank as a kid helped me hear new birdsongs, so living my life in a more conscious and quiet way as an adult helps me discover new facets of myself. Noise truly does bring confusion; when we're busy and rushed we hurtle forward and miss the nuances of our story, the insight into our behavior and our patterns. And sometimes we miss the very obvious, big themes as well. It's like running through a museum looking at all the Impressionist paintings close up, then complaining they don't show anything. If we only slowed down, stepped back, and gazed at them from a distance, we'd see each scene with clarity and understanding. Sometimes to see what's right in front of your eyes, you have to separate a bit.

Once you begin to get into the habit of looking before reacting, you are able to change on a deep level. Breathing calmly, meditating, and proactively cutting off the stress response are all techniques that will help you cultivate a healthy degree of detachment and earn some lucidity. You stop connecting to the symptoms of life—the dramas and the daily highs and lows—and you avoid getting taken on such a wild ride by your emotions. If your style is to dig in to daily dramas—turning toward the problems, getting deeper inside them, and trying to fix bad feelings with all your might—getting quiet will help you detach from those dramas instead. Silence helps you see the truth of what is going on in front of you, not whatever story you have laid on top of the situation from emotional habit.

If, when things are hectic or unpleasant all around you, you simply stop reacting for a moment and become very present in your body—breathe, close your eyes, get quiet—you realize that in fact you are not stuck to the circumstances nor are you defined by your emotions. You are you, and the circumstances that are going on are simply events happening all around you. Those emotions that are powerfully running through you? They are not you either. They are temporary bursts of energy that will be different in an hour. When you get quiet, you can kindly reconnect to the you that is always there, regardless of the momentary circumstances: the you that is calm, capable, and confident.

That's what is meant by separating: you become an observer to your own life, able to watch the dramas unfold in front of you instead of being stuck inside the drama. Almost like being a witness to your own behavior, you can observe how you act in the context of your family or your career or your friends, and you notice how you might habitually repeat certain behaviors or patterns that don't serve you any longer. You can gain some insight into where those patterns come from—perhaps your upbringing or your parents imprinted them on you, and they aren't true to who you are

today. It's not uncommon to feel imprisoned by bad habits, but the fact is, once you observe your patterns, you can often just let them go. With a healthy degree of detachment comes the awareness that bad habits are no more stuck to you than the pencil you're holding is stuck to your hand. You realize that you have a choice: often, you can simply let go of the thoughts or emotions that keep you from being as joyous and healthy as you want to be.

For years, as I've mentioned, I felt stuck with the burden of my early experiences and fear about my family legacy. My silent practices helped me to become conscious of who I am in a much deeper way; I am more than the circumstances of my upbringing. I was able to separate from my history by seeing that it was just a collection of memories and that memories aren't attached to me—nor can they actually hurt me, as painful as they seem. To get to this point, I had to understand my behavior and accept it and then kindly ask myself if I could change certain habits, as gently as dropping a pencil from my hand. Finding self-acceptance was an epiphany, the start of the journey toward becoming a balanced and conscious person. Accepting who you are is the beginning of healing; it is also the beginning of the ability to let go of what no longer serves you in life.

■　■　■

LIKE MANY OTHER PEOPLE, I often fall into old patterns of behavior. I believed over the years that I must have always done something to get me in trouble and that things are always my fault. Today I understand that belief came from my childhood. Nobody ever explained to me why my family was so unhappy; all I knew was that we took our gourmet meals to the TV room and my father went away a lot on fishing trips. I didn't know that my sisters' drug problems caused huge rifts in my parents' marriage and that my mom's anger at my dad was due to her feeling abandoned by her first husband's early death. Children who grow up with this kind of tension often feel that in some way it is their fault. Perhaps I was not being as good as I could be, and therefore I was *in some way the cause of their pain and proble*ms. I had begun to sleep next to my mother when she had cancer to care for her in the night, and in doing so I saw that my dad wasn't there. I blamed myself for that but was too scared to leave my mother's side because deep down I was afraid she was going to die.

I put so much misguided blame on myself at such an early age that the habit of believing I am the cause of all the disharmony in life became ingrained in me. It still plays out three decades later; whenever I sense tension with my husband I have a habit of asking him, "Are you okay? Did I do something?" But the difference is that now contemplation and quiet are helping to break that pattern. When that thought starts to come or the words are in my mouth, I stop, get quiet, and ask myself one question. Instead of jumping to an age-old reaction, I ask, "Is this true?" In taking a

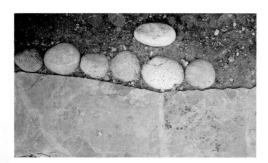

moment to get quiet, I find my harmony and usually realize quickly that not everything has to do with me—the tension is coming from a completely different source. The best response I have to tension now is to break the negative thoughts by asking the question, and then to take any feelings that may still be ruminating to my meditation corner. I go into a seated silence, and during my session I breathe and watch the thoughts dissipate and lose their power. That is how I retrain my synapses and work toward my personal freedom.

In these moments of quiet I am able to see myself in the situation and observe that I am reacting to my childhood instead of to the experience at hand. Other times I observe that I am acting like my mother did, frustrated or even resentful of my daughters' goofy exuberance, for when they were young they had a freedom of expression I never had at their age. I used to get mad at them for giggling at the dinner table, so envious was I of their carefree spirits. The moment would always end with me in tears, hating myself for acting like Jekyll and Hyde—loving one moment, hypercritical the next. When this happens, I press pause on my reaction by quietly asking myself, "Is this true? Is this the way I really am?" and I remember that I am no longer my mother's little girl and her habits needn't be my own. Instead of being miserable, like she was, I can let myself enjoy my daughters. I was able to be a better parent when I finally saw that my reactions to my daughters' frisky behavior were based on my upbringing, not on who I am. In the silence of observation I change the patterns in my life.

■   ■   ■

is derived from my habit of observing life as it's happening. I have found that it is indeed a practice—something that one needs to do on an ongoing basis. When I practice being as quietly present as possible during the very ordinary moments of my life, like getting up in the early morning, going downstairs, feeding the dogs, noticing the day outside, making the tea, and so on, I build my ability to see what's going on in more complex situations when my emotions threaten to cloud the issue in front of me. Practicing mindfulness at ordinary moments of the day can make your whole life a moving meditation. It is an excellent example of taking peace and awareness off the yoga mat and into the real world.

MINDFULNESS

One simple principle you can apply to anything you do, whether work or leisure: You can either check out of the task that you're engaged in and do it with half a mind, or you can do it with full attention. When you practice doing the latter, bringing your whole mind to the task at hand, you retrain the brain to stay with the present experience and you stop the habit of spiraling off into tangential thoughts. This state of quiet concentration is known as mindfulness, and when you develop it in small ways throughout your day, it is an excellent remedy to the frazzled feeling that can come from constant busyness and multitasking. When you can simply draw your attention back to the act that you're doing right here, right now, let go of the inner monologue that runs on a constant loop, and ignore the impulse to switch to a new task, you are teaching yourself to stay in the present. This is the essence of all meditative practices. I like the way that my friend, author and teacher Hale Dwoskin, puts it: "Do what you're doing while you're doing it; don't do what you're not doing while you're not doing it."

It sounds faintly absurd to tell adults that they must learn how to pay attention to what they're doing—didn't we hear enough of that in grade school? The fact is that we do need to relearn it. We've become so used to doing a hundred things at once and consequently not doing any one thing well. In fact, doing lots of things with half a mind rather than fewer things with full awareness only serves to make us anxious and less effective, not least because we're left feeling that the little jobs aren't quite completed.

Mindfulness is about trusting in the power of doing one thing well: starting a single task, noticing it as you're doing it, and completing it with a sense of satisfaction. Even when applied to the most mundane daily activities, mindfulness is calming because it slows down the pace of the day, allows you to take stock of where you are, and reins in the runaway-life feeling that strikes so many women—the fear that we've never quite done "enough" and we're always catching up with a list of to-dos.

To practice mindfulness, you take the basic components of Exercising with Intention from the previous segment and apply those techniques to daily duties. The mundane chores that you do every day are a great time to practice being here now. Since you don't need to think hard about them, you can just drop into the experience.

Silence

Exercise: Menial Mindfulness

This week, pick one ordinary task that you do each day that is fairly short in duration and does not require active problem-solving skills. It could be washing the dishes, brushing your teeth, making the bed, chopping carrots (or any repetitive cooking job). Each time you do it, you will use those few minutes very deliberately to slow down and drop into your quiet mind. Take a moment before you begin the task to set the intention: "I am practicing how to be here now." Make it your purpose to stay with the experience at hand. Notice the situation before you (an unmade bed, a pile of vegetables). Purposefully begin the task while practicing the three intentional techniques:

1. **NOTICE YOUR BREATH.** Breath awareness is your way in to being present in all activities. Don't try to do anything fancy; simply turn your attention to the way you're breathing. If you notice your breath is shallow and fast, can you alter the pace and slow it slightly?

2. **OBSERVE** what is happening without having complex thoughts about it. Just observe how the experience looks, feels, smells, and sounds—the vibrant hue of the carrots, the satisfying chop of the knife against the chopping board. Notice how it feels to hold the knife in your hand. Notice how you are holding your body and how your feet feel against the floor. Don't start an internal dialogue about it; just feel as much as you can about the experience.

3. **ASK** yourself a question from time to time if you feel thoughts start to drag your attention away from the task: "Can I allow myself to stay with the experience?"

When you've completed the task, even if it was two minutes long, pause and notice what about the situation has changed in front of you (a neatly made bed, a saucepan full of carrot slices). Acknowledge that you have finished your task satisfactorily.

Once you feel comfortable doing this exercise with just one task a day, apply it to other things that may take a bit longer, such as driving to work, taking a bath or shower, or playing with your kids. (Playing with your dog or cat makes a good substitute.) All these experiences change when you start with a quiet external environment, make the intention to focus on the task or game before you begin, and bring yourself back to the present again and again throughout. Granted, you won't be in a focused state the whole time, or even for very much of it. But practice the three techniques, and notice the brief moments when your thoughts about what else you should be doing drop away and you enter the flow of the experience. Doing daily activities in this conscious way is a form of moving meditation. The quality of the experience improves—you accept life as it is right now and get more pleasure from it (as do your kids and dogs and cats). And it is a salve to an anxious or scattered mind.

One way to slow down and stay present through the day is to designate something a mindfulness trigger. This very simple exercise helps you to check tendencies to rush and stress.

Exercise: Mindfulness Trigger

For one day, turn some ordinary sound or sight into your reminder to breathe. It could be every ring of the phone or every time you arrive at (and stop at) a yellow light while driving. It could be every time the e-mail pings. Or it might be every time your kid asks you something. Each time the trigger goes off, breathe fully before responding, moving, or acting. After breathing, then respond. If you feel resistance to taking a slow and deliberate breath, notice the feelings that push you to answer the telephone on the first ring, to rush through yellow lights, or to check the e-mail instantly. Why would rushing to respond faster make the experience any better? Can you let go of whatever is making you rush?

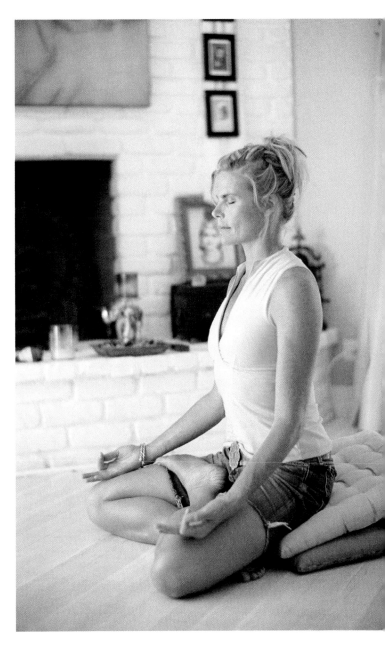

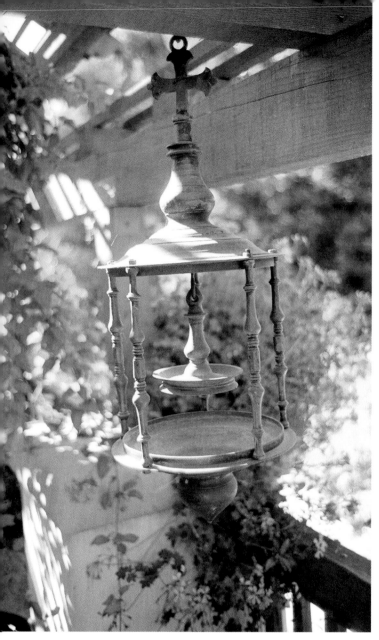

my inner monologue, and it changes my attitude. I lose the resistance to the chore and find some pleasure in the quiet harmony of my mind and actions, both focused on the same goal. Pull back the sheets, smooth them forward, plump the pillows, and tuck in the corners. I am able to use the moment as a moment of respite and to breathe my way into calm. For working women who come home from work and then have to keep house, doing your chores as a moving meditation practice brings a new kind of benefit. You clean your mind and spirit as you clean your house.

In Praise of Low-Tech Hobbies

Getting into the flow of the moment is easiest when you are doing things that you enjoy. Activities that might seem monotonous to some, such as sewing, knitting, gardening, painting, or doing handiwork around the house, can be wonderful ways to practice mindfulness because they get you focusing on a single task while doing a repetitive action with your body. As you may have discovered through walking with intention, any repetitive physical activity can quiet the mind and create a hypnotic rhythm that keeps you engaged in the present moment. Our forebears knew it instinctively; my grandfather on my mom's side was known as "Whittlesticks" because he found solace in

DOING CHORES isn't my favorite way to spend an afternoon. But sometimes if I'm making the bed, I think, "You know what, I'm doing a service for my family I want to do this nicely, so let me see if I can do this really well." I focus deeply on the task at hand and drop carving wood and enjoyed sitting quietly alone for hours while working his hands. But we have become so focused on the extremes of high-action leisure pursuits, on the one hand, or passive TV watching, on the other, that we sometimes underestimate the value of pastimes that fall in the middle and allow for quiet, soft focus of the mind. These kinds of repetitive hobbies can allow the active beta waves in the brain to slow down and give way to the relaxed alpha wave mode—and possibly even to theta waves, accessed by deep meditation and prayer. It's worth posing the question next time you are about to wind down with some entertainment at the end of the day: Could you wind down with a calming hobby instead?

■　　■　　■

FROM MINDFULNESS comes understanding. From understanding comes loving-kindness and compassion. When you are mindful in relationships, you become a better listener. It also makes you take more responsibility for your actions because they are intentional, not accidental.

This is how practice becomes such an empowering tool—because the key to living successfully with other people, such as your partner or kids, is taking responsibility. It's your life and your patterns—and once you see that your patterns were created (perhaps by your upbringing, perhaps by you), you also see that you can change them. With that knowledge comes the responsibility to improve our attitude when it is off. It's a reversal of the regular way of dealing with difficulty. Instead

of wishing that your partner wasn't a jerk or your kids weren't so trying, you focus instead on yourself. For the beauty—and the challenge—is that ultimately the only control you have is over your own attitude. Instead of, "Change my circumstances!" the silent plea should be, "Change me." Instead of getting frustrated about what's wrong with the other person, we can recognize, "I have an issue, so I better go sit over there and calm down on my own." Whatever the other person has done to drive you crazy, they're just exhibiting their own patterns, and you're probably not going to change them through an argument. That's why when things get tense on the home front, I might retreat to my meditation or go for a long hike. Rather than go round and round in a dispute, I say, "Give me the space to change my attitude," and I step away so that I can see the true cause of the tension. With time, I almost always find I can resolve it and return feeling better and more willing to compromise.

It is more work and more effort to do things this way, but it breaks the lazy tendency to think we are the victims of our circumstances. Even when my marriage is not harmonious and I don't know if I can make it, I do know that if I change my attitude—even if I'm "right" about something, or think I'm right—then it doesn't really matter. This more spacious response also improves my relationship to my kids. When their behavior is at odds with what I think is right, I always ask whether or not I need to change them or if I can accept that they are who they are. When my girls were in their middle teenage years, moody and sometimes verbally attacking, I'd have to pray

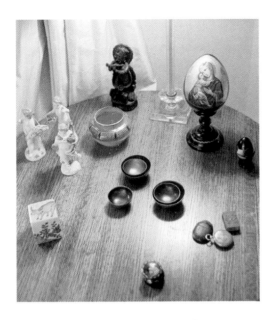

figure out how to maneuver in this world. In the quiet, realizations about what it meant to be a teenager came to find me, and my patience taught me how to respond.

■ ■ ■

MOST OF OUR PAIN is not here in the present. It's attached to the past or the longing for the future. It's attached to some way we were taught to deal with situations. In silence, we can shed the negative beliefs by asking if they are really true. "Am I really less than so-and-so, or am I less deserving than he or she is?" No. "Are we created equal, and do I have the ability to feel joy just like anyone else?" Yes. Once you begin to ask for truth, you break down that self-imposed prison that keeps you away from your birthright of joy. You begin to see the absurdity of all your problems and realize that most of the time, they are there to show you something about yourself. The less weight you put into their power, the more you feel joy.

for strength. I turned toward my own silence so that I could listen, listen, listen to them—a hard one to learn because no one in my family ever listened to me when I was their age. I listened and gave myself the time and space to ask, "What can I learn from this?" I tried to remember that this mood would pass and this frustration needed to be expressed in order for them to feel better about themselves and

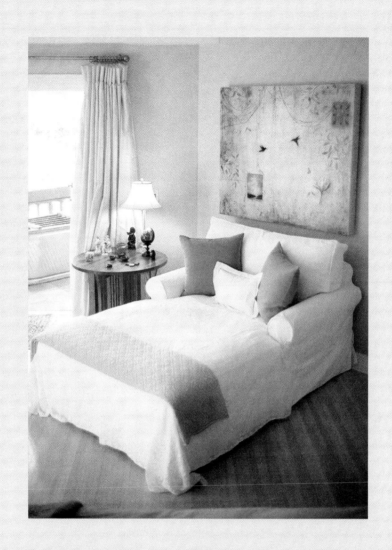

Food

Silence

Exercise

PART FOUR

Home

Home

QUESTION: WHEN YOU GET INTO BED AFTER A LONG DAY,
HOW DOES IT FEEL TO BE IN YOUR BEDROOM?

> A. Not that different from any other room in the house, except that I'm tired and in my pajamas.
>
> B. As if the outside world has dropped away and I am in a cozy, rejuvenating retreat.
>
> C. A little bit off; I've never quite felt as peaceful as I could be in there, and I'm not sure why.

THE SURROUNDINGS THAT I FIND MOST SOOTHING TO MY SENSES ARE:

> A. Cozy and classic, featuring plush furniture, full drapes, and neutral or pastel colors.
>
> B. Minimalist and modern, featuring concrete floors, metal fixtures, and sleek wooden furniture.
>
> C. Exotic and eccentric, featuring spicy colors, ethnic furniture, and patterned carpets.

YOUR EXTERNAL SURROUNDINGS profoundly influence your internal state; if they promote comfort and calm, you will be supported in making the right choices throughout your life. Making your home environment right is integral to your journey toward health and balance. There's no magic formula for an ideal home, but when you clear out any excess and tune in to what works for you, the surroundings that serve you best will start to take shape.

For much of my adult life, I lived in white spaces. Wherever I lived, I had white walls, white sofas, white rugs; it was pristine, clean, and minimal. Looking back, I now understand that during those years I was scared to commit to my life and enjoy it. I see that I was desperately seeking security and clarity through all my disciplined habits—reflected in my spare, white environment. After my husband, two babies, and five dogs entered the picture, the white interior became another excuse to be tense and disciplined because it couldn't accommodate any imperfection. It required constant cleaning—in fact, It was never clean enough for me. Needless to say, it didn't add to my happiness or stability.

As I got older, though, and began to enjoy life and find peace inside myself, my external environment transformed to match. I learned that as your life changes you have to look at your environment anew and see what is needed. My house became colorful; today every room is a different hue. Decorative objects, art, and small statues that are significant to my husband and me adorn walls and surfaces. The newest addition is water: small, tabletop fountains placed here and there create a pleasant sound that makes my home feel alive. The house feels so good now. It's my sanctuary and my shelter: when I walk in I feel safe and serene. I know that I am in a good place to refuel my body, restore my spirits, and rest. I know that my husband is in a good place to maintain his health and that our daughters stick around more than normal for kids their age because the atmosphere embraces them. Just as important, other people feel comfortable in our home. It is not perfect, interior-designer chic, but it is warm and welcoming and I love the way it feels.

To make your life more balanced, you need to examine your environment in the same way you evaluate your eating, exercise, and quiet habits. Ask if your home is nurturing every aspect of you and promoting healthy habits or if it is getting in the way of you finding your peace. We can get stuck in an unhealthy environment just like we get stuck eating the same old food. We can get stifled in a cluttered environment without realizing it, just like we get stifled through shallow breathing. It can be tempting to dismiss the external stuff—to think it's a bunch of superficial details that can wait until later. But the living environment we create will either support us on the path to well-being or produce obstacles that get in our way. If the success, happiness, or calm you seek isn't arriving, try clearing out some things you don't need and playing around with your living space. Sometimes changing one thing sparks other changes.

■　■　■

NOW IT'S TIME to turn your focus from the world within you—the one you are improving through food, physical motion, and a quiet mind—to the world around you. When it comes to creating balance, understanding your relationship to the environment in which you live is an essential piece of the puzzle. Do you look forward to slipping into your bedroom at the end of the day? Is the room soothing and conducive to a quiet state? When you walk through the front door after an exhausting afternoon, does your space invite you to breathe and unwind, or do you feel overwhelmed by objects and mess? Is there a special spot in your home that is just for you, to which you can retreat without being disturbed, or would that be considered a luxury in your busy household? In other words, is your home environment supporting you in your pursuit of health and happiness? Perhaps because it takes tremendous effort to set up a home that fulfills our basic needs (not to mention the needs of kids, partners, and even pets), we often forget to ask the subtler questions, such as, "How does this space make me feel?" "Do I feel comfortable?" "Do I enjoy being in my home?"

If it's challenging to keep your household running in a (somewhat) sane and efficient manner, then to even ask these questions may seem a little froufrou or self-indulgent. Who has time to worry about how a living room makes you *feel* when in practical terms it's going to take forty minutes to vacuum and clean it? Yet these questions are fundamental. The external environment you create is simply another way of making choices that either help or hinder you in the quest for balance. Home is not an afterthought; it is one of the four cornerstones of the balanced life because it is has a direct effect on your internal state—your energy, mood, and frame of mind. When your home environment is out of balance, for example by being cluttered, you will feel out of sorts. Or if the lighting, colors, or even furniture arrangement in your rooms are at odds with what you find to be peaceful, your ability to relax and recharge will be compromised.

Yet when all is calm and ordered in your environment, and when the way it looks reflects your individual idea of what is pleasing, then home becomes the stage on which you can best accomplish the work in this program, a place to take stock of your existing habits and behaviors, and a tranquil setting in which to introduce some new routines. When you are conducting your life in a supportive setting, it's surprising how much easier it is for new behaviors to flourish—a spacious, uncluttered, and appealing environment invites you to cook nourishing food or roll out the mat for yoga far more readily than an unappealing, claustrophobic, or soulless environment, not least because you actually want to spend the time there.

Therefore, consider enhancing your home environment to create the conditions for success, both in this program and in the rest of your life. It's critically important because home is the place in which the practices of eating

better, treating your body more consciously, and acting more mindfully come together. They stop being exercises in a book and over time become a lifestyle. In this final section of the program, you are creating the space in which to practice and enjoy all the new skills that you learned in the preceding sections.

MAKING HOME A HAVEN

QUESTION: JUST HOW IMPORTANT IS A BUILDING, ANYWAY?

Consider this: Has there ever been a period when you didn't have a reliable home base? Perhaps you were between apartments or on a long trip out of town, or you were a student or going through a life change. How did it affect your body and mind to not have a safe and consistent place to start and end each day? How did it affect your ability to focus and achieve things?

Even if you have long been installed in a home of your own, try to remember a time when you didn't have one. For most people it is much harder to maintain healthy habits, not to mention a positive state of mind, if they do not feel grounded in the physical world. Commitment, confidence, and clarity suffer when you lack a living environment that you trust. That's why building sensitivity to the way your current home serves you is crucial. In order to achieve balance, it helps to have solid roots.

Women in particular tend to nest. We like familiarity; it makes us feel peaceful and safe. Yet the demands put on us by busy lives mean that sometimes we feel like caretakers in our homes, constantly on cleanup duty and chaos control. (Even if you live alone the dishes, laundry, and unopened mail can suck up your whole evening after a long day at work.) Factor in the way that lifestyles today are more materialistic than ever before, with average home sizes increasing and houses filled with more possessions than our parents ever had need for, and the result is a growing domestic workload for women. Instead of home being a sacred place to reboot our systems and nurture our spirits, it can seem like a purely functional place where we work hard—and get drained of energy, not filled with it.

Obviously, we can't suddenly change the way our household is run or give up key duties that keep things together. Whether we have a job outside the home or are busy raising a family and holding down the domestic front, chances are, we are the center around which the household rotates. But without doing anything drastic, we can find ways to redress the balance a bit so that home becomes a restorative place, not just an arena for doing chores. We can find ways to make home more of a haven, a place that feeds us with good energy and shelters us from the dramas and demands of daily life.

Making a home a haven doesn't mean doing a radical overhaul or redesign. It's not about turning your two-bedroom apartment, your townhouse, or even your dorm room into a spa or stand-in for a boutique hotel. It comes down to incorporating some changes that pacify the senses rather than agitate them and that boost your spirits rather than depress them. The modifications may be fairly minor: shifting things around so that your sofa faces the light-filled window, not the dark front door, or adding warm-toned curtains or softer lights to a bedroom to make it feel cozier. Perhaps it's as simple as removing the TV from your bedroom and bringing in some plants. But these small gestures can be powerful because they are done with a specific intention. Just as with exercise, when you work with intention, the limitations of your space, your budget, or your time are not a problem; instead, they help you stay focused because they keep your project doable and achievable. (In comparison, redoing a whole home can be overwhelming.) Your work is also satisfying because the few changes you make to foster calm in your space will deliver immediate results that you can see, touch, and sometimes—in the case of a few fresh-cut flowers placed on a nightstand—smell.

A home becomes a haven when it is filled with things that you love arranged in a way that pleases your soul. Your environment then becomes an expression of who you are and what you care about. This aspect of the program is fun because enhancing your living environment is a creative process and an opportunity for self-expression. You get in touch with something deep in yourself when your project is to make your surroundings more you. The expressions may be subtle, particularly if you live with someone else and need to take their taste into account, or they may be out there and attention grabbing. But even the simple act of making your own sacred corner, as we will discuss in Step 2, is enough to put your signature on your space.

In much the same way that feeding yourself whole, fresh foods is an act of kindness to yourself, as is moving your body through yoga postures, making a few modifications to your environment so that you feel the best you can when you're in it is also an act of kindness. The way we think and talk about our living spaces can be so utilitarian and practical—

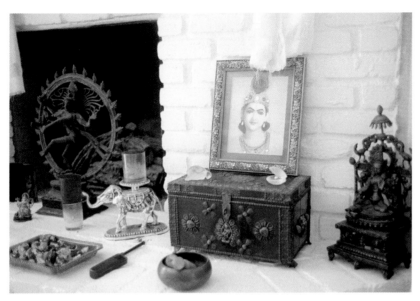

"How many square feet is the kitchen, and could we convert that closet to a bedroom?"— that sometimes we forget to act from the heart. But when you ask the subtler question—*"What will make me feel better in my space?"*—you give yourself the opportunity to slow down and act from the heart by making one or two kind choices that might be neither functional nor logical but instead just feel right to you. Bringing a few touches of warmth and sacredness into your home will help slow down your life: it will soothe your spirit and make you feel more balanced. Even if sleep accounts for much of your time spent at home, the atmosphere of your environment is affecting you all the time that you're inside it, so it's got to be right.

Becoming conscious of the effects of your environment means paying attention not just to the way it is physically arranged, but also to the way you act in your home. Do you treat the living space like the special place it is? Do you throw open the curtains in the early morning to let in natural light? Do you make the bed so that you leave your bedroom as beautiful as you want to find it later? Do you create a calming atmosphere in the evening with music, scent, or lighting, or if you work from home, do you deliberately shut down technology and close the door on your home office when you're finished, and leave the work behind? These things too are small gestures that express your intention to make home a haven. They are small expressions of who you are and what you care about. Actions, just as much as new carpets and paint jobs, transform your home. After all, people put an energy into a place that can be felt and identified. When this energy is warm and welcoming, you can't help but want to pull up a chair and stay a while.

Thinking of environment in this inclusive way—incorporating both the aesthetics of the space and the actions you do within it—means that everything you do in your home, even the most mundane little thing, can become a creative act. When I put out food for my family, I might spontaneously select the funky plates that my daughters made at the local pottery store when they were ten and twelve, brightly colored and beautiful in their imperfection. This choice reflects how I feel at the moment: joyful and maternal. Another night may find me serving delicate spring rolls on a geometric white platter, decorated with a flower that I plucked from my garden, because the mood of the food calls for something more clean, spare, and graphic. Later, while washing the pots and pans after dinner, I look at my kitchen window ledge, upon which a few of my favorite objects sit: a delicate and intricate om symbol carved from wood; a small, stone Buddha; a gurgling water fountain that plugs into the wall; a vibrant, green succulent plant. Because they're placed right above the sink, they help create a condition of quiet focus in which I can mindfully do the dishes. Some might think it oddball to have a Buddha above the sink; I love it because I've deliberately designed an aspect of my environment to facilitate my own awareness and calm.

The small gestures like these that I make throughout my environment serve to anchor me in my life. They help me find satisfaction in what I have: when I walk into my bedroom, with its soothing blue-gray walls and white-washed floorboards, any frustration I'm feeling about life, career, or family gets tempered. Each time I pass my sacred corner—the small collection of treasured objects and inspirational pictures in my bedroom where I meditate—its beauty and simplicity remind me that all that I have in my life right now is *enough.*

I may not be an interior designer or an artist; I don't paint canvases or make sculpture. Yet to me, my environment is just as much a creative act as any of those things. When I change something in my home or create a new atmosphere in a room, I am exploring something of my inner self and getting to know what motivates me. In that way each of us can be an artist in our own lives.

When your home is a haven, it is not only a place that encourages your creativity, it is also a healing place. By that I mean a place where every day you can shed your fatigue or stress, feed and care for your body in a positive way, and lift your spirits so that you experience sustained well-being. It's a place where you can tend to yourself if you feel the beginnings of imbalance and where you feel unapologetic about the need to let yourself rest. Should you fall ill, or should life hit one of the rocky periods and start throwing hard challenges at you, the good energy you have put into your environment will support you in finding your way out of the difficulty and will make you feel safe.

When home is a healing place, it not only brings harmony to your own existence, it also promotes harmonious interactions with your family and friends, who will feel more welcome and more relaxed there as well. You can't control the lifestyle choices that anybody else makes—your partner, kids, or roommates—but even if they don't acknowledge it, they are as sensitive to their environment as you are. By creating a calmer, slower home—one that is slightly quieter and conducive to reflection and mindful behavior—those you live with and love will often begin to pick up healthy-living cues themselves.

Work with What You Have

No matter where you live or how much or little you have, you can make your home a haven. Comfort has almost nothing to do with how big a space is. Nor is it relevant whether you own your home or occupy a temporary rental. Wherever you live, right now, is your home and merits making into a space that feels great to you. Even when I am living in a hotel room or rented apartment for a few weeks during a movie shoot, I make a few simple modifications to create an environment that will support me, such as shifting furniture around, throwing colored shawls or soft fabric on top of bare dressers, and even putting together my own homemade water fountain—a drum of water with an aquarium motor in it. (You may call that bizarre; I prefer the word *innovative*.)

The point is, your intention can make any place special, and intention can exist in any kind of home, be it humble or grand. Too often people put off improving their environment until they get the better apartment or finally buy their dream house. Don't fall into that trap. Take an honest look at your current living space—even if you're a student with one room to work with—and do a bit of experimentation.

Few of us are ever going to live in a perfectly serene home—I tried to do that with my all-white house, and it didn't work. The idea is to create an environment that offers spots of serenity within the busyness and occasional chaos (in my case, teenage daughters who ride skateboards through the kitchen and the twenty muddy paws belonging to our dogs) so that peace is available when you need it.

I will never forget the time I stayed at the home of a friend who happens to be one of the most wise and expert yoga practitioners I've met. Having known him for years without ever visiting his house, I expected that it would be an airy, minimal temple, as pure and graceful as the yoga postures for which he is famous. How surprised I was to find that in fact it was something of a zoo: kids and their many toys strewn around, half-finished coloring projects left here and there, plates piled up in the sink. Nor did my friend arise at dawn, as I'd always imagined. He woke up at eight, like many other mortals do. Yet he went straight to his beautiful sacred corner to meditate, sitting among the lovely things that bring him peace, and quietly began his morning that way as he did every day. It showed me that there is no template for the right environment. We all have within us ideas of what is secure, safe, and nurturing, and a peaceful home looks different to different people. More important, even if the space isn't absolutely

PICKING UP THE SIGNALS

When it comes to making the most of your home, you can find innumerable books and advice magazines on the topic and thousands of professionals who revamp interiors for a living. And every expert has their list of dos and don'ts demanding your attention. But you don't need to turn to outside opinions in order to figure out how an environment feels. Everyone has an instinctual response to space: you might walk into a beautiful home that doesn't feel comfortable or welcoming, and even if you're not sure why, you know you don't want to sit on the chairs or hang out for long.

ideal, when you bring in one component that is special to you and invest it with personal meaning, it can have a powerful effect on your state.

In this final section of the program, you will look at your living environment with fresh eyes and introduce a few elements to enhance it. In Step 1, you will "Clear the Clutter" in order to get rid of stagnant energy and quiet the visual noise. Then, in Step 2, you'll "Create Your Sacred Space," your very own sanctuary for contemplation and reflection. In Step 3, you will "Slow Down Your Home" with physical changes that make one room more relaxing and restorative. In the same way that changing your eating habits is easier if you start with one meal, modifying a single room is a reasonable and doable goal that will inspire you to make changes elsewhere in the home when you have time. The bedroom is a great place to start, as it is a space that is so significant in your overall wellness: it's where you start and end the day and where you get your rest. However, if your bedroom is exactly as you like it already, take on a different room, such as the living room or a home office. And finally, you will "Protect Your Reserves." By becoming more conscious of your needs to rest, recharge, and refuel, you learn how to come "home" to the natural state of balance within.

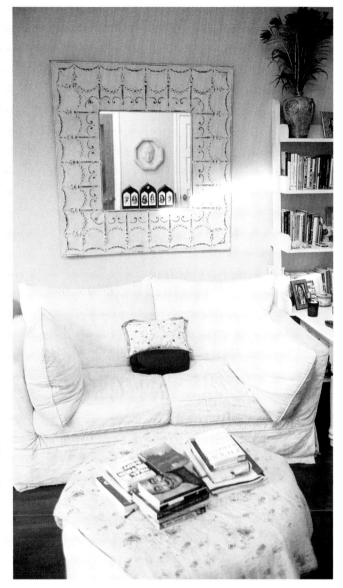

Likewise, you can walk into the next home on the block and cherish the warm and soothing atmosphere you find there. It's "something in the air"; it's the way the place invites you to breathe, to be instead of do, and to let down your defenses.

The first stage of enhancing your environment is turning that instinct, which is so easy to tap in to when you're in other people's homes, toward your own environment. It's a simple matter of stepping back for a moment and developing sensitivity to the way the external environment affects you. It doesn't require any expertise, just awareness. In order to connect with this guiding instinct, it is helpful to take a mental inventory of your home.

Home

Home Inventory

Sit for a moment in a quiet place in your home and ask yourself, "Where do I spend no time in my home?" Which parts of your home do you avoid? Is there a room or area of a room that you circumvent out of habit or simply never use? It could be a corner of a room that is wasted space or a hallway that you've never bothered to decorate. Go stand in it, and feel what you feel. Ask yourself, "Do I feel comfortable in this space?" You will pick up an energy from the space. There's nothing psychic about sensing energy; it's simply a case of noticing the source of your physical, mental, and emotional reaction. Maybe you sense discomfort there, and it comes from the fact that the room is dark or depressing or the light is too harsh; maybe it comes from the view you see outside or the lack of windows. Maybe the cause is something as subtle as an annoying vibration or hum from a piece of machinery.

Or perhaps the negative energy you feel there has emotional roots. Are sad memories connected to that space? Does it still look exactly the way it did when you were in a dark period or in an old relationship? Is it filled with possessions from a phase of your life that you left behind long ago? Notice if your body feels uncomfortable there. What is off in this space, and why?

Next ask yourself, "Where in my home do I feel most vibrant?" Where do you love to be most, whether to curl up with a book, to be active with a hobby, or to spend time with friends? Walk into that space, and notice which elements make you feel vibrant there. Is it thanks to the colors, the lighting, the furniture, the textures, the sound or lack of sound? Does it have to do with what happens in that space, the way you go about things when you're there? Simply observe what feelings come up in that good space, and look for their sources. Chances are, you've made some choices in your surroundings that serve you well, so notice what they are. Or, if you don't have a space in your home where you feel particularly good, note that as well. Are you always going out when you want to relax, hanging out at the coffee shop, gym, or friends' houses instead? Let that be your motivation for making a few changes to your personal space (even if you've got multiple roommates who don't know the meaning of serenity). If you are more comfortable at your local café, then visit the café and look at it critically: what about that space says "comfort" to you? Could you incorporate some of those elements into your own space?

This inventory is entirely subjective and instinctive; there is no right or wrong answer. Yet often several people sense the same kind of energy in a space. It's an instinctual feng shui, a nontechnical version of the time-honored Chinese practice dedicated to bringing balance into your home and thereby into your life. According to feng shui principles, your living space mirrors your life—and the way your space is arranged can affect your life for better or worse. A peaceful environment that permits the free flow of energy will encourage a peaceful life full of good fortune and opportunity; likewise, a living space that is somehow off will compromise your success and progress.

I've absorbed some of the classical feng shui rules into my home over the years, but much of what I've done has come from pure instinct and awareness of my emotional response to my home. In any space, if you get quiet you will know what is right for you, or at the very least, you will be able to feel what is wrong.

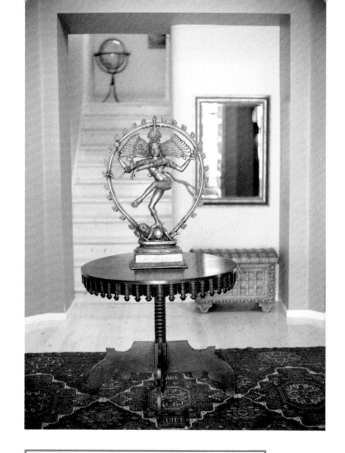

Feng shui is a fascinating tradition in which the flow of natural energies inside the home are balanced and harmonized to create positive effects in all aspects of your life—from your financial situation to your romantic relationships to your health and charisma. Feng shui is a complex discipline that examines the interplay of universal energy between people and places, and a true practitioner takes account of your personal astrology as well as the history and geology of the land under your home when offering suggestions for improving your space. Nevertheless, there are some quick fixes you can apply to encourage a better energy in your home. Start making a few changes here, and if you enjoy the way your environment feels, explore feng shui further through books.

TREAT YOURSELF: *Hire a feng shui expert to do an evaluation of your home. He or she may direct you to modify your furniture arrangements, switch rooms around, and add elements such as water, metal, earth, and wood to the property. Ask at your local health food store, yoga studio, or holistic wellness center for recommendations.*

Quick Fix #1: Love at the Front Door

Put some love into your front door area. If your home is like the body, the front door is the mouth; it's where energy comes in. You want to invite it, in the best way possible, to come in. Make sure the outside area is clean, clear, and unblocked by large trees and shrubs, though plants placed near your entrance will make it more appealing. The door, doorbell, and number should be well maintained, and a light should make your door visible at night. If the door has a glass panel, hang a piece of fabric on the inside so you feel supported and protected by your home.

Home

Clear the Clutter

A BALANCED ENVIRONMENT is built on moderation. It is neither excessively minimal nor filled with too much. It should support you in attaining comfort yet not suffocate you with stuff. You attain that balance when you apply the same approach to your home as you do to your diet: strip away excess, tune in to what works for you, then construct your surroundings with only those things that serve you and satisfy.

Decluttering your space is an important first step. It's like turning down the volume on your surroundings: objects that don't serve you disrupt the potential for peace. When you clear them out, or organize them in a simpler way, you gain not just a clean environment, but calm and clarity within. Empty space, like silence, is conducive to a more meditative state of mind.

Decluttering can also be inspiring. Because it is a process of physical transformation, it can usher in a sense of opportunity and optimism, which will support you in making changes throughout your life. (Think how cleaning your kitchen when you're in a funk can help to wash away the blues.) Just like a diet overloaded with junk can drain you of your mojo, an environment overloaded will things that don't serve a purpose can make you stuck in the mud. Clearing them out can have a cleansing effect on your whole life: it reveals open territory into which fresh ideas and fresh directions can arrive. When you put energy into "out with the old," then "in with the new" often comes with little effort.

WHAT IS CLUTTER?

Clutter falls into two categories: visual noise and stagnant energy. Visual noise comes from disorderly objects that are distracting or irritating. Perhaps it's a bookcase that is overflowing with paperbacks, so glaring in their messiness that you can't help but notice them every time you walk into the room. Perhaps it's the pile of shoes in the hallway or jumble of coats on a coat rack that in their disarrangement silently communicate chaos every time you enter the front door. Maybe your kitchen countertop has become a catchall for everything that doesn't have a home—keys, coins, mail, and pens. These are all minor infractions, but they still create interference, like static on the radio. What is calming to the eye are smooth surfaces, a sense of order, and certain amounts of empty space.

Out of sight does not mean out of mind: if T-shirts are tangled in knots in your dresser drawers or stacks of outdated fashion magazines are stored under your bed to save space, they add to the subtle sensation of overload. You might not see them every day, but your psyche knows they're there. It's always surprising how much better you feel after streamlining even these unseen areas.

Quick Fix #2: Clearing Front-Door Clutter

Clutter left by the front door should be the first to be cleared. Not only does it set the tone for the whole home—it's the first thing people see upon entering—it also (according to feng shui practitioners) blocks the flow of chi, or energy, into the home. Adding some boxes or baskets for shoes and outerwear, a decorative tray for odds and ends on a front-hall table, and ensuring all coats are hung up in a closet will turn negative into positive.

Stagnant energy comes from anything that is taking up space without serving a purpose. Everything that you make the effort to include and care for in your home should be

Quick Fix #3: Deal Now

Deal with things as they come up. Open mail and deal with it immediately, and put envelopes and junk in recycle bin. Read the newspaper when it arrives, and don't keep it another day. Answer any e-mails when they come in, filing those you need and deleting those you don't. All these things not only take up space (literally or digitally), but they also disturb your peace of mind because the more they accumulate, the more you have to catch up on.

either useful or beautiful. If a hulking couch dominates your living room and forces you to constantly move around it, it's not as useful as it could be. If plants have wilted on your windowsill or flowers have passed their prime, they're neither useful nor beautiful. Anything broken or nonfunctioning? Not useful. A wall painted a color that makes you wince? Not beautiful. You only have a certain amount of space in your home and a certain amount of physical energy to care for things. When your home contains things that do not serve a purpose, your energy is in small ways depleted.

That's why in order to refresh your environment and lighten the load, you must also examine whether you simply have too much. Does the sheer amount of possessions in your life outweigh your ability to use them? It's a tricky thing to look at; after all, today's culture prizes consumption over introspection, and a lot of effort goes into planning for, purchasing, and thereafter taking care of belongings. Yet the tendency toward too much in the home reflects the tendency toward extremes in every part of life: too much food, too much stimulation, too much noise, and so on. When you have too much of anything it becomes a stress on the body and mind, and if you are going to stay in balance, some kind of shedding has to occur. Could it be that possessions have the same effect?

In order to live a more intentional life—one in which each action has a purpose and contributes to your well-being—it pays to become intentional with belongings and recognize which things truly serve you today and which do not. When you pare down the ones that don't contribute to your healthy, happy life today, you will find that your load is lightened—because "stuff," be it clothes, accessories, appliances, tools, toys, and even cars, takes up not just physical space in closets, garages, and living rooms, but psychic space as well. All possessions require your energy and attention to some degree (hands up if you've said you "don't have time" to exercise or to read a book yet still found time for online shopping). And stuff almost always carries some emotional investment, by making you feel safe, symbolizing your success, or reminding you of something from your past.

The message of moderation doesn't mean giving up all the possessions you love, it simply means stepping back, taking a critical look at what fills your world, and asking, "How much do I really need?" It means asking if you are losing time to things you don't truly care about, such as spending days shopping for clothes you don't end up wearing or cleaning rooms in your house that barely get used.

By focusing attention on those possessions that serve you today and lightening your load of little-used objects, you are enhancing your ability to stay present in the now. Holding on to clothes that come from a time when you were happy or skinny or sexy is a way of holding on to the past. Displaying furniture that your mother gave you but that you've never liked might remind you of old family tensions. Keeping exercise equipment that you've never used is like staking your hopes on tomorrow ("Maybe I'll use it next week . . .") instead of recognizing what you're realistically going to achieve now.

Part of creating a lighter, calmer, more peaceful life is being willing to release old habits you no longer need; part of creating a lighter, calmer, more peaceful home is being willing to release old belongings you no longer need. Ask yourself, "If my house were to burn down, what would I want?" Be willing to give away things that have lost their meaning for you. What do you think really matters? Give those superfluous objects to charity, and let somebody who needs them benefit. When you scale back, you free up energy for practices that give you more peace and pleasure and bring some simplicity into your world.

In my own life, I think of clutter as the enemy of clarity and peace. I can pretty much guarantee that I'm on some downward emotional spiral or I'm missing too much meditation time if I find that my personal areas in the home look cluttered. Clutter is a clue that life is tipping off balance. I know there is some-

Releasing the Resistance

As much as this book is about change, it is also—as you've realized by now—about overcoming emotional resistance to change. Resistance is when that inner two-year-old wants to have a tantrum and just yell, "No!" Anyone who practices yoga, at any level, becomes very familiar with this state; you learn to trust the fact that your higher self got you to the yoga mat for a good reason and to accept that the physical, mental, and emotional resistance is your less-grown-up self acting out, trying to sabotage the good feelings. Then you let the breath power you through the resistance to the end of your practice. Meditation could be called the act of looking at resistance; you simply observe where you resist the act of sitting still in silence, and then you try to refrain from reacting.

Clearing your environment and seeing it with new eyes can be equally testing. Even the most well-intentioned person can suddenly feel huge resistance about reorganizing and changing things around. If you find that you resist making space more streamlined or enhancing your home to make it cozier, accept the resistance but decide to power through it. Do some self-inquiry: try to examine the source of the resistance. Is it coming from a perception that you don't have the time or energy, or is it coming from a deeper emotional place? Maybe your parents were always hard on you about picking up your stuff and you're still rebelling by maintaining disorder. If so, get over it because the only person who suffers now is you. Perhaps you don't feel settled in your home or in your relationship, so you are staying noncommittal about making it more special and acting like you don't care. Since your home is in many ways a mirror of your soul, any issues that come up with regard to transforming it can be quite revealing.

Chronic clutter often reflects fear and low self-worth: letting stuff pile up around you might feel comforting and safe at first, but it can perpetuate a cycle in which you feel ashamed of your home and don't invite others in to share it. As you work on streamlining your life and connecting more powerfully to how you feel in your body and mind, you will step out of that cycle. You realize that stuff doesn't give you safety; the sense of grounding and security you seek can only come from within. Let your surroundings support you in getting to that point by encouraging you to live mindfully instead of insulating yourself with possessions. When you free yourself of the physical clutter, just as when you lose excess weight that you may have gained as a protective shield, you begin the process of freeing up more space in your emotional life.

thing going on in my head that needs to be addressed because for some reason I am letting my world swallow me up. I try to nip that negative state in the bud. As soon as possible, I devote some time to working in the area that's gone awry, and almost always the action involves some internal assessing of where I am and what I'm doing.

That's why I think one of the most refreshing and empowering things you can do in your environment is to clear it of excess objects and impose order on chaos. It not only allows you to feel new in your home, it is one of best ways to get your head together. It shouldn't be a once-a-year thing; it is a tool you can use any time to gain a sense of renewal and fresh energy for your purpose and goals. When your home is driving you crazy, don't freak out that you need to move and change everything about your existence. Try tackling a particularly cluttered corner of your environment and see how creating order in a tangible way helps calm your mind.

TIP If you are clearing out things that have had some value to you, don't simply toss them in a bag and take them to the charity store. Spend a moment acknowledging what their importance was to you and how they served you, and then set the intention that you want to retrieve the energy that these dead-weight objects may have been taking while in your space. If that sounds too "woo-woo," then simply say to yourself, "Out with the old, in with the new."

Exercise: Clear the Clutter

Pick three things in your home that for years have served no purpose, and remove them. It might be a stack of clothes and shoes or just one outdated overcoat; it might be kitchen equipment, old magazines, a doormat, an old video recorder, or a pile of makeup that you never touch. It could even be an unfinished project sitting in your office or living room, and if you are honest you know you won't complete it. If you can donate any of these things to charity or a friend, all the better. How does it feel to get rid of these items? If you are wavering about getting rid of an object that has some value but that you just don't need, put it aside for three days and then see if you still feel so attached. Remember, what you don't like or don't remember, you don't need. If throwing out three things feels good, keep going.

Attack! Common Clutter Spots

- **IN THE LIVING ROOM:** Old magazines and newspapers that need to be tossed. Media in disarray or too visible (CDs, DVDs, and books). Visible tangles of electric cords from media and technology. Wilted plants.
- **IN THE BEDROOM:** Chaotic clothing and accessory closets and drawers. Objects stored under the bed.
- **IN THE HOME OFFICE:** Poorly filed paperwork. Old research or source materials that could be recycled or chucked. Chaotic supply cabinet. Badly organized computer files.
- **IN THE KITCHEN:** Recyclables and trash waiting to be taken out. Disorganized crockery cupboards. Food cupboards containing jumbled-up and expired products. Crowded countertops and tabletops.
- **IN THE BATHROOM:** Product-covered countertops. Jumbled under-sink area. Towels stacked messily (roll them instead for an instant spa look).

CREATING A CLUTTER-FREE environment doesn't mean you need to run around making sure your house is in perfect order at all times. That obsessive behavior is something I've had to curb in myself. When my daughter Dree turned thirteen and I saw that there was no chance that I could control the disgusting nature of her room, I decided that my controlling impetus was one little thing that I should let go in order not to make myself crazy. I could close the door, run past her room, and refuse to deliver laundry or anything else near her room. Since then I've been much happier in my home. She is eighteen now and still challenging in this area, but I know that because I don't harp on the small stuff, she is home still and loving our house and being with me.

I had to learn that part of finding balance in my environment was surrendering a little control. It's been a hard one because I am so invested in having a neat, harmonious atmosphere for my own peace of mind. Ironically, I have often meditated about letting there be more chaos because letting the chaos happen is part of having a family. I've trained myself to let go and let things fall apart a bit, to allow my daughters to make a mess and be responsible for cleaning up even if it's not the way I'd do it or on my schedule. The house will not be a

pigsty forever, and giving my family respect and the trust that they can do things on their own is often empowering and encourages great results. Today I recognize that although my elder daughter is a notorious mess, she also has a great ability to organize, and when it counts she does show up and clean up. Periodically she does a massive overhaul of her room; without me ever saying it, she instinctively knows that when she's overwhelmed, cleaning her room helps her get her head straight. Once in a while, when I let go of the reins enough to give her some slack, she gets a deep pleasure in showing me how well she can clean.

Quick Fix #4: No More Junk Mail

Spend an hour researching the numbers you need to call or addresses to write to in order to get off junk mailing lists and unsolicited marketing call lists. If you receive a lot of mail-order catalogs, write to them directly to be removed from their mailings. This will be significant in reducing the amount of noise in your home.

Create Your Sacred Space

You must have a room or a certain hour of the day or so where you do not know what is in the morning paper. A place where you can simply experience and bring forth what you are and what you might be. At first you may think nothing's happening. But if you have a sacred space and take advantage of it and use it every day, something will happen. Your sacred space is where you can find yourself again and again.

—JOSEPH CAMPBELL

M Y FAVORITE SPOT in my house is my sacred corner. It is in my bedroom, around a nonfunctioning, stone fireplace that I have painted white. The fireplace sits slightly off the ground and features a large ledge just a few feet above the floor. I've taken over that ledge and placed on it a collection of objects that have the most significance to my spiritual practice. It is like my own personal shrine, a small version of the decorative altars I have seen in temples of many religions around the world. There are miniature stone statues of gods and goddesses that I find beautiful, images of Paramahansa Yogananda, the Indian mystic and author of *Autobiography of a Yogi,* who created the particular meditation technique I follow, one or two candles, metal bowls, and tiny vases with fresh flowers. The combination of all these things is incredibly pleasing to me: each thing I've selected brings peace to my spirit and pleasure to my eyes.

I pass by this corner many times a day, and because it sits diagonally across from my bed it is one of the first things I see upon waking and last things I see before turning out the light at night. Its purpose is not simply decorative: it is a useful prop that helps me slow down and live more mindfully. When I am moving too fast and caught up in my thoughts, my sacred corner invites me to take a time-out— even if it's only for two minutes of calming breathing or just ten seconds to carefully place some fresh-cut blossoms in the pretty vessels. It gives me permission to put down my to-do list and pause the rush of thoughts. As I place the flowers there or sit gazing at my pictures, I breathe, I remember to acknowledge how I'm feeling, I remember to be grateful for all that I have. My sacred corner is a large-scale mindfulness trigger; looking at it inspires me to carry through the important practices in my life—to find fulfillment in quality, not quantity; to do the small things in life as creatively and beautifully as I can.

Not surprisingly, I use this spot to sit in meditation. Since I created it specifically to resonate with all that my deepest self finds peaceful, simply sitting in front of my corner helps to orient my mind inward. I deliberately placed it in an area that has plenty of space all around, so this combination of decorative beauty and emptiness holds a certain energy that I find tranquil and conducive to inner quiet—similar to the way I've felt in Hindu or Buddhist temples, where the beautiful altar is surrounded by plenty of space that invites you to come closer. By having a dedicated spot for reflection and contemplation, my act of sitting still is invested with more significance; I commit to my practice because I have committed to making a space for it.

Even though it is quite small, the effect that my sacred corner has over the rest of my environment is powerful. Because my little shrine stands for consciousness, creativity, and beauty, it sets the tone for my whole home. It helps my environment feel like a haven.

Everyone can benefit from having a sacred corner somewhere in the home. It's a simple way to create a slower-paced, more intentional feeling in your environment. When something is sacred, it means dedicated to a higher purpose and worthy of respect. By devoting a bit of space to whatever idea you consider sacred, you set the intention to fill your life and your environment with the spirit of mindful living.

Some people create an entire sacred space—a whole room devoted to mindful practices such as yoga, meditation, prayer, or journal writing, scrapbooking, and crafting—where they can close the door and "find themselves again and again." That's great if you have the space, but you can get the same effect from devoting one small shelf in a relatively quiet section of your home, plus some empty floor around it, to the same purpose. It does not necessarily have to contain objects of a spiritual or religious nature, of course, but it should hold a few things that are symbolic of whatever makes you feel calm and makes you smile. Your collection may start with one or two special things that have personal meaning, like a card from a loved one and a candle, positioned in a deliberate and attractive way. And it can grow from there. You add objects that represent what you love in your life and where you want to go, or the values you want to stay in touch with.

When you create your own sacred space, no matter how simple or how complex, you are expressing your creativity in undiluted form. The objects you select and the way you arrange and display them is unconditionally your own; you are acting from somewhere deep within, and nobody else's opinion of what looks good matters at all. That's important, especially if you share your home with others. As adults, we rarely have "rooms of our own" in the family home; although it's a given that kids need their private space when possible, we downplay our grown-up needs. By creating a small patch of personal space and using it for quiet times alone, even if it is in a shared bedroom, you are carving out some privacy and expressing your uniqueness.

Exercise: Create Your Sacred Corner

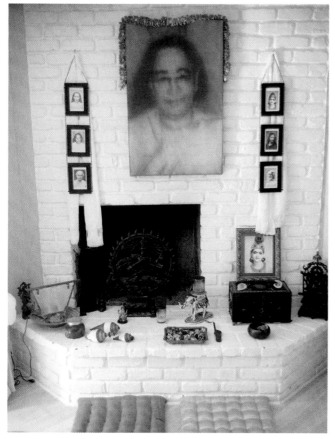

This is a fun exercise to do after you have made some headway on clearing the clutter in your home. First, pick a spot to create this small installation. It should be an area that is quiet, out of the way, and feels good. Look for an existing shelf, table, or ledge. Perhaps you could clear one bookshelf or use the top of a dresser. Using a shelf inside an armoire is an option as well; opening the doors to access it lets you "step in" to your special area. There should be space to sit opposite this surface, on a cushion on the ground or in a chair, if that is how you like to meditate. Consider using unexpected areas like a garden or deck if you live in warm climates (you can always move your location in harsher seasons), and scan spare rooms: perhaps there's an unused alcove or nook that could be given new purpose with some paint and better light. To create more privacy, you could bring a folding screen into the space to cordon off your area when you are using it for quiet sitting, thereby creating the feeling of seclusion.

If there's no ledge or surface available, you'll need to get one. A simple solution is to purchase an inexpensive child's step stool, which you can paint or decorate if necessary, to create a low, small shelf. Or look for a small cheap table at a flea market and cut the legs off to make it the appropriate height. This will become the foundation for your little shrine.

Now you're ready to create the arrangement. Let your creativity take flight. You can go as simple or as fantastic as you like. I've seen minimal, Japanese-style corners with just three beautiful objects—a rock, a bowl of water, and a plant—displayed on a piece of wood, and I've also seen Mexican-influenced altars featuring vivid colors, kitschy knick-knacks, and chili pepper Christmas lights that throw red light into the room. The question is, what type of space will encourage you to connect with the comfort and peace within?

Start simply and allow your style to emerge over time. This is a work of art that will always be in progress; you can change or modify this space as much as you want. Laying down a strip of beautiful fabric is a good way to begin because it makes an ordinary surface more special and marks this as a separate space. Look for a color or texture that delights you. Shimmering silks in vibrant hues such as purple or orange have a spiritual appeal, while red is warm and sensual. Or, neutral textiles in taupe or white will create a clean and minimal backdrop for your arrangement. Next, gather a few objects to display. The idea is not to simply decorate the surface with things that look cute together but to combine objects that create a sensation of "ahh." I find a combination of elemental objects—things that represent earth, fire, water, and air—with personal objects works well. The only criterion is that they appeal to your sensibility and feel right.

Elemental items can ground your sacred corner because they are tangible, visible things that connect you to the physical world. One or more of the following may be used:

■ TO REPRESENT EARTH:

some polished rocks, pebbles, or sand

■ TO REPRESENT FIRE:

a candle

■ TO REPRESENT WATER:

a small bowl of water with flower petals in it; a plug-in
water fountain

■ TO REPRESENT AIR:

incense or a scent stick

Now add in a few items that have emotional and spiritual
significance, meaning that they reflect your personal passions
and interests and connect you to your truth. They may be me-
mentos and treasures, pictures in carved or decorative frames,
postcards, letters, small statues, or figurines. Small bells and
bowls, reminiscent of Buddhist shrines, can be beautiful. Animal
figures may have significance for you. If there's a place that you
find inspiring, include a photograph. You may want to leave
photos of your family or friends for other parts of the house; this
spot is devoted to a very personal and introspective state, and
images of those you have relationships with can bring up a lot
of thoughts. Let nature be your source: try adding in attractive
shells, feathers, small plants, and flowers. If fresh flowers aren't
available, choose silk flowers over dried ones, which can have a
dusty, dead energy.

Arrange the items in the way that best pleases your eye. Try
making something the focal point: a statue, a beautiful candle,
a picture, or a plant. Around this focal point, balance the other
components so the total effect feels complete and whole. Keep
changing the mix or modifying it as time goes by, adding new
elements according to the season or the things that you want to
focus on in your life. You may want to completely reinvent your
corner from time to time—know that there's no reason you have
to stick with one setup for long. Above all, let this little installation reflect your personality, taste, and dreams. Add any extra
decorative elements that enhance the area above or around your
sacred corner.

TIP In order to create harmony in relationships or invite a new relationship
into your life, include pairs of objects, such as two
shells or two candles.

After you have created it, notice how this sacred corner
makes you feel. Does it change the atmosphere of the room it
is in? Does it inspire you to make other changes in the home?
Are there colors or textures you've used here that could be
added to other rooms? Let this be the spot where you do your
short meditation practice; lighting a candle is a wonderful way
to add an element of ritual to the habit, and gazing at a flame
or a beautiful object before shutting your eyes will help induce
a meditative state of mind.

The more you use this corner, the more meaning it ac-
quires. It acts as a reminder to honor some of the blessings
that you already have: a home to shelter you; your health,
which is only getting better; the love of other people; your
faith; the grace of nature—even the curiosity that has driven
you to this book and this program deserves a moment of
recognition. In a world that so often drives us to seek more,
more, more and to fret about all we haven't yet achieved or
accomplished, a sacred corner acts as a ballast. For a moment or two we can feel grounded, rein in those fears and
desires, and recognize that the fact we are conscious of our
breath, calm in our body and mind, and on the way to feeling
even better every day is indeed enough.

BONUS: MORNING/EVENING RITUAL.

If the idea of meditating in front of your sacred space every day
doesn't work for you, simply try to incorporate the space into a
ritual for three days in a row, whether it's as simple as putting
on your shoes or brushing your hair in front of it, or spending a
few minutes to set your intention for the day. It's all too easy to
create the space and then get too rushed to acknowledge it.
These small habits will incorporate your sacred space into your
everyday life so it becomes a mindfulness trigger.

TIP Some people create their own small
rituals, such as writing words represent-
ing things they want to achieve on a small slip of
paper and placing the paper in a bowl on their
shelf, or burning slips of paper containing words of
things they are ready to let go of and allowing them
smolder into ashes (do this in a metal or ceramic
bowl for safety).

■ ■ ■

IF YOU LIVE ALONE and your home is already tranquil, having a sacred corner is still powerful. It can be a place where you focus your attention inward in ways you don't elsewhere in the house, and, through displaying symbols of things you want to achieve, you can set your intentions so you invite those things into your life. Regardless of what your life situation is, you will find that your sacred corner helps turn new techniques, like short meditations or spells of relaxing breathing, into rituals that you love to include in your day.

■ ■ ■

I HAVE ALWAYS HAD AN ALTAR SPACE in the bedroom, but at a certain point I realized I'd added so many things, it was getting cluttered and undefined. I didn't like it but didn't quite know what to do. So I removed everything and went back to zero. I divided up all the objects: those that still moved me and those that no longer did it for me. I sifted through the things to settle on the few that truly mattered. Then I put back the selected items in a way that delighted me, and the things that didn't make the cut, I moved to the garage and soon gave away. It proved to me that nothing is ever fixed or final: you can evaluate and re-evaluate what's working with you in all areas of

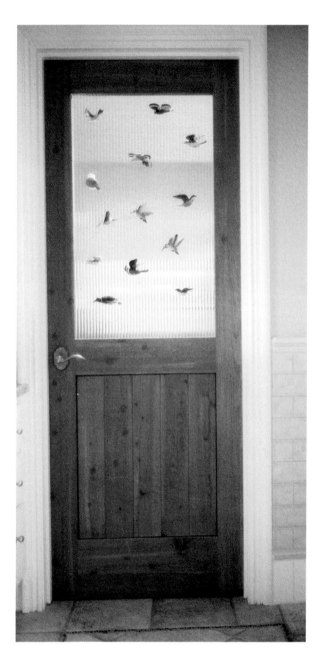

life and constantly make small readjustments. Balance is attained through noticing what's around you and how it makes you feel on a day-to-day basis.

Slow Down Your Home

NOW THAT YOU'RE TUNING IN to how your environment affects you, it's not as hard as it might seem to create an environment pervaded with a sense of serenity and peace. The key is to start small: focus on just one room at first, and modify it with a few manageable elements. Because unlike what you might see on makeover TV shows, a real home grows o rganically, changing color, shape, and look as your life takes its twists and turns. Pick one room that could use some work, and think about developing an atmosphere in the room—one that is welcoming, warmer, and more nurturing—rather than trying to impose a brand-new redesign on it. Just as making one or two different food choices today might lead to your eating a radically different diet a year from now—and feeling and looking infinitely better—simply becoming more attuned to your environment and making a few different choices in it today might lead to a transformed home, without much effort on your part, twelve months down the road.

A "slower" home doesn't mean one in which nothing gets done; it means one that is comfortable for your body, mind, and soul. It provides more than simply comfortable armchairs for physical rest. The way it is arranged and the details you choose for it promote a free flow of energy and a harmonious atmosphere, thereby promoting your mental and spiritual rest as well. Our senses are being stimulated all day long by the world outside our homes, and our minds must stay constantly active. Coming home becomes a pleasure when our personal space is a rejuvenating antidote to the outside world. Achieving a slow home doesn't require any decorating knowledge; it starts by asking the question, "What will make me feel better, calmer, and more rested in this space?"

QUESTION: BASED ON WHAT CAME UP WHEN YOU TOOK THE INVENTORY OF YOUR HOME, PICK A ROOM OR AREA THAT YOU'D LIKE TO TRANS- FORM AND ASK YOURSELF "WHAT WOULD MAKE THIS SPACE MORE COMFORTABLE?"

IT COULD BE one of the spaces that you avoid because it has a negative energy, or it could be one of the places that instinctually feels

Home

good and that you want to develop to make even better. Whether it's your bedroom, your living room, your kitchen, your bathroom, or an office space, ask yourself, "What is the true purpose of this room, and what do I want to feel in here? Peace, mental focus, creativity, well-being, sociability?" Sit in the room for a bit, and ask if it serves you in the best way it could.

- If you pick the bedroom, is the bed in a position that feels good, is there nice light in the morning, or does the sun hit you harshly? Is the lighting cozy at night? Is there enough air flowing and enough space around your bed?
- If it's the living room, does it encourage winding down and interacting with family or friends? Or is all the furniture clustered around the entertainment center?
- If it's the kitchen, is it friendly enough that you're inspired to spend the time it takes to prepare, cook, and possibly eat food there? Or is it too utilitarian, with no signs of your personality and interests?
- If it's the bathroom, does it welcome you first thing in the morning when you are most vulnerable and soothe you late at night as you shed the stress of the day? Does it encourage your self-care and well-being?

QUESTION: WHEN IT COMES TO THAT PARTICULAR SPACE, WHAT IS YOUR IDEA OF COMFORT?

FOR SOME PEOPLE, opulent, plush rooms invite a peaceful state while for others, streamlined, minimal rooms create inner tranquillity. Spend a few minutes considering what type of environment best soothes your senses—relaxed and sunny, sleek and spare, or perhaps rich with color and texture. Looking through magazines is a great way to figure out what you like, but don't get caught up in the idea that your place should be designer-home perfect, or you will never start.

Then read the following ideas for how to make the space feel better, and pick one, two, or three of them to implement in the space. Focus on enhancing the space from your sense of delight and comfort, and don't worry about whether what you're doing adds up to any kind of "style" or not. Your creativity will start to express itself naturally because with this program, you're expanding your awareness through ordinary things—tuning in to the way you breathe, eat, and move. This puts you in touch with your instincts and opens the creative channels. Discovering what you like comes organically: as any clutter or ugliness is removed from a space and you listen to the way a room feels, you get a clearer and clearer picture of what will work in the space.

When we were kids, it was natural and instinctual to change our rooms around, put new stuff on the walls every month, and shift the furniture into new configurations on a whim. Allow some of that spontaneity to resurface now; it didn't ever go away, even if you haven't used it for a while. Sometimes what we need to do most when it comes to our environment is to loosen up a little. We can get so set in our ways about how each room "should" look that after a while it can become frozen in time, never changing an inch over years and years. Turning things on their head can be invigorating: in the bedroom, flip the bed the other way around; borrow a carpet from the living room; swap some lamps, and change where the pictures are hung. Only by experimenting do you come up with the right balance.

Don't forget that modifications can be very small, and they allow you to change your environment on a daily basis. Creating a beautiful flower arrangement and displaying it prominently, making a fire in winter, lighting up an aromatherapy atomizer to diffuse lovely smells, even selecting some great music to shift your mood can be effective ways to bring things back into balance when you feel tested or tried. Not only do others who walk into the house feel that my family and I are welcoming them with thoughtfulness and attention, it also helps me find fulfillment in the little things of life instead of perpetually seeking the new.

I spent a lot of my younger years always hungry for the next high—the next meal, the next endorphin rush of exercise, the next trip away. It's a little addiction that many of us have: hankering after the next big surprise that may be just around the corner, and grinding through today while we hold out for the vacation that will come tomorrow, meanwhile complaining that we're bored with our lives. But is it that our lives are boring, or is it that we're not present while we're living them? Through bringing more attention to the small details of life, we can make every day creative and get more pleasure from what we already have. Frustration with what's in front of you comes from wanting to experience something new; I'm learning we can feel new any time we want. Instead of wishing for that new home, new car, or whole new life, we can create a new experience within and without so easily— through exercise, eating something that bursts with flavor and goodness, or changing the way our home feels.

Exercise: Reinvent Your Room

Enhance your chosen room by picking two of the following eight ways to slow your home. You needn't spend money on this; use what you already have in other rooms or your closets, attic, or garden. Remember that flea markets and secondhand stores offer infinite options and can be a great way to get creative juices flowing. (Feel free to do more than two of the options if you like.) Your room most likely won't come together completely in one week, but start the process now, and keep refining it over time.

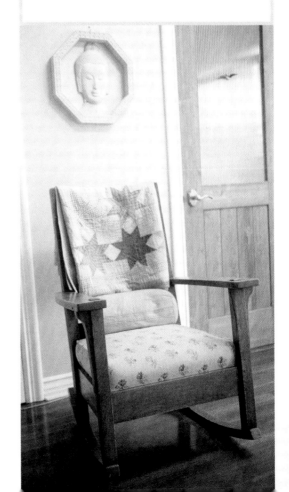

EIGHT WAYS
TO SLOW YOUR HOME

1 ARRANGEMENT

Separate out or conceal any objects in the room that do not fit the room's purpose. For instance, a bedroom is for two things: sleeping and intimacy with a partner. It's not for working, fielding phone calls, or zoning out with entertainment. Anytime you do these things, such as bringing your laptop to bed, it sends mixed signals to your brain, telling it that the bedroom is a place for mental activity. Winding down and getting sleepy becomes harder. Create an environment in which all your senses pick up the message that the purpose of this room is to rest and to connect with your partner, if you are in a relationship. Try to make your bedroom a technology-free zone, leaving your computer outside; to take it a step further, leave all phones outside too. Cover or hide the TV when you're not watching it, for instance by draping a beautiful fabric over the top or placing it in an armoire, and if you are used to watching movies and late-night shows in bed, train yourself to watch them outside the bedroom. When you do the Sacred Morning, Sacred Evening exercise in Week 4, you will refrain from watching anything just before sleep, as doing so stimulates the brain. Get a head start, and try doing that as early as Week 1.

If space constraints mean you can't put things like computers, entertainment centers, or even workout gear outside the bedroom, conceal them with folding screens when you're not using them so that your awareness of their presence during resting time is lessened. Make this room a private retreat; if it opens directly onto a public area such as living room or entrance hall, keep the door closed so that only those who are invited in may enter. A bed placed directly opposite a door can make you feel vulnerable when you sleep; likewise, a bed directly under a window can make you feel unsettled. Position the bed diagonally across from the door if possible so you can see the door but are not in line with it. Cover any window directly above the bed with fabric.

No matter which room of the home you are working on, take a good look at whether the room supports its purpose, and make adjustments accordingly. Pay attention to the placement of the major pieces of furniture in the room. Does the arrangement feel right to you? Make some changes to the physical objects in the room, and see if it helps your experience in it.

TIP

Too much symmetry can be a downer. The ancient Indian science of design and architecture, called *vatsu*, says asymmetry is instinctively more comfortable to us because it echoes the patterns in nature; our bodies are asymmetrical, plants are asymmetrical, and so on. A room in which everything is perfectly aligned may benefit from a bit of disruption: throw off the matchy-matchy look by moving furniture around, balancing square shapes with circular, breaking up shelves of neat books with a vase or statue.

There are physical health reasons for removing excess electronics from your bedroom. Electromagnetic fields (EMFs) produced by electrical wiring have been shown to produce sleep disturbance, nervousness, allergies, inability to focus or concentrate, fatigue, and headaches. Switch electric alarm clocks and radios to battery-operated ones, or move them far from your body. Do not use electric blankets or heating pads while you sleep. Stereos and other equipment should also be positioned far from your bed.

2 LIGHTING

Notice whether you could take better advantage of daylight in the room by moving furniture to catch more of it, swapping too-heavy drapes for sheer fabric panels in summer, or simply placing plants or decorative objects in the sun to play with the light. Colored glass vases on a window ledge are a beautiful way to call your eye to the morning sun. If you have a pretty view outside, maximize it by keeping drapes pulled back by day. Notice how the atmosphere of the room changes as daylight fades. Is the nighttime lighting conducive to cozy feelings? Changing the lighting can provide an instant face-lift to a room. Most overhead lighting tends to be harsh, so lamps set invitingly on tables are often a better choice for room lighting. Adding a dimmer switch to overheads avoids excessively lit rooms, which are overstimulating and unsettling.

Candlelight instantly promotes a soft and tranquil environment without your having to buy new furnishings. Though more expensive, natural beeswax or soy wax candles burn better than conventional candles, which are made of paraffin and release toxic substances when burned and often have wicks made of lead, which can cause lead exposure.

3 COLOR

The effect that color can have on your mood is well known. Color is the perception of the frequency of light, meaning that what you are seeing when you look at color is essentially different vibrations of energy. Notice whether the colors in your room energize you, calm you, or seem off in some way and make you feel uncomfortable. You could repaint a whole room, paint a wall, or bring in furnishings, throws, cushions, or accents with colors that suit that room's purpose. My living room was cream colored until one day I got inspired and painted the whole room deep red. The intense color is balanced by comfy furniture and Eastern objects, which make it a warm space that invites conversation and hanging out. Now it is much more fun to be in.

Within each color, you can find multiple shades and hues that can vary from uplifting to depressing. A good way to find a shade that pleases you is to start collecting colors you see that instantly resonate positively with you. A bag that you love, the wall in a store near you, the cover of a book: make note of the shades that please you, and let your collection narrow down the field of colors and choose

Home

the ones that fit your home. Use these general rules to inspire you, and play with finding a particular shade that affects you positively.

- **RED:** Powerful and stimulating. Energizes, inspires passion, activity, and movement. Can be overwhelming.
- **ORANGE:** Brings joyous energy, conducive to happy gatherings; convivial, optimistic.
- **GREEN:** Promotes calm and active energy at once: a color of balance, healing, and harmony. Refreshing.
- **YELLOW:** Inspires clear-headed thinking, intellectual activity, clarity. Not great for a room dedicated to rest.
- **BLUE:** Calming, meditative, soothing, a cool color. Balances the nervous system. Might be too cool if you feel lonely in your home.
- **PURPLE:** Spiritual, supports intuition. Deep shades are intense, but a very light lavender or violet may be right.
- **WHITE:** Uplifting and purifying. The effect can be sterile if there's too much of it.

TIP Often overlooked for bedrooms, a color palette that reflects the skin tones of all races creates a very sensual and soft environment. Consider beige, taupe, peach, apricot, tan, cocoa, with subtle yellow and pale violet for contrast. Accent colors from the skin tone family, like cinnamon, burgundy, gold, and bronze, can add to the warmth. If you prefer cool colors like blues, grays, and greens for a bedroom, check that they don't get too cold; you may want to add accents of warm shades here and there through textiles, artwork, or furniture to maintain a cozy feel.

Adjust the color palette of your chosen room in a deliberate way, whether through painting it or adding colored fabric to windows, to the bed, or draped over furnishings or through accent pieces such as cushions, pictures, and decorative objects.

4 SOFTNESS

One of the easiest ways to introduce warmth into a room is to add furnishings and textile elements that create softness. Touch is a very important sense; we should cater to it and feed it with nice experiences. Much of the day spent in cars, at desks, at computers, or on our feet mean our bodies yearn for the relaxation of pleasant touch sensations. Add an element of softness to your room. It doesn't have to mean buying sumptuous new furniture. Add plump pillows with soft covers to the sofa, or include giant cushions on the floor. Consider putting in a textured rug where there was none before, draping delicate table runners on surfaces, or softening windows with drapes instead of blinds. Notice how even a bare wooden table can have softness, the sleek feel of polished wood under your fingers. A decorative fabric wall hanging instead of a framed picture will also instantly telegraph softness. If you prefer a minimal room with clean lines and edges, simply contributing one or two soft elements will make a subtle but strong impact.

For affordable curtains and textiles, check eBay.

5 HEAVINESS

A few weighty features can ground a room and make it feel significant, thereby contributing to the stability of the home. Add a deliberate

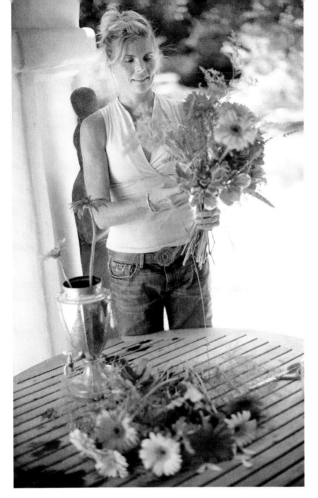

feel of a space and needn't be difficult to care for. Because plants are living objects that grow slowly and enhance your well-being through helping you breathe (literally, through delivering oxygen and consuming carbon dioxide), they embody the slow-home principles. Even adding one small one to a bedroom is a gesture of self-care. (Place an aloe plant by your bed as it gives off oxygen by night, the reverse of most plants.) Try adding large, dramatic plants such as spiky succulents or ficus trees. Almost like having a Christmas tree in the room, they have a definite presence, which will affect your spirits. Flowers, when lovingly arranged in nice vases, are like a gift to your house; by placing

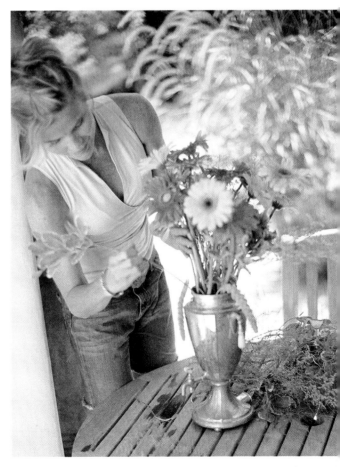

heavy element to your room. Make a few bold gestures with heavy objects like small statues, oversized vases, or even dramatic pieces of furniture. In my living room I have Indian and Chinese statues; they balance the soft furnishings, temper the sensuality of the red walls, and provide a focus for the eye and make it a room that demands respect. Your nature component, below, may fill this need, especially if you use stones or wood.

6 NATURE

Bringing the outdoors in, with green plants or fresh flowers, is refreshing and soothing. Plants and flowers can instantly transform the them in areas that they'll be seen and appreciated by all, you are celebrating your home and thanking it for sheltering you.

Other ways of bringing in objects from the natural world are to use organic elements like shells, stones, and pieces of wood for decoration instead of store-bought knickknacks. They can contribute an ancient presence that counters the modern world's rush and artificiality. Arrange thoughtfully to showcase their preciousness. A shallow, woven basket of similar-shaped small stones, placed under a glass coffee table, is soothing to the eye and calming to the spirit. Likewise, a platter holding large shells, displayed on an entrance hall table or dining table, is a connection to the sea; try contrasting the shells on an antique metal platter or dish to enhance their beauty. Even beautiful chunks of driftwood are soothing.

TIP In the kitchen, take dry foods such as cereal, pasta, and rice out of boxes and store them in glass jars; put fruits and vegetables that don't need to be refrigerated into bowls (thick-skinned items like bananas, avocados, and grapefruit.

Creating a floral display is a meditative act that not only soothes you, it brings peace and beauty to your home. Either pick some plants and flowers from nature, or go to a flower store and select individual stems and greenery that appeal. Take a good half hour to cut the stems, lay out your individual components, and arrange the individual elements into a whole. Follow no rules but your own idea of what looks pretty. Try to achieve a balance between colors and between flowers and empty space. It is nice to do this in silence and to tune in to your breath. Allow your eyes to take in the colors and textures and your nose to take in the scent. Place the finished product somewhere in your home where you will enjoy it the most. Bring the arrangement into your bedroom at night.

For something more permanent, gather a few nature elements to create a decorative piece for your room. Decorative objects don't have to come from fancy architectural or design stores. Check out garden and home supply stores for components, or if possible gather items from a seashore, forest, or riverbank. Arrange your chosen stones, shells, or wood to create an appealing arrangement.

7 WATER

Most Western homes keep water in very utilitarian places: the sinks, toilet, and shower. But when you add water features in more decorative ways, you can bring a beautiful feel into the home. Water is used extensively in feng shui because it is an important element that promotes sustenance, abundance, charisma, and the flow of life. It is brought into the home through fountains or aquariums full of brightly colored fish. Or you can bring it to your front door or yard with a horse trough and a pump.

Add a small water fountain or aquarium to your chosen room. Small tabletop fountains are easily found online and need not be expensive. The water should always be in motion: you not only see the water moving, you hear it and benefit from the negative ions released into the air. The placement of fountains is done on a calculated basis in feng shui, and if you like the effect of this exercise, investigate feng shui rules further to find the perfect spot for water in your house. (For example, when properly placed in your bedroom, it is said to encourage romance.) Adding water has dramatically changed the feel of my house so that now it is more vital, more alive—more "charismatic," as the feng shui experts would say—while at the same time providing a soothing sound track to our lives.

Smells and the sound of a river bring me home wherever I am. I have fountains in my house to bring me back to that feeling of a loving past, to Mother Nature's embrace. In California I get the smell of my roses in late summer that smell unreal in the evening when the cold strikes. The lemon-tree blossoms are so scented and wonderful, I often go back to the plant to see if the smell is real. It is intoxicating. In late spring, the night jasmine scent wafts into my bedroom from the garden—what else do I need to be happy?

8 SCENT

Use scent to instantly transform the mood of your home. The simplest and most natural way to create a scent effect is to use essential oils—pure plant extracts obtained through distillation—which are the basis of aromatherapy. When heated in a small diffuser, their aroma is released into the air, changing the feeling of a room. Essential oils have been therapeutic agents for thousands of years; you can also add a few drops to a bath, or add to a carrier oil (such as almond oil) and massage onto your body.

Different scents have different effects:

- Early morning, for uplifting: grapefruit, lemon, lime
- Midafternoon, for awakening: peppermint, geranium
- Evening, for calming: lavender, chamomile, jasmine

TREAT YOURSELF: *Ceramic diffusers use a tea-light candle or electricity to heat a dish of water sprinkled with a few drops of essential oil. Diffusers and oils are easy to find online.*

TIP If you use commercial air fresheners, particularly the plug-in kind, your environment may be filled with strong smells without your even realizing it. We get used to smell when it is around us all the time, but our senses are nonetheless being exposed to the stimulation. Consider removing all artificial air fresheners to create a clean slate in your home. Then, if you like, use essential oils or gently perfumed candles from time to time to introduce a mood when you choose. Consider also going smell-free with your personal care products for a day, to quiet down the noise of multiple perfumed products on your body.

DETOX YOUR HOME

Just as it pays to lower your exposure to chemicals in your food, it pays to become conscious of the amount of chemicals that you are exposed to inside the home. You are probably interacting with more chemicals than you realize every day, through common cleaning products, personal care products, dry cleaning, and even pet care products. All these things contain toxins that, little by little, accumulate in your body (and in your children's bodies) and can cause symptoms like headaches, rashes, and breathing difficulties. Many health advocates are making the link between the synthetic chemicals in our in-home products and diseases like cancer and asthma as well as hormonal, reproductive, neurological, and immune disorders. Just as with food, it is simply good common sense to lower the load of chemicals in your environment. You don't have to go completely natural overnight; make a few different choices to lower the load. If you normally buy extra-strength kitchen cleaner, try a toxic-free one from a natural products brand. If you have bought the same brand of feminine hygiene products for decades, for one month, try a brand made with unbleached cotton.

Top Ways to Reduce Your Toxic Load

CLEANING PRODUCTS: Look for cleaners, detergents, and dishwashing products that are earth friendly. The packaging should include the following words: *non-petroleum-based surfactants, chlorine and phosphate free, nontoxic, biodegradable.* These products are often comparable in price to those made with synthetic chemicals, and if they're hard to find in stores, they are easy to buy online. Try a brand like Seventh Generation.

DRY CLEANING: The chemicals used in conventional dry cleaning have been linked to cancer, birth defects, and central nervous system damage as well as short-term effects like dizziness, nausea, and shortness of breath. Though they are supposed to evaporate from your clothes, these chemicals can easily get trapped in the plastic wrapping, so if you must use a dry cleaner, always be sure to air out clothes. Alternatively, seek cleaners that use nontoxic or "green" methods; they are becoming increasingly common nationwide.

PERSONAL CARE PRODUCTS: When you use antiperspirants, your body absorbs aluminum, which has been consistently linked to Alzheimer's disease. Antiperspirants are also considered by many to be connected to breast cancer, particularly when used in combination with underarm shaving. An easy step to safeguard your health is to use natural deodorants, which are aluminum free and can be quite effective (however, do check that there are no parabens in the ingredients). Feminine care products, whether tampons or pads, are another product to switch: conventional ones made of bleached cotton expose you to highly toxic chemical dioxin, which is a known carcinogen. Look for brands that don't use chlorine to bleach. Other products to consider switching include sunblock, hair dye, toothpaste, and fragranced body and hair products. Health marts and online drugstores typically carry a good selection of alternative brands.

PETS AND GARDENS: Reduce your exposure to pesticides by using nontoxic flea treatments for your pets as well as natural pest-control solutions and insect sprays in your garden where possible. Organic fertilizer is also a healthful option if gardening is your hobby.

PLANTS: Plants filter the air of toxic chemicals as well as release fresh oxygen into the environment and contribute to balanced humidity. When it comes to pollution, indoor environments can be worse for you than outdoors because the paint, carpeting, textiles, and appliances in homes contain formaldehyde, acetone, and other chemicals that release vapors into the air. Strategically selecting plants that absorb these chemicals is a great way to counter the toxic effect. Consider adding plants such as areca and reed palms, gerbera daisies, Boston ferns, English ivy, chrysanthemums, spider plants, and golden pothos. Two or three plants are needed to clean the air of an average living room. Caring for plants is not rocket science; plus, it is a meditative, spirit-boosting act.

TIP Fresh air is a great tool for countering the pollution that is inherent to every home; it's easy to find and free. Throw open the windows whenever possible to get clean air in your home, especially when cleaning, and keep bedrooms ventilated at night.

TREAT YOURSELF: *An air purifier is a great addition to your space, particularly if you have pets. If someone smokes in your home, consider it an invaluable investment.*

My friend, the feng-shui expert David Cho, came to do a full evaluation of my environment and tell me what he discovered about the energy of my home. In classical feng shui, many sets of complex calculations are done to check not just the setup of the interiors, but also the positioning of the house on the land and even the geology below it. Needless to say, I thought that by now, after all my introspection and adjustments, I'd get a straight-A report. Yet to my surprise David told me that the office room in which I work had the worst energy for getting things done. I'd always wondered why it was so hard for me to mentally focus there; he said I should be using it for meditation and spiritual practice. He directed me to try the formal living room downstairs for working in because it had much better potential in this area. With just that one simple suggestion—one I would never have thought of—I found new opportunity within my own home. I made a nonfunctional room into a highly usable room. It used to be the typical living room untouched by everyone except the pooch placing his muddy feet on the couch. It was my mother's living room, the everything-in-its-place room, the don't-touch-a-thing room. Now it is a light-filled energy source for me. I love it. Because I am a neat freak, I know it will never become too messy. I added two huge trees for my own sense of warmth, and then I set my computer up on the desk that we had built into the shelving unit on the wall years ago. We never quite knew why we had added that desk, but now I know.

David, meanwhile, said that other rooms are wonky in their energy, like my husband's and my bedroom. He insisted that the bedroom is in the wrong part of the house, facing the wrong way, and we should be sleeping elsewhere. Yet I love that room! I always sleep wonderfully in it! So again, just as with diet and all the choices you make in life, you may not always follow the experts but instead take some tips from them when they feel right, and go with your gut. So while I refused to change my bedroom to another part of the house, as he insisted, I incorporated many of his suggestions, such as adding some water fountains and metal, while keeping true to my own taste as well. My bedroom feels fantastic now.

Negotiating with a Partner

One of the delicate issues that comes up with changing your environment, if you have a family, is that you have to consider how to make the environment work for everyone else. I fought compromise for a long time. In fact, it pissed me off when my husband had opinions about what I was doing to the home. As a wife and mom, I was the one who was home most of my time, so setting up the space the way I liked was "my job," and I also probably thought my taste was better than his, which just made him resentful and made the space a lot less happy than it could be. A lot of men don't care about the decor or style of the home, but since my man did, I had to learn to have an open attitude and talk about it as our collective space. It helps to communicate; it's crucial to start a discussion. "I don't always feel comfortable in here; how do you feel?" If your partner doesn't mind that the kids leave their stuff all over the living room, and you hate to see their clutter, then how can you together make a space that suits you all? Through communicating, you can find a creative solution, such as giving the kids their own low coffee table in the living room. Then everyone knows it's okay for them to leave their stuff there, and you won't get stuck in that battle in which Mom plays the resentful housekeeper role, always picking up after them and being mad about it.

Protect Your Reserves

SOMETIMES THE CHALLENGES OF WORK, LIFE, AND FAMILY combine to sap my energy completely and I know to watch out—I'm on the cusp of getting sick. Those first signs of fatigue, moodiness, and off-color feelings are a sign that I have been overstimulated and overdoing it, and it's time to press pause and take care of myself. That's when I let the home environment I've created nurture me a bit. Recently, I was exhausted mentally and emotionally from doing something I love, but the nature of the job—shooting twelve yoga videos in two days—was too much, especially as it came right on the heels of flying to Vancouver for one project while I was still recovering from the movie shoot in New Zealand. Emotionally, I was dealing with anxiety about leaving my family yet again while adjusting to fall weather and dark skies. All of it pulled at my energy and got me down and triggered the beginnings of a cold. Yet thankfully, I gave myself permission to slow down and take care of myself. Rather than keep plugging through a hundred tasks like a maniac, I allowed myself to have a very quiet day, retreat to my beautiful bedroom, and restore what was lost by doing too much.

When my health feels compromised, I know that I am responsible for staying well. Yet it's a challenge to dial down the voice that says, "There are things to be done!" I battle the guilty fear that I'm being useless on the family and work fronts, yet I remember that the world can go on without me and others can in fact fend for themselves. I talk myself out of doing the ironing (even though my husband needs his shirts). I let the girls go to the store alone and trust they can make their own meals. I resist cleaning up after my older daughter, as tempting as it may be, and I give myself permission to meditate whenever my energy can focus. As for food, I take it very easy. If my appetite is screwy, I eat very little and keep drinking warm water with lemon. After a quiet day like this, my balance is often restored and whatever illness was circling me has been blown out like bad weather. My appetite returns, and I feed myself the plain, steamed veggies that taste clean and soothing to my stomach. I let my bedroom act as my healing spot: being in it soothes me and makes me feel better. Anytime I am laid up, it teaches me the beauty of slowness and the need for doing nothing in particular; it reminds *me that I am a success without doing and there is nothing that I am doing that is not right here in this moment. These are my lessons, and my breath gets me back to it.*

When you pick up the first signals of fatigue or find yourself fighting too much in your body and mind, stop, listen to your instincts, slow down your thinking mind, and give yourself permission to do whatever your body is telling you it needs to get back to balance, even if that may mean just lying around for a while. It's not being unproductive; it's taking responsibility for your own health. One of the hardest lessons we have to learn is to protect our own well-being like the precious resource it is.

■   ■   ■

IT'S TAKEN ME FOUR DECADES to see the obvious: I must take care of myself first or I will spend a great deal of effort trying to care for others without the resources I need. As a teen, I was the caretaker to my mother during her final illness and was constantly wracked with worry that I wasn't tending to her enough. As a young mom, I would push and push myself to be superwoman: super-fit, super-hardworking, and super-available for my kids as well. I would get to whatever film or TV set I was working on extra early and pal around with the cast and crew all day long because I wanted everyone to have a good time. I'd get out of bed ridiculously early to power through a workout on an elliptical machine at home;

and any free time I had at the weekends was all about the kids. I don't think I ever slowed down long enough to feel how tired I was (hence my ever-larger doses of caffeine). In fact, it didn't even cross my mind that it would be okay to take time for myself unless I was using it to work out hard or prepare some special kind of food. Take some downtime for resting or recharging? I didn't need that! I was the woman who ran vertical mountain trails and jump-roped her way through three episodes of *Taxi.*

Yet I was kidding myself. My energy was shot much of the time because sheer will-power overruled any subtler sensitivity to how I was really doing. I didn't know that if I took more quiet time for myself during those busy days on set—like retreating to a trailer to meditate as I frequently do today—and if I focused more on the quality of time I spent with my daughters rather than just logging quantity, we would all have been happier and healthier. During many of those years, even though to everyone else I was sparkling with spirit, I was actually fatigued and struggling to find peace with my life.

Many women, whether or not they work outside the home or have a family or live alone, run on empty. Yet pushing yourself to the max is an unsustainable approach. Eventually, your ability to function at optimum level gets lower and lower until body, mind, and spirit are sapped. Today I've found a middle ground. Did something major have to get sacrificed in order to free up hours of time? No. I became more aware of my energy levels from day to day and moment to moment, and I am more careful about protecting my reserves.

So far, this program has directed you to become conscious of how food affects you, how exercise changes your state, and how busy your mind might be when you sit in silence. In this final section, as you look at the sanctuary of your home, you can think about how the energy in your home relates to your overall energy levels. It's clear how stresses on your system can come from the noisy stuff: the sugars and stimulants in your food, the toxins in your environment, and the constant stream of information and technology. Yet stresses also come from too little sleep, too little time in nature, or tensions between family members in the home. To achieve balance, it's important to develop sensitivity to the ways in which your energy might be unnecessarily expended so that you catch the first signs of imbalance. We need to practice energy conservation in our homes and appliances, and we need to practice it in our bodies and minds as well.

QUESTION: WHERE DO YOU TEND TO GET "STUCK" IN YOUR HOUSE?

SITTING IN ONE AREA OF THE HOUSE for too long can get your body and mind stuck in a rut and drain you of vital spirit. If you're watching a movie or TV or working at your computer and you feel yourself slumping into lethargy, then mix things up a bit. Move to a different place, lie on the floor for a while, or get up and moving during the commercials or a self-imposed break: all will prevent you from getting to that fogged-out state where you're more likely to reach for comforting or stimulating food or drink.

Taking care of ourselves in this way is important because as a society, we tend to wait until we are sick to make corrections in our habits. Our health-care system is oriented toward dealing with disease; it still prioritizes intervention over prevention and promotes pricey pharmaceuticals much more loudly than natural, health-building habits. In fact, there's such a focus on the diseases and treatments that await us that we may have lost faith that we can take responsibility for our own well-being. Yet we must trust our own abilities. There's no guarantee that we won't get sick, but we can ensure we are fit for life when we put more importance on the small acts that keep us rested and well.

If you're an overachiever, you may have to retrain your brain so that you regard taking time for yourself and your wellness not as a waste of time but as an investment in yourself. Do you secretly subscribe to the belief that if you're pushed to capacity, you're more needed or important or valued? Whether you're a stay-at-home mom or a CEO, you may find it easy to fall into that thinking. Do you think you should push on because you can, even when your body is lagging and it's become a struggle?

In my case, mental busyness and anxiety clearly manifested in physical fatigue, low immunity, and more than a little crankiness with my husband and kids. I had to develop awareness of when I was overdoing things and scale down my activity so that I didn't lose my physical balance and my emotional balance as well. I'm healthier and happier today in my midforties than I was during much of my twenties and thirties because I am grounded by my body's own wisdom: I respond kindly to what my body and spirit truly need rather than obeying what my mind—in other words, my ego, vanity, and insecurity—try to instruct me to do. Instead of trying to achieve so much, I accept how much I can accomplish and don't always try to go the extra mile.

That's why, hand in hand with tuning in to the energy of the home comes the skill of tuning in to the energy within yourself. Pay attention to when you have a lot of it and when you are depleted. Each person has only a certain amount of energy available to her each day, and just as it's easy to waste water by leaving a tap dripping, it's easy to lose your energy through mindless habits. Scan your typical day for little things that are not critical and that, while they may be fun, could get the chop so you could have more empty space. Millions of us bring work home with us; is it absolutely critical to be doing homework when you give so much at the office already? Notice if you have let boundaries between home and work get too blurred. Or do you lose time in softer ways: reading gossip magazines, stopping for tea to go when you could make it at home, watching television that doesn't particularly excite you? Make these things a treat the way you make certain food a treat: turn to them selectively rather than indulging in them frequently. If you make several phone calls a night to friends who talk your ear off, ask yourself if you are spending precious time on something that isn't critical.

When you're accomplishing the twentieth task of the day that could in fact probably wait a while, check in and ask, "Am I being kind to myself?" When you're staying up late to watch a silly movie, ask, "Am I doing what I could to maintain optimal energy?" Everything you are doing during this month-long program is

reorienting you toward building and maintaining a better core of energy than you've ever had before. The following four healthy habits will round out your set of tools.

FOUR SMART HABITS FOR MIND-BODY BALANCE
1. Get Better Sleep

QUESTION: WHAT IS YOUR ATTITUDE TOWARD SLEEP?

- A. I feel like I always need more of it and am slightly resentful that I'm not getting enough.
- B. I make it a priority to get the right amount and get to bed at around the same time every night.
- C. It's up and down. Sometimes I value it, and other times I squeeze by on bare minimum.

WHY IS BEDTIME SUCH A RITUAL for little kids—"Please tuck me in. Please read me that familiar story," and "Leave the nightlight on"—but such an overlooked detail for adults, who typically flop into bed, exhausted, at whatever time the tiredness hits? It's because kids instinctively crave structure to the day and consistent habits; it grounds them and makes them feel safe. We move away from that as we get older (the teen years in particular are a time to rebel with erratic sleep patterns), yet our human nature is to want that stability, and it serves us to weave it back into our daily life.

Sleep is both a critical element for physical health and an important daily ritual. When you make sleep a priority, not an afterthought, you benefit on all levels: regular sleep heals physical imbalances and soothes emotional ones as well. It should be the easiest health benefit in the world to claim, yet people today have trouble with it: one disturbing sign that we are out of balance is the fact that sleeping pill prescriptions have grown 55 percent in the last four years. The way we deal with sleep is emblematic of the way we deal with the rest of our health: making changes in habits and improving food, drink, and exercise in order to achieve better sleep is always better than going straight for medication.

The point was powerfully driven home for me when my husband was interviewing the Dalai Lama for a documentary. His Holiness was adamant there was one healing thing above all else that Stephen should do now that his cancer was in remission: "Sleep. Sleep. Sleep!" Any time you're under stress, allow extra rest.

QUESTION: DO YOU TEND TO FALL ASLEEP ON THE COUCH IN FRONT OF THE TV?

THAT'S A BAD HABIT to get into. Wean yourself out of stretching out late at night with a blanket to watch the box; if you are that tired, wind down your activity and prepare yourself for bed.

The number of hours of sleep you get does clearly affect how you feel. Everyone's different, but seven hours is often about right when you are at optimum health. (Don't beat yourself up if you need longer, especially in winter months, when the body craves more.) No matter how long you need, one of the best

things anyone can do for their overall wellness is to get to bed by about 10:30 every night. That's because the body does most of its recovery and restoration during the hours of 11:00 P.M. to 1:00 A.M. If you are not asleep during that window of opportunity, you miss out on the prime time for bodily repair. Our bodies are programmed to wind down after sundown, much like other animals; when we fight those rhythms, we are compromising the natural state of wellness that is our birthright, for abnormal sleep patterns can throw off other bodily functions like hormone production (which affects your appetite, mood, and reproductive function). The advent of electricity, and subsequently our modern, twenty-four-hour culture in which many people work late into the night, has thrown nature a curveball because now there is no impetus for us to be asleep when our body most needs it. It's up to each person to make a choice: sleep is more important than Letterman, Leno, or one more blog that's waiting to be read. (If you work the night shift at your job, and your health is subpar, you should research this subject further as night-shift workers have been shown to suffer from their consistently abnormal sleep patterns.)

Getting to bed by 10:30 also serves to make your bedtime more of a ritual, albeit without the stories and night-light of childhood. If you have been modifying your bedroom to make it more of a haven, this will come naturally. To prepare my room for sleep prior to bedtime, I turn on a soft light or two, take the decorative cushions off the bed, fold back the comforter, and plump up the pillows. I fold back my husband's side too. (I stop short of putting mints on the pillows, but sometimes I'm tempted.) I might light a candle to perfume the air, or open the window if the room needs it. With these small gestures, which sometimes happen a couple of hours before bed, I set my intention: tonight my partner and I will rest well, and tomorrow we will wake up feeling new.

Simple as it sounds, this is a sacred act. It brings a deliberate close to the day; when I get into bed to sleep, I take a few moments to run over all that's happened that day and to check whether any intentions I set for myself at the start of the day or during a meditation have manifested. (You may find this a good time to write in a journal and put anything in your head down onto paper.) Like all the rituals in this program, I find this one comforts me when there are bigger issues stressing me out; by returning to the same action day in and day out, I touch solid ground and slow down my whirring thoughts.

The improved diet, exercise, and quiet-mind practices you are doing in this program, as well as creating a calmer bedroom, will all help you to get better sleep. But if good sleep is elusive, try the following:

■ Go to bed on a regular schedule, and before 11:00 P.M.
■ Don't drink caffeine in the afternoon or evening, and know your personal balance with food: some people benefit from lighter dinners while others sleep better having consumed more protein and fat. Experiment.

■ If you tend to need to urinate in the night, don't drink fluids for two hours before going to bed.
■ Take a hot bath or shower before bed. Your body temperature will rise and then fall, which encourages sleep.
■ Try herbal teas made for sleep: chamomile teas and special blends based on chamomile can have a powerful effect in tipping you toward sleep. Avoid any sugary beverages or snacks.
■ Keep the room temperature mild (below 70 degrees), and crack the window. Notice if your bedcovers are warm enough and stay on you neatly through the night.

TIP Pay attention to the way you wake up. Many indigenous cultures believe that sleepers should never be abruptly wakened but instead drawn slowly out of sleep so as not to shock their spirit. If you use a shrill alarm clock to wake you (or, worse, a cell phone alarm), consider how the sudden noise might be setting you up for a cranky morning. Try a gentler alternative, such as a clock that quietly chimes over several minutes to draw you gradually to a waking state or one that gradually brightens the room to simulate the sun. This can profoundly alter your first impressions of each day.

TREAT YOURSELF: *A Zen Alarm Clock pulls you gradually out of slumber by chiming slowly and quietly over a ten-minute period so that each day dawns with gentle serenity.*

Exercise: Better Sleep for a Week

- **OPTION A:** If you are a night owl, commit to one week of going to bed by 10:30 P.M. and waking up by 6:00 or 6:30 A.M. It may mean curtailing your social schedule if you go out a lot or changing when you do your work, but just do it as an experiment. Notice if you feel more rested and ready to get out of bed in the morning.
- **OPTION B:** Commit to one week of preparing your bedroom in a deliberate way for sleep by entering the room prior to bedtime and setting it up in the most inviting way. Add whatever small sacred touches you can to make going to bed a more reverent act (journal writing, reading inspirational or calming texts, prayer, and so forth).

Getting on a good sleep schedule may mean trying a few different things until something works, so don't give up.

I am a big believer in setting an intention not just for each workout session but also for each day. Before falling asleep every night, I reflect on what I want to achieve the next day or how I want to feel, and I state it to myself in a deliberate way: "I will be energized and enthusiastic about my job." "I will be calm and patient with my children." "I will look and feel beautiful, radiant, and sexy." This imprints the intention to be new tomorrow in the mind, where it can take root overnight. It might sound a bit wacky, but it is powerful. As a Sikh teacher I met told me, "In dreaming, we rehash our old patterns over and over. So unless we consciously declare that we want to be different, we will wake up and repeat what we already do." When you wake up, try to remember that intention. Checking in with yourself like this nicely bookmarks the day and will counteract the sensation of days rushing by and blurring into each other. I believe that it will subtly shape your life the way you want it to be. Thought can have a magnetic power: holding the thought of what you want in your mind attracts it to you because you are more conscious of possible choices.

EXPRESS EXERCISE

Set Your Next Day's Intention

For the four weeks of this program, commit to setting an intention for the next day each time your head hits the pillow. It may be about the program, such as, "I want to enjoy my short yoga practice tomorrow and feel more connected to my body." Or it may be about the way you want to feel about yourself or act toward others. It may be an intention for the world at large. Upon waking, restate the intention. It may help to put a note or sticker by your alarm clock to remind you.

TIP Sometimes it can be hard to leave the concerns of the day behind when you head to bed. Try this technique to get better rest. At the end of the day, as you go into your bedroom to get ready for sleep, stand by your door and draw a line with your toe where the closed door would be. Say out loud an affirmation, such as, "I am now entering my sanctuary of rest and tranquillity," or "I am entering a space of peaceful dreaming." Step across your threshold, and shut the door (your phones, computers, and any reminders of workaday concerns should be outside). Some say that 80 percent of an affirmation's power comes from your tone of voice; if you don't feel totally wacky, speak these words aloud in a peaceful tone!

✸ IF YOU ARE FREQUENTLY VERY TIRED, can't sleep, or are anxious or depressed, have your doctor do a blood test and check your hormone balances and your thyroid function. Hormone function in general is a huge issue for women, especially as we age, and treatment can radically shift your energy and outlook. Personally, I am not into synthetic hormone replacement therapy, but I have found great success with bioidentical hormone therapy, a natural way to address hormone imbalances. Some in the natural health field say that you should do nothing for hormone imbalance and let nature take its course, but maybe it's because they haven't experienced the aches, pains, and tiredness themselves (not surprisingly, they're often men). It's also important to remember that today we live in a highly polluted world that harms thyroid function. An underactive thyroid or even a hyperactive thyroid

can throw you way off balance. Whether you follow treatment or not is up to your personal discretion, but it is worth investigating if you are uncharacteristically down.

2. Step into the Sun (Carefully)

Like plants, humans need water, food, and a bit of downtime at night to rest our petals. We also need the sun. It's controversial to suggest that sunlight is anything but extremely hazardous these days; too much sun prematurely ages your skin, and skin cancer rates have risen precipitously for women in recent decades, with melanoma incidences increasing faster than any other forms of cancer. Most—but not all—skin experts trace the cause to extreme sun exposure and sunburns. Yet the vigilant sun-avoidant habits that we have been taught to practice may be doing us more harm than good because humans need a sensible dose of sunlight on their skin in order to make the essential nutrient vitamin D. The vast majority of our vitamin D has to come from sunlight; food and supplements deliver much lower amounts, no matter how smartly we eat. Without vitamin D, the health of our bones is seriously compromised, and osteoporosis as well as chronic bone and muscle pain (frequently misdiagnosed as fibromyalgia) can be the result. Vitamin D makes calcium absorbable by the body; no matter how much calcium you consume in food, it can't be utilized unless your D levels are good. Research now shows that we need the vitamin to guard against many forms of cancer, including breast, colon, and ovarian, as well as depression and other diseases (without enough of it, many people especially in northern latitudes experience the wintertime blues known as seasonal affective disorder). Many adults and children in America today are seriously deficient in vitamin D, and because the darker your skin, the more sunlight you need, African American women are the most lacking. The truth is that sun is a healing ray; while too much of it is dangerous, too little of it is equally bad for our health. As with everything good, the message is once more *moderation.*

So what to do? Advocates of sensible sun exposure say it's important to get direct sunlight on your skin daily to build up your vitamin D stores. The amount of minutes to get will depend on your skin shade, the time of year, and the latitude of your home, but the baseline for those with Caucasian skin that burns fairly easily is about five to ten minutes of sun exposure in the prime hours (between 11:00 A.M. and 3:00 P.M.) on about a quarter of your body at a time. African-Americans with dark skin may need considerably more time to benefit: up to fifteen times as long. Use sunblock on your face if you like, but let your body absorb the light, and do not wear sunglasses. If you plan to stay out longer than that, add sunblock afterward (preferably a natural one that uses the mineral titanium dioxide to reflect rays rather than synthetic compounds that are thought to be toxic). If there is little sunshine where you live, careful use of tanning beds can be an option, as are vitamin supplements, but the best bet is to get some sun during the months when it is available to tide you over the gloom.

TIP For detailed information, have a look at the book *The UV Advantage* by Dr. Michael Holick.

TREAT YOURSELF: *A light bath (also called a light box) can stand in for sun over winter months or in climes where there are just too many clouds.*

Exercise: Say Hi to the Sun

If sun is available and you are comfortable with the idea of sun exposure, allow yourself fifteen minutes three times this week to soak in the rays if you have light skin and thirty minutes three times this week if you have very dark skin, following the parameters above. If you are staying out longer, follow up with normal safeguards such as sunblock, sunglasses, hat, and so on.

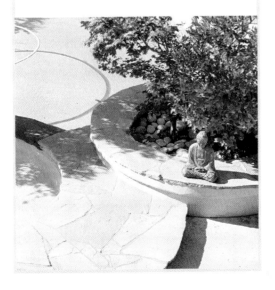

Home

Dive into Nature

If you don't get some nature in your life, you lose touch with your life. When you're cut off from nature, your natural instincts get muffled; I think you're more likely to make poor choices in diet or leisure activities when you don't regularly feel the vital energy that comes from being in nature. Deprive yourself of experiencing the green trees, expansive spaces, and fresh breezes outside, and it becomes harder to feel those sensations inside. The primal urge to eat natural foods, to walk for miles in clean air, and to stand quietly in yoga's Tree Pose, doing nothing but respiring and swaying in the breeze, subsides. That's why connecting to nature on a fairly regular basis is one of the best gifts you can give yourself: it makes all the healthy habits in this program come more easily.

I'm fortunate that a love for nature was solidified at such a young age; a childhood spent running up mountain trails and hurtling down snowy slopes imprinted the message on every cell in my body: *I am nature and nature is me.* When it comes to finding balance in life, tuning in to this message is an exceptionally potent tool, albeit one that is hard to convey. All it takes is getting out there more—literally, putting yourself in nature's way from time to time and absorbing some of that chi, prana, good vibes, or whatever you choose to call it.

Just as having plants in your home can fill it with a slower energy, spending time outdoors will harness you and bring you back to a more realistic pace of life. The size and scale of nature will humble you and restore your perspective on what really matters. You don't have to be an extreme adventurer. All kinds of recreation—picnics in the park, playing games with the kids outside, or walking the

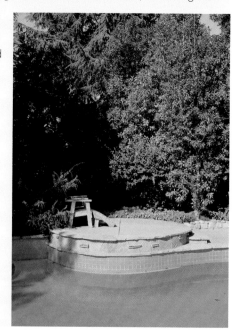

dog—will uplift the spirit and boost the body. If you can get to nature's spectacular spots—the epic mountains, thrilling canyons, and exhilarating beaches—your reward is nourishment that fills your physical and spiritual tanks to the brim. Enjoying time in nature is a way to forget your cares, wipe the slate clean, and come back home to what is simple and true. If we tune in to the rhythms of nature, we are tuning in to our greater heartbeat. It is one of our greatest teachers.

During this program, try to take some of your walks in spots that feel far from the urban environment, or take your friends and family out for a group walk. Use the Sense the Moment technique (described in the Exercise section), and allow yourself to absorb the sensations, sounds, and smells of nature.

TIP Don't overlook the rejuvenating effects of water. When I'm stuck or in a low-energy funk, sometimes the most effective tool for shifting my state is a hot shower. As with exercise, I almost always feel different after it. Others have their most introspective moments in the bath. It's a good reason to apply some of the Slow Down Your Home practices to the bathroom and make it look and feel like a place that heals.

WANT TO STAY HEALTHY while traveling by plane? Try carrying a small vial of raw sesame oil with you and dabbing it inside the nostrils from time to time. It is a natural antimicrobial agent and will help protect you from germy recycled air as well as preventing your nostrils from cracking.

3. Surround Yourself with People Who Support You

Though we might be on our solitary paths toward health and balance, we don't live in isolation. We work with other people or live with them or socialize with them, and their moods and attitudes do have a considerable effect on our progress toward health and happiness. Your family, friends, and colleagues exert a constant push and pull, and your challenge is to calmly hold your ground. While the goal of this program is to build your own foundation from within, there's no denying that the people around us become part of that foundation; when they are invested in our success, we are empowered. When the people around you live and act in ways that are at odds with what you want in your own life, staying on track is more of a challenge because you have to be your own team, coach, and cheerleader at once. If you feel too alienated on your journey—unsupported by those who understand why you are eating differently or taking time to yourself to sit in silence—the temptation to turn to self-soothing behaviors, like eating for comfort, might be harder to fight.

That's why part of protecting your energy reserves means noticing how the people around you either add to them or sap them. First, take stock of just how much of your energy you are putting into relationships: Are you talking to friends on the phone (or e-mailing them) so much that it drains time from your day or evening? Are there too many people in your "inner circle" who expect you to check in on them and listen to their problems? Finding more time for yourself may mean honestly evaluating where you can make more space in your world. It doesn't mean suddenly dropping friends like hot potatoes, but sometimes it's smart to ask, "Which relationships are truly nourishing me, and which are just contributing more noise?" It's important to have those friends who understand you and are rooting for your success, your harmony. Your goals may not be their own—they may think it's a bit nuts to put a water fountain in your living room—but if you say to them, "This is who I see myself as," they should support you. Notice who is frequently telling you all their problems and asking for help; can you realistically serve that person, or is she or he becoming a drain? Setting limits can also help keep things in check; rather than having long phone chats with your close confidantes, set a date to spend time in person and leave the catching up until then.

When you're a mom, it can seem almost impossible to set limits, particularly if your family is used to your being on call all the time. But from my experience, when you ask clearly and calmly for what you need (time alone, quiet, help with the home) rather than being passive-aggressive and resentful that you're deprived, family members step up to the plate. It doesn't have to be much more complex than that: by allowing you to have what you need to live a little calmer, your family is supporting you.

Second, ask whether the people you spend time with both at work and socially encourage you or distract you from your goals. It's impossible to pick who you are paired with on the job, but you can be bold in your choices about who you spend time with after work. If someone is always trying to get you out to a bar or instigate a juicy gossip fest about others when you're trying to cultivate more compassion for yourself and everyone else, perhaps you're not on the same page. There are no rules saying you have to be sociable with everyone; set the boundaries for yourself, and let work relationships stay at work unless you feel you'll be enriched by inviting people into your personal space. Proactively look for those who share similar aims: seek people who want to eat healthily at lunch or who want to take a power walk after work; seek those who understand why eating quietly under a tree might be more rejuvenating than discussing the latest office rumors. And then, when you have free time, try to connect with people who support you in this healthier lifestyle—friends who enjoy similar habits, similar foods, or are curious about what you're learning. Perhaps you have time to find new acquaintances: if you enjoy the yoga sequence in this program, perhaps finding a local yoga studio will encourage you on your healthy path. Or consider joining a walking or hiking group.

Make a strong commitment to surround yourself with people who support who you are now and who you want to be: healthy, happy, and peaceful in body and mind. Write it in your weekly e-mail at the end of the fourth week of the program. It's funny how when you make those decisions, even at the subtle level of thought, things can fall into place. When you make up your mind—*this is how I want to focus my life*—it opens a door: new people, new possibilities will cross your path, as they always do, but now you will be able to see them and grab them.

4. Boycott Bad Thought Patterns

Throughout the program, we've focused on practicing self-acceptance alongside practicing new habits. The two are inseparable: kindly accepting where you are today is imperative to safeguarding your energy reserves and knowing when they are running low. When you regularly ask the question *"How much can I reasonably do today?"* you become a better caretaker to yourself and you move closer to finding satisfaction. If you answer that question honestly, you begin to turn off the relentless sound track in your mind that says,

"Do more, do more, do more!" and you get more comfortable with the idea that from time to time simply *being,* not doing, is enough. It's a critical component of finding balance—being able to find satisfaction in what you have right here, right now, rather than always focusing on what else could be out there. Society says it's the big things we should strive for—the bigger house, the new car, looking like you're twenty when you're forty. But if your daily life is not focused on your daily life, you're going to miss out on living it. Your life will go by before you notice it: time will pass, the kids will be grown, and there will be no getting your life back. If there is one thing this project is about, it's about being in your life as it unfolds, feeling the best you can feel.

If living in the present is tricky, practicing *self*-acceptance—acceptance of the person you are now and the person you are becoming—is even trickier. It means looking a little deeper at what old wounds, old stories, and old habits you are bringing to the table and clearing them out if they no longer serve you. Practicing self-acceptance means peeling back the layers of the onion and cleaning out some of the noise in our hearts. Almost every woman I know regularly launches little mental missiles into herself—barbed thoughts about her looks or her success, love life, or potential—and, though silent, they can be powerful obstacles to peace and harmony. Often, these thoughts are so automatic and habitual, we barely register we're thinking them. But were we to say them to a friend, we'd recognize their intolerable cruelty. Chances are, you have a few of them in your repertoire—I know I do.

"Gee, you look haggard this morning."

"Wow, those pants make your thighs look fat."

"You haven't achieved any kind of success compared to your friends."

"How are you ever going to find love—you're going to be alone forever!"

These thoughts are symptoms of the tragic flaw that lies within almost all of us—the deeply held negative beliefs that resurface again and again to get in the way of practicing true kindness to ourselves. Exercise, as we've seen, is one way to release the power of negative thought when it builds up too much (see "Shedding the Schlock," described in the Exercise section).

It's also important to notice the small repetitions of negative thoughts as they skitter across our minds throughout the day: start noticing just how often you are harsh on yourself when you look in the mirror every morning or night. Breaking free of my own negative thought patterns is an ongoing practice for me. I frequently find that my mind conjures some harsh evaluations of myself, and before I know it I'm believing what it tells me and sliding down a slope of pain and self-doubt. *"I'm old! I'm over! I look terrible! My thighs are enormous!"* What I've learned is that when these pop up, I consciously draw my attention to them. I acknowledge what I'm doing: "Oh, look at me being judgmental of myself again, look at me being cruel again." And I sit with that acknowledgment for a second.

Denying that I have the horrible feelings only makes them stronger because trying to resist anything only makes it into a bigger monster; it slams into you, trying to get your attention. Then I ask myself, "Would I ever say that to my friend? To my daughter? To the old woman down the street?" The answer is always no. I see that those words would certainly not work to motivate or better someone else, and therefore why am I using them on myself? Through simply noticing myself having the thought and asking if it's helpful, it is often divested of its power.

If these thoughts come up during a hike or a quiet moment, I frequently find that my mind roams free and hits upon their trigger point, or source. It's like discovering that the emperor has no clothes: these beliefs that hold me back are rooted in some tiny moment that happened years ago. I realize that memories can't hurt me. They don't even exist unless I give them power. With each moment of self-inquiry, I am closer to self-acceptance. It doesn't happen overnight because problems are repetitive; yet when we have the tools to chip away at them, we start to dissolve our own suffering and find our freedom.

Yes, it takes work to notice bad habits. It takes awareness to change them. But this is what "taking it off the mat" is all about. To create the yogic attitude in the rest of your waking life—calm and balance inside and out—you have to be conscious not just about the simple preventive methods outlined in this program, but also conscious of how you think about

yourself. You have to take responsibility not just for healthy eating and exercise habits, but for healthy thought patterns as well. In order to start and end the day from a place of optimism and calm, you have to give up more than just junk food and constant cell phone calls; you have to give up on the thinking that sabotages your harmony.

It's a choice to go into those dark places. And it is hard to get out of them. When a thought is consuming, or when I feel a deep pain or hurt in me from sorrow or anger, I acknowledge it; and then I acknowledge the space around it—the space that doesn't hurt or doesn't offend me. I see that there is another way to feel. Expand your awareness to a space outside yourself, and it is like an automatic letting go of all that is squeezed up inside.

A good way to take care of yourself when you're frustrated with yourself and you're in one of those dark places we all go to is to focus on someone else. Focus that energy on doing something kind for somebody else, and I guarantee your mood will shift faster. Sometimes you have to trick yourself—*"I'll come back to you later, horrible thought"*—but in the interim, you almost always get to a new place by practicing care and concern for someone you love.

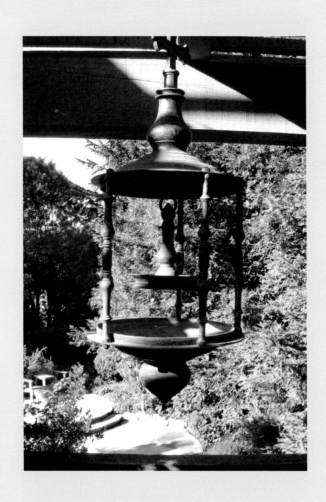

The Quickstart 30-Day Program

YOU'VE READ THE BOOK THROUGH, and now you're ready to begin making the changes that will have you looking great, feeling renewed, and living a radiant life. Here's how it works. The 30-Day Program begins with a Friday or Saturday of planning and making sure you are set up to tackle the next four weeks. Review the exercises, and look at what you will need to have ready in order to eat well, exercise, and make time for yourself. You'll see that certain tasks are to be done every day that week, while others are to be done once, twice, or three times a week. In addition, there are a number of Express Exercises, which require just a few minutes of introspection and awareness. Every exercise has been fully explained on the corresponding page in the preceding chapters, so you can turn back to read the details in full.

During the preliminary weekend, map all the exercises for the first week onto your calendar so that you are creating an itinerary that works with the demands of the week. For instance, if you know you have a lunch meeting on Tuesday when you won't be able to choose your food, don't select it as a day for introducing a new lunch; if you know you'll have a quiet household on Thursday evening, block that night to build your sacred space. It helps to write even the express exercises onto your itinerary as well so that each day you have a selection of different activities to perform. If you know your schedule for the subsequent weeks, go ahead and map out a provisional schedule for the whole thirty days. If not, map each week out on the Sunday before it starts so you are ready to roll on Monday morning.

Once you've made the chart for each week, you can stick it up on your fridge as a reminder of what you need to do that day. Crossing off each exercise as you go is a good way to keep track. (You'll notice that each week comes with certain phrases already stamped on it. These are there to motivate you, remind you of some core principles, and keep you on track.)

When it comes to eating, each week builds on the week before it. Once you have introduced three new breakfasts in Week 1, add in three new lunches in Week 2—and keep eating healthy breakfasts as well, at least three times that second week and more if possible. In Week 3, add in three healthy dinners to your three (or more) breakfasts and lunches. After you add in new snacks in Week 2, keep eating new snacks throughout.

TIP It's a smart idea to photocopy the blank weekly calendars several times over so that if you repeat this program again in the future, you have clean pages to work on.

If this sounds a lot like a summer camp schedule, well, it is! Except that this schedule should be integrated into your existing life as best as you can so that it is doable and maintainable. You may need to make certain compromises, such as missing a regular social event, in order to fulfill all the tasks. You may need to book a babysitter or ask a friend to watch your kids here and there to give you time for certain assignments. That's why taking the time to map out the week ahead is invaluable. And after you have made a visual itinerary, it is easier to commit to the tasks ahead.

But let's get back to Sunday night. For the four weeks of this program, spend a few moments that evening to take stock of what you need to do for the week ahead. Notice what food is in your fridge and what you will have to pick up in order to eat well. Make a shopping list. Then write the weekly e-mail to yourself. This is a good way to gather your thoughts, reflect on how you're feeling right now about your life, your body, your mental and emotional state, and put in writing what you would like to achieve in the week ahead. Send this e-mail to yourself, and save it in a designated folder for reading at the end of the program.

First Friday/Saturday: Before You Begin

In addition to planning out your calendar, use your free time on these preliminary days to get set up. You will need a few basic items ready in order to start the program. The more prepared you are in advance, the more likely you will be to follow through on all the tasks.

- Comfortable workout clothes and sneakers
- A yoga mat
- Ingredients for the breakfast recipes, including substitute foods for your noisy foods (green tea instead of black tea, and so on). If possible, order your pantry essentials online before you begin.
- Ideas of where you can safely and energetically walk in your neighborhood, depending on the season. Can you take to the streets, or do you need to go to a gym and use a treadmill?

Week 1

This week you will start to turn down the internal noise by cutting at least one kind of noisy food, you will introduce new breakfasts into your diet, begin the walking and yoga practices, and initiate a short mediation practice.

To download the weekly calendars go to: www.marielhemingwayshealthyliving.com

This Week's Program

Sunday E-mail

Flip back to the introduction, and type out the contract shown there in an e-mail, then send it to yourself. If you don't have e-mail access, simply write it out in a notebook that you keep exclusively for the purpose of making notes during this program. Add a few lines under the contract. Why are you embarking on this program? How do you feel right now? What would you like to achieve?

Plan Ahead

Mark times for your workouts on the calendar, even if they end up changing. Look into getting spring water delivered.

Daily Missions

- Three-minute meditation (S, pages 201–207). At least once this week, do it after a vigorous workout.
- Turn Down the Volume. Pick at least two of the following (F, page 48):
  - Option A: Downgrade caffeine consumption by one degree.
  - Option B: Downgrade sugar consumption (any added sugar, sweet treats, soda, fruit juice, alcohol).
  - Option C: Cut processed food completely.

Remind Yourself to

- ✿ Drink more H2O.
- ✿ Set your intention for each workout.
- ✿ Do you need to watch that TV show?
- ✿ Have you eaten fresh vegetables?
- ✿ Practice using, "Could I let it wait?"
- ✿ Veto soda and fruit juice.

Personalize Your Program

3x a week

- Eat a new breakfast (F, pages 64–68).

2x a week

- Walk: 20 minutes, focus on breathing in concert with movement and on sensing the moment (E, pages 116–117).
- Yoga: Do the sequence straight through (E, pages 134–175).

1x a week

- Spring Cleaning for Your Fridge, Archeology Mission, and Check Your Food for Vital Stats (F, pages 50, 44, and 30) (under 1 hr.).
- Buy Two New Foods (F, page 79).
- Breathe Through Your Morning (E, page 107).
- Home Inventory (H, page 228) (15+ mins.).

Key

- ■ Food
- ■ Exercise
- ■ Silence
- ■ Home

Sunday

Sunday E-mail
- Three-minute meditation (every day)
- Turn Down the Volume (every day)

- ❑ Eat a new breakfast (3x)
- ❑ Walk (2x)
- ❑ Yoga (2x)
- ❑ Spring Cleaning for Your Fridge (3x)

- ❑ Buy Two New Foods (1x)
- ❑ Breathe Through Your Morning (1x)
- ❑ Home Inventory (1x)

Monday

- Three-minute meditation (every day)
- Turn Down the Volume (every day)

- ❑ Eat a new breakfast (3x)
- ❑ Walk (2x)
- ❑ Yoga (2x)
- ❑ Spring Cleaning for Your Fridge (3x)

- ❑ Buy Two New Foods (1x)
- ❑ Breathe Through Your Morning (1x)
- ❑ Home Inventory (1x)

Tuesday

- Three-minute meditation (every day)
- Turn Down the Volume (every day)

- ❑ Eat a new breakfast (3x)
- ❑ Walk (2x)
- ❑ Yoga (2x)
- ❑ Spring Cleaning for Your Fridge (3x)

- ❑ Buy Two New Foods (1x)
- ❑ Breathe Through Your Morning (1x)
- ❑ Home Inventory (1x)

Wednesday

- Three-minute meditation (every day)
- Turn Down the Volume (every day)

- ❑ Eat a new breakfast (3x)
- ❑ Walk (2x)
- ❑ Yoga (2x)
- ❑ Spring Cleaning for Your Fridge (3x)

- ❑ Buy Two New Foods (1x)
- ❑ Breathe Through Your Morning (1x)
- ❑ Home Inventory (1x)

Thursday

- Three-minute meditation (every day)
- Turn Down the Volume (every day)

- ❑ Eat a new breakfast (3x)
- ❑ Walk (2x)
- ❑ Yoga (2x)
- ❑ Spring Cleaning for Your Fridge (3x)

- ❑ Buy Two New Foods (1x)
- ❑ Breathe Through Your Morning (1x)
- ❑ Home Inventory (1x)

Friday

- Three-minute meditation (every day)
- Turn Down the Volume (every day)

- ❑ Eat a new breakfast (3x)
- ❑ Walk (2x)
- ❑ Yoga (2x)
- ❑ Spring Cleaning for Your Fridge (3x)

- ❑ Buy Two New Foods (1x)
- ❑ Breathe Through Your Morning (1x)
- ❑ Home Inventory (1x)

Saturday

- Three-minute meditation (every day)
- Turn Down the Volume (every day)

- ❑ Eat a new breakfast (3x)
- ❑ Walk (2x)
- ❑ Yoga (2x)
- ❑ Spring Cleaning for Your Fridge (3x)

- ❑ Buy Two New Foods (1x)
- ❑ Breathe Through Your Morning (1x)
- ❑ Home Inventory (1x)

Week 2
This week you will continue to eat several healthy breakfasts and now introduce three healthy lunches during the seven days. All your snacks should now be wholesome ones. You will continue to downgrade your chosen noisy foods, or, if it was easy to cut the chosen habit last week, now try to cut a second one. Tune in to your personal food balance by asking the series of investigative questions after your meals. You will lengthen the meditation practice slightly and add some funk to your yoga session. If there's sunshine available, give yourself short spurts of light to boost your health. And there are two creative assignments this week: make dinner into a ritual by slowing it down and adding some special elements. And create your sacred space—the area of the house that encourages contemplation and reverie.

This Week's Program

Sunday E-mail:
How are you feeling about yourself after Week 1? What was the hardest challenge last week? What went well? What would you like to achieve this week?

Plan Ahead:
Start thinking what area and objects you can use for your sacred space. Gather any objects to set your table for your Ritual Dinner.

Daily Missions:
- Five-minute meditation: At least once this week, do it after a vigorous workout.
- Turn Down the Volume (F, page 48)
  Pick at least two of the following:
  - Option A: Downgrade caffeine consumption by two degrees in the first half of the week, three degrees in the second.
  - Option B: Continue to cut sugars, and now minimize grains.
  - Option C: Cut processed food entirely.

Remind Yourself to
- ☼ Use your sacred space.
- ☼ Am I experiencing true symptoms of hunger?
- ☼ Are you eating anything in a plastic package? Don't!
- ☼ Are you using your Exercise Quick Fixes?
- ☼ Set your intention for each workout.
- ☼ Are you breathing?

Personalize Your Program

3x a week
- New lunch (F)
- New snack (each time you snack) (F)
- Say Hi to the Sun (optional) (H, page 261) (15+ mins.)

2x a week
- Walk: 20 minutes, focus on breathing, observing, and asking questions. (E)
- Yoga: Add funky five-minute music. (E)
- Ritual Dinner (F, page 84)

1x a week
- Buy Two New Foods (F)
- Create Your Sacred Corner (H, pages 238–239) (1+ hr.)
- Mindfulness Trigger (S, page 213)

Key
▢ Food	▣ Exercise
▢ Silence	▢ Home

Do all daily missions in yellow band | Personalize your program by scheduling these missions

Sunday

Sunday E-mail
- ▢ Five-minute meditation (every day)
- ▢ Turn Down the Volume (every day)

❑ Eat a new lunch (x)
❑ New snack (each time you snack) (x)
❑ Say Hi to the Sun (optional, 3x)
❑ Walk (2 x)
❑ Yoga (2 x)

❑ Ritual Dinner (x)
❑ Buy Two New Foods (x)
❑ Create Your Sacred Corner (x)
❑ Mindfulness Trigger (x)

Monday

- ▢ Five-minute meditation (every day)
- ▢ Turn Down the Volume (every day)

❑ Eat a new lunch (x)
❑ New snack (each time you snack) (x)
❑ Say Hi to the Sun (optional, 3x)
❑ Walk (2 x)
❑ Yoga (2 x

❑ Ritual Dinner (x)
❑ Buy Two New Foods (x)
❑ Create Your Sacred Corner (x)
❑ Mindfulness Trigger (x)

Tuesday

- ▢ Five-minute meditation (every day)
- ▢ Turn Down the Volume (every day)

❑ Eat a new lunch (x)
❑ New snack (each time you snack) (x)
❑ Say Hi to the Sun (optional, 3x)
❑ Walk (2 x)
❑ Yoga (2 x

❑ Ritual Dinner (x)
❑ Buy Two New Foods (x)
❑ Create Your Sacred Corner (x)
❑ Mindfulness Trigger (x)

Wednesday

- ▢ Five-minute meditation (every day)
- ▢ Turn Down the Volume (every day)

❑ Eat a new lunch (x)
❑ New snack (each time you snack) (x)
❑ Say Hi to the Sun (optional, 3x)
❑ Walk (2 x)
❑ Yoga (2 x

❑ Ritual Dinner (x)
❑ Buy Two New Foods (x)
❑ Create Your Sacred Corner (x)
❑ Mindfulness Trigger (x)

Thursday

- ▢ Five-minute meditation (every day)
- ▢ Turn Down the Volume (every day)

❑ Eat a new lunch (x)
❑ New snack (each time you snack) (x)
❑ Say Hi to the Sun (optional, 3x)
❑ Walk (2 x)
❑ Yoga (2 x

❑ Ritual Dinner (x)
❑ Buy Two New Foods (x)
❑ Create Your Sacred Corner (x)
❑ Mindfulness Trigger (x)

Friday

- ▢ Five-minute meditation (every day)
- ▢ Turn Down the Volume (every day)

❑ Eat a new lunch (x)
❑ New snack (each time you snack) (x)
❑ Say Hi to the Sun (optional, 3x)
❑ Walk (2 x)
❑ Yoga (2 x

❑ Ritual Dinner (x)
❑ Buy Two New Foods (x)
❑ Create Your Sacred Corner (x)
❑ Mindfulness Trigger (x)

Saturday

- ▢ Five-minute meditation (every day)
- ▢ Turn Down the Volume (every day)

❑ Eat a new lunch (x)
❑ New snack (each time you snack) (x)
❑ Say Hi to the Sun (optional, 3x)
❑ Walk (2 x)
❑ Yoga (2 x

❑ Ritual Dinner (x)
❑ Buy Two New Foods (x)
❑ Create Your Sacred Corner (x)
❑ Mindfulness Trigger (x)

Week 3

This week you will add in three new dinners to your repertoire of wholesome meals. Continue with your healthier breakfasts, lunches, and snacks, and move toward making them daily norms. Please also continue with the Ritual Dinner exercise, even in the most simple way. You will find a new provider of wholesome food in your area, to see where else you could shop. A big focus this week is sleep, and you can choose between two options to improve your sleep. And you will lighten up your life: you will reduce physical clutter, do a basic mindfulness exercise every day during some very ordinary activity, and take a day without a cell phone or e-mail so as to quiet your mind. In both yoga and walking, the focus is on breath this week—when you walk, try to push yourself a little harder and test your edge.

This Week's Program

Sunday E-mail:

How are you feeling about yourself after Week 2? What was difficult about last week? What went well? What would you like to achieve this week? And what is your relationship to silence—do you get enough of it in your week? Are you comfortable with it?

Plan Ahead:

Organize your evenings so you can wind down and get to bed early. Block out an hour or two to clear the clutter. Pick the menial activity for your mindfulness exercise. Ask friends where they shop for food, or do some research in your area to find new shopping spots.

Daily Missions

- Seven-minute meditation (S)
- Better Sleep for a Week: Option A or Option B (H, page 259)
- Menial Mindfulness (S, page 212)

Remind Yourself to

- ☼ Drink more H2O!
- ☼ Tune in to your personal food balance.
- ☼ Remember: no more noisy foods or drinks.
- ☼ Can you lengthen your walk or yoga session?
- ☼ Are you breathing?
- ☼ Set your intention for each workout

Personalize Your Program

3x a week

- Eat a new dinner (F)

2x a week

- Walk: Either 30 minutes at moderate pace or 20 minutes faster pace/steep terrain or 30 minutes fast pace/steep terrain. (E)
- Yoga: Add Ujjayi breathing. (E, page 125)
- Ritual Dinner (F, page 234) (1+ hr.)

1x a week

- Get Fresher (F, page 78) (1+hr.)
- A Day Without a Cell Phone (S, page 188)
- Clear the Clutter (H, page 234) (1+ hr.)
- Buy Two New Foods (F)

Key	
■ Food	■ Exercise
■ Silence	■ Home

Sunday

Sunday E-mail
- Seven-minute meditation
  (every day)
- Better Sleep for a Week (every day)
- Menial Mindfulness (every day)

- ❑ Eat a new dinner (□x)
- ❑ Walk (2x)
- ❑ Yoga (2x)
- ❑ Ritual Dinner (2x)

- ❑ Get Fresher (□x)
- ❑ A Day Without a Cell Phone (□x)
- ❑ Clear the Clutter (□x)
- ❑ Buy Two New Foods (□x)

Monday

- Seven-minute meditation
  (every day)
- Better Sleep for a Week (every day)
- Menial Mindfulness (every day)

- ❑ Eat a new dinner (□x)
- ❑ Walk (2x)
- ❑ Yoga (2x)
- ❑ Ritual Dinner (2x)

- ❑ Get Fresher (□x)
- ❑ A Day Without a Cell Phone (□x)
- ❑ Clear the Clutter (1x)
- ❑ Buy Two New Foods (□x)

Tuesday

- Seven-minute meditation
  (every day)
- Better Sleep for a Week (every day)
- Menial Mindfulness (every day)

- ❑ Eat a new dinner (□x)
- ❑ Walk (2x)
- ❑ Yoga (2x)
- ❑ Ritual Dinner (2x)

- ❑ Get Fresher (□x)
- ❑ A Day Without a Cell Phone (□x)
- ❑ Clear the Clutter (1x)
- ❑ Buy Two New Foods (□x)

Wedneday

- Seven-minute meditation
  (every day)
- Better Sleep for a Week (every day)
- Menial Mindfulness (every day)

- ❑ Eat a new dinner (□x)
- ❑ Walk (2x)
- ❑ Yoga (2x)
- ❑ Ritual Dinner (2x)

- ❑ Get Fresher (□x)
- ❑ A Day Without a Cell Phone (□x)
- ❑ Clear the Clutter (1x)
- ❑ Buy Two New Foods (□x)

Thursday

- Seven-minute meditation
  (every day)
- Better Sleep for a Week (every day)
- Menial Mindfulness (every day)

- ❑ Eat a new dinner (□x)
- ❑ Walk 2x
- ❑ Yoga (2x)
- ❑ Ritual Dinner (2x)

- ❑ Get Fresher (□x)
- ❑ A Day Without a Cell Phone (□x)
- ❑ Clear the Clutter (1x)
- ❑ Buy Two New Foods (□x)

Friday

- Seven-minute meditation
  (every day)
- Better Sleep for a Week (every day)
- Menial Mindfulness (every day)

- ❑ Eat a new dinner (□x)
- ❑ Walk (2x)
- ❑ Yoga (2x)
- ❑ Ritual Dinner (2x)

- ❑ Get Fresher (□x)
- ❑ A Day Without a Cell Phone (□x)
- ❑ Clear the Clutter (1x)
- ❑ Buy Two New Foods (□x)

Saturday

- Seven-minute meditation
  (every day)
- Better Sleep for a Week (every day)
- Menial Mindfulness (every day)

- ❑ Eat a new dinner (□x)
- ❑ Walk (2x)
- ❑ Yoga (2x)
- ❑ Ritual Dinner (2x)

- ❑ Get Fresher (□x)
- ❑ A Day Without a Cell Phone (□x)
- ❑ Clear the Clutter (1x)
- ❑ Buy Two New Foods (□x)

Week 4
You're on the last leg! This week you may be feeling quite different from when you started. The majority of your meals should be wholeful ones now, or incorporating natural elements whenever possible. Your walks will be slightly longer, and you should be moving quickly enough to hear your breath and feel your body working. Cultivate peace in the home this week: start and end each day with a half hour of calm and quiet. Get out into some sunlight if you can. The two longer assignments this week are unusual and uplifting. You will revamp one room of your home to make it as peaceful and nurturing as it can be, and you will give your body a break by doing a modified version of a dietary cleanse. By the end of this week, you are going to feel great in body, mind, and spirit.

This Week's Program

Sunday E-mail

How are you feeling about yourself after Week 3? What was difficult about last week? What did you notice about yourself? What went well? What would you like to achieve this week? And how do you feel about your home: is it peaceful, nurturing, and supportive to this lifestyle you are creating? What could be better?

Plan Ahead:

Block out an afternoon or evening to work on your chosen room. Consider where you might pick up some new items that will improve it. Stock up on vegetables for the one-day cleanse.

Daily Missions

- ■ Ten-minute meditation (up to 20 minutes) (S)
- ■ Sacred Morning, Sacred Evening (S, page 188)

Remind Yourself to

- ☼ Discover new places to walk.
- ☼ Remember to veto fruit juice and soda.
- ☼ Ask yourself, "What kind of workout is right for me today?"
- ☼ Don't watch TV or read or work on the computer while you eat.
- ☼ Set your intention for each workout.

Personalize Your Program

3x a week

- ■ New breakfast, lunch, and dinner (3 times each) (F)
- ■ Say Hi to the Sun (H, page 261) (15+ mins.)

2x a week

- ■ Walk: 30 minutes fast pace and/or steep terrain. Bonus: Can you get out into nature? (E)
- ■ Yoga: Start playing with Freedom Yoga (E, page 125)

1x a week

- ■ Add Your Food Treat (F, page 88)
- ■ Reinvent Your Room (3+ hrs.) (H, page 243)
- ■ Spring Cleaning for Your Body (one-day veggie cleanse) (F, page 50)
- ■ Buy Two New Foods (F)

Key	
■ Food	■ Exercise
■ Silence	■ Home

Sunday

Sunday E-mail
- Ten-minute meditation (every day)
- Sacred Morning, Sacred Evening (every day)

❑ New breakfast, lunch & dinner (x)
❑ Walk (2x)
❑ Say Hi to the Sun (x)
❑ Yoga (2x)

❑ Add Your Food Treat (x)
❑ Reinvent Your Room (x)
❑ Spring Cleaning for Your Body (x)
❑ Buy Two New Foods (x)

Monday

- Ten-minute meditation (every day)
- Sacred Morning, Sacred Evening (every day)

❑ New breakfast, lunch & dinner (x)
❑ Walk (2x)
❑ Say Hi to the Sun (x)
❑ Yoga (2x)

❑ Add Your Food Treat (x)
❑ Reinvent Your Room (x)
❑ Spring Cleaning for Your Body (x)
❑ Buy Two New Foods (x)

Tuesday

- Ten-minute meditation (every day)
- Sacred Morning, Sacred Evening (every day)

❑ New breakfast, lunch & dinner (x)
❑ Walk (2x)
❑ Say Hi to the Sun (x)
❑ Yoga (2x)

❑ Add Your Food Treat (x)
❑ Reinvent Your Room (x)
❑ Spring Cleaning for Your Body (x)
❑ Buy Two New Foods (x)

Wednesday

- Ten-minute meditation (every day)
- Sacred Morning, Sacred Evening (every day)

❑ New breakfast, lunch & dinner (x)
❑ Walk (2x)
❑ Say Hi to the Sun (x)
❑ Yoga (2x)

❑ Add Your Food Treat (x)
❑ Reinvent Your Room (x)
❑ Spring Cleaning for Your Body (x)
❑ Buy Two New Foods (x)

Thursday

- Ten-minute meditation (every day)
- Sacred Morning, Sacred Evening (every day)

❑ New breakfast, lunch & dinner (x)
❑ Walk (2x)
❑ Say Hi to the Sun (x)
❑ Yoga (2x)

❑ Add Your Food Treat (x)
❑ Reinvent Your Room (x)
❑ Spring Cleaning for Your Body (x)
❑ Buy Two New Foods (x)

Friday

- Ten-minute meditation (every day)
- Sacred Morning, Sacred Evening (every day)

❑ New breakfast, lunch & dinner (x)
❑ Walk (2x)
❑ Say Hi to the Sun (x)
❑ Yoga (2x)

❑ Add Your Food Treat (x)
❑ Reinvent Your Room (x)
❑ Spring Cleaning for Your Body (x)
❑ Buy Two New Foods (x)

Saturday

- Ten-minute meditation (every day)
- Sacred Morning, Sacred Evening (every day)

❑ New breakfast, lunch & dinner (x)
❑ Walk (2x)
❑ Say Hi to the Sun (x)
❑ Yoga (2x)

❑ Add Your Food Treat (x)
❑ Reinvent Your Room (x)
❑ Spring Cleaning for Your Body (x)
❑ Buy Two New Foods (x)

Fourth Sunday E-mail:

You've made it to the end of four weeks of changes. Congratulations! Please take a few moments on the last Sunday to reread your earlier e-mails to yourself and write a final one. How are you feeling now? Which aspects of this program did you like the most, and which the least? Where could you continue to make improvements? Write a few lines about which new habits you can easily keep going from now on. Which are going to take more effort? Were you kind to yourself throughout this program, or did you find yourself getting critical or tough?

It doesn't matter whether your life looks radically different or not after these four weeks, but ask yourself: Have you experienced the possibility of doing a few things differently? Have you touched a few new ways of eating, exercising, relaxing, and restoring? Have you discovered the place of balance within? It is my heartfelt wish that you have. Come back to the advice and exercises in this book any time you need, for reminders, for inspiration, or for motivation. May you continue on your journey with health and happiness, and stay equipped with this set of useful tools at your side.

Index of Products

Food

Oxygen water: www.hiosilver.com

Rishi tea: www.rishitea.com

More teapots: www.adagio.com

Chemical-free decaf coffee: www.swisswater.com

Teeccino herbal coffee: www.teecchino.com

Yerba maté: www.guayaki.com

Reverse osmosis filtration system: www.gaiam.com and
    other vendors

Fruit and vegetable wash: www.environne.com

Vita-Mix blender: www.vitamix.com

Pantry Essentials:

Stevia and xylitol: www.xlearinc.com

Whey protein powder: www.jayrobb.com

Coconut oil: www.mercola.com

Flaxseed powder and flax oil:at any health food store

Fish oil or cod liver oil: www.nordicnaturals.com or
    www.carlsonlabs.com

Bulk raw nuts: at any health food store or www.
    bobsredmill.com or Authentic Foods (800) 806-4737

Exercise

Yoga mats: www.gaiam.com

Masai Barefoot Technology sneakers:
    www.swissmasaius.com

Swopper stool: www.swopper.com

Silence

Meditation cushion or bench:
    www.gaiam.com

Home

Water fountain: www.gaiam.com

Ceramic diffuser: www.gaiam.com

Nontoxic cleaning products and
    personal care products:
    www.seventhgeneration.com

Air purifier: www.tryfreshair.com or
    www.gaiam.com or
    www.mercola.com

Zen Alarm Clock: www.now-zen.com

Light bath or light box: www.gaiam.com or
    www.mercola.com

Water purificaation system:
    www.ecoquestintl.com

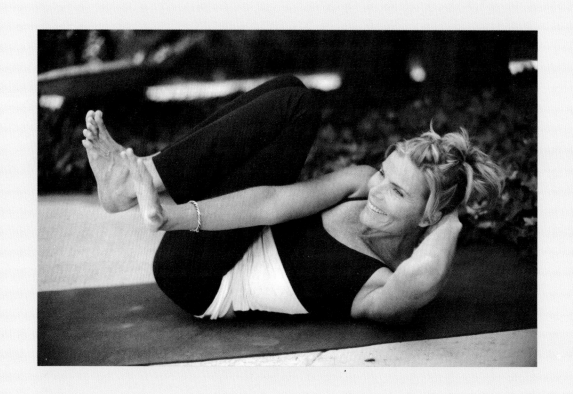